KV-376-012

NURSE'S DICTIONARY

originally compiled by
HONNOR MORTEN

Revised by
JOAN M. MARTIN
B.Sc., Dip.Ed., S.R.N., S.C.M., R.N.T.

Twenty-ninth edition

FABER AND FABER

London   Boston

Twenty-eighth edition 1976
Twenty-ninth edition 1980
Published by Faber and Faber Limited
3 Queen Square, London WC1
Set, printed and bound in Great Britain by
Fakenham Press Limited, Fakenham, Norfolk
All rights reserved

British Library Cataloguing in Publication Data

Morten, Honnor
  The nurse's dictionary—29th ed.
  1. Medicine—Dictionaries
  2. Nursing—Dictionaries
  I. Title II. Martin, Joan M.
  610'.2'4613   R121

  ISBN 0–571–18007–8

PREFACE TO THE TWENTY-NINTH EDITION

As medical and technological advances accelerate, so do the problems of keeping books such as this up to date. The changes in this edition concentrate largely on removing material that is now obsolete. Some may feel that there is much left behind that is old-fashioned, but not all nurses will be working in a totally up to date environment.

The International System of Units (Systeme International, SI) has been introduced and a list of the commoner physiological values used in medicine has been given.

The resultant volume is somewhat slimmer and, thereby, a more truly 'pocket' dictionary.

My thanks are due to the professional friends and colleagues who have given me help and advice in preparing this edition.

J.M.M.
1979

CONTENTS

ABBREVIATIONS OF LATIN TERMS AS USED IN PRESCRIPTIONS, &c.

(The use of abbreviations in prescriptions is a dangerous practice and contrary to the policy of the DHSS)

Abbreviation	Latin	
a.c.	ante cibos	before meals
ad.	adde	up to
ad lib.	ad libitum	to the desired amount
alt. dieb.	alternis diebus	every other day
aq.	aqua	water
aq. dest.	aqua destillata	distilled water
aurist.	auristillae	ear drops
b.d.	bis die	twice a day
B.N.F.	—	British National Formulary
B.P.	—	British Pharmacopoeia
bal.	balneum	bath
c.	cum	with
comp.	compositus	compounded of
crem.	cremor	a cream
dil.	dilue	dilute
ext.	extractum	extract
gutt.	gutta or guttae	drop or drops
haust.	haustus	a draught
inj.	injectio	an injection
lot.	lotio	lotion
mist.	mistura	mixture
mit.	mitte	send
noct.	nocte	at night
oc.	oculentum	eye ointment
o.d.	omne die	every day

Abbreviation	Latin	
o.m.	omni mane	every morning
o.n.	omni nocte	every night
p.c.	post cibos	after meals
pig.	pigmentum	paint
p.r.	per rectum	by the rectum
p.r.n.	pro re nata	as occasion arises
pulv.	pulvis	powder
p.v.	per vaginam	by the vagina
q.d. } q.d.s. }	quarter die	four times a day
q.s.	quantum sufficit	as much as is required
R.	recipe	take
rep.	repetatur	let it be repeated
sig.	signetur	let it be labelled
s.o.s.	si opus sit	if necessary (to be given once only)
stat.	statim	immediately
syr.	syrupus	syrup
t.d. } t.d.s. }	ter in die	thrice a day
tinct. } tr. }	tinctura	tincture
ung.	unguentum	ointment

COMPARATIVE WEIGHTS AND MEASURES

WEIGHT

Metric System

1 kilogram (kg)	=	1,000 grams
1 gram (g)	=	1,000 milligrams
1 milligram (mg)	=	1,000 micrograms
1 microgram (μg)	=	1,000 nanograms (ng)

Conversions

Imperial System		Metric System
1 pound (lb.)	=	453·59 grams
1 ounce (oz.)	=	28·34 grams
Metric System		**Imperial System**
1 kilogram (kg)	=	2·2046 pounds or 35·274 ounces or 15,432 grains

VOLUME

Metric System

1 litre (1) = 1,000 millilitres
1 millilitre (ml) = 1·000028 cubic centimetres (cm³)
(The millilitre and cubic centimetre are usually treated as identical.)

Conversions

Imperial System		Metric System
1 pint (pt.)	=	568·25 millilitres
1 fluid ounce (fl. oz.)	=	28·412 millilitres
1 minim (m.)	=	0·059192 millilitres

Metric System		Imperial System
1 litre (1)	=	1·7598 pints or 35·196 fluid ounces
1 millilitre (ml)	=	16·894 minims

A 1 per cent w/v solution means:
1 gram solute dissolved in solvent to make 100ml solution (1 ounce in 5 pints is approximately 1%)

LENGTH

Metric System

1 metre (m)	=	100 centimetres
1 centimetre (cm)	=	10 millimetres
1 millimetre (mm)	=	1,000 micrometres
1 micrometre (μm)	=	1,000 nanometres (nm)

British System

1 mile	=	1,760 yards
1 yard	=	3 feet
1 foot	=	12 inches

Conversions

Metric System		British System
1 metre (m)	=	39·370 inches
1 centimetre (cm)	=	0·39370 inches
1 millimetre (mm)	=	0·039370 inches
1 micrometre (μm)	=	0·000039370 inches

British System		Metric System
1 mile	=	1609·344 metres
1 yard	=	91·44 centimetres
1 foot	=	30·48 centimetres
1 inch	=	2·540 centimetres

COMPARISON OF CELSIUS (CENTIGRADE) AND FAHRENHEIT THERMOMETRIC SCALES

Boiling-point = 212° F = 100° C

Freezing-point = 32° F = 0° C

Normal temperature of the body = 98·4° F
   = 37° C

To convert degrees F into degrees C deduct
   32, multiply by 5, and divide by 9.
   e.g. 104° F to centigrade,
      104 − 32 = 72 × 5 = 360 ÷ 9 = 40
   ∴ 104° F = 40° C

To convert degrees C into degrees F multiply
   by 9, divide by 5, and add 32 to the result.
   e.g. 36·6° C to Fahrenheit,
      36·6 × 9 = 330 ÷ 5 = 66 + 32 = 98
   ∴ 36·6° C = 98° F

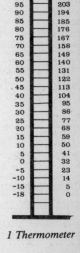

C	F
100	212
95	203
90	194
85	185
80	176
75	167
70	158
65	149
60	140
55	131
50	122
45	113
40	104
35	95
30	86
25	77
20	68
15	59
10	50
5	41
0	32
−5	23
−10	14
−15	5
−18	0

1 Thermometer

SOME USEFUL EQUIVALENTS IN CLINICAL THERMOMETER READINGS

Fahrenheit		Celsius
107·5	↔	41·9
107	↔	41·7
106·5	↔	41·4
106	↔	41·1
105·5	↔	40·8
105	↔	40·6
104·5	↔	40·3
104	↔	40
103·5	↔	39·7
103	↔	39·4
102·5	↔	39·2
102	↔	38·9
101·5	↔	38·6
101	↔	38·3
100·5	↔	38·1
100	↔	37·8
99·5	↔	37·5
99	↔	37·2
98·4	↔	36·9
97·8	↔	36·6

A GUIDE TO PRONUNCIATION

After each entry in the dictionary the pronunciation is found in
brackets. The stress mark ' shows where the emphasis should be
made in a word of more than one syllable, and these are divided by
hyphens.

The basic vowel and consonant sounds are listed below:

Vowel sound	Example
a as in bat	cataract (*kat'-a-rakt*)
a as in mate	flatus *flā'-tus*)
ah as in father	after (*ahf'-ter*)
ar as in far	carbon (*kar'-bon*)
ā-r as in air	aerosol (*ā'-rō-sol*)
aw as in fall	audiometer (*aw-dē-om'-et-er*)
e as in get	electric (*e-lek'-trik*)
ē as in been	ether (*ē'-ther*)
ē-r as in ear	sclera (*sklē'-ra*)
i as in bit	nicotinic (*ni-kō-tin'-ik*)
ī as in bite	eye (*ī*), hydro- (*hī-drō*)
o as in hop	optics (*op'-tiks*)
ō as in hope	isotopes (*ī-zō-tōps*)
oo as in soon	croup (*kroop*)
or as in for	orbit (*or'-bit*)
ow as in how	sound (*sownd*)
oy as in boy	boil (*boyl*)
u as in cup	tongue (*tung*)
ū as in mute	cubit (*kū-bit*)

Consonant sound	Example
f the sound of ph as in phobia (*fō'-bi-ah*)	
j the sound of g as in dermalgia (*der-mal'-ji-a*)	

A GUIDE TO PRONUNCIATION

Consonant sound	*Example*
k the sound of c	as in catalyst (*ka'-ta-list*)
ks the sound of x	as in X-ray (*eks'rā*)
kw the sound of qu	as in quintan (*kwin'-tan*)
s the sound of c	as in lucid (*loo'-sid*)
shon the sound of tion	as in ablution (*ab-loo'-shon*)
zhon the sound of sion	as in invasion (*in-vā'-zhon*)

A

a- or **an** (*ā or an*). Prefix denoting absence of, *e.g.* achlorhydria, absence of hydrochloric acid; anuria, absence of urine, etc.

ab (*ab*). A prefix signifying from, away from, *e.g. Abenteric*, situated away from and not in the intestine, etc.

abalienation (*ab-ā-lē-en-ā-shon*). Mental derangement.

abdomen (*ab-dō'-men*). The belly. The body cavity immediately below the thorax, bounded above by the diaphragm, below by the pelvis, behind by the lumbar vertebrae, and in front and at the sides by muscular walls. It contains many important organs, including the stomach, intestines, liver, kidneys, spleen, pancreas, bladder, uterus and ovaries. It is lined with a serous membrane called the peritoneum,

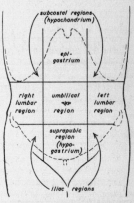

2 Areas of the abdomen

which is reflected onto many of the organs in the abdomen (*see* illustration).

abdominal (*ab-dom-in-al*). Pertaining to the abdomen.

abdomino-perineal (*ab-do-mi-nō-pe-ri-ne-al*). Used to describe operation of excision of rectum, utilizing approach from both abdominal and perineal incisions.

abducent nerves (*ab-dū'-sent nervs*). The sixth pair of cranial nerves, activating the external rectus muscle of the eyeball, which rotates the eyeball outwards.

abduct (*ab-dukt'*). To draw away from the mid-line.

abduction (*ab-duk-shon*). The act of moving a limb away from the middle line of the body.

abductor (*ab-duk'-ter*). A muscle which draws a limb from the median line of the body, *e.g.* deltoid.

aberrant (*ab-er-ant*). An anatomical structure, generally a blood vessel or nerve, which does not follow its normal course.

aberration (*ab-er-ā'-shon*). Deviation from the normal. In optics, defect in focus of a lens. *Mental A.* Mental disturbance or peculiarity.

ablation (*ab-lā'-shon*). Removal or detachment of a part; or procedure that results in total loss of function of that part.

ablution (*ab-loo'-shon*). Cleaning by washing.

abnormal (*ab-nor'-mal*). Irregular, unusual.

abort (*a-bort*). To terminate a process before the full course is run, especially applied to pregnancy.

abortifacient (*a-bor-ti-fā'-si-ent*). A drug taken for the purpose of procuring abortion.

abortion (*a-bor'-shon*). Discharge of the gestation sac from the pregnant uterus before the fetus is viable. Abortion may be *complete* or *incomplete*; it may be *threatened* or *inevitable*, according to the cervical canal being closed or open. Finally it may be *missed*: that is, the fetus may be dead, but may not be discharged immediately. *Tubal A.* When an ovum developing in the Fallopian tube becomes detached, and is thrown off through the abdominal ostium of the tube into the Pouch of Douglas.

abortus fever (*ab-or'-tus fē-ver*). An undulant fever, also called brucellosis, caused by infected cow's milk.

abrasion (*ab-rā'-zhon*). A superficial injury to the skin or mucous membrane.

abreaction (*ab-rē-ak'-shon*). A state of mind brought about during the process of psychoanalysis. The patient lives again through past painful experiences which may unconsciously be causing the neurosis.

abscess (*ab'-ses*). A collection of pus in a cavity, the result of inflammation. *Alveolar A.*

One which develops in the socket of a tooth. *Blind A.* One with no external opening. *Cold A.* One which develops slowly, without inflammation, as in tuberculosis. *Ischiorectal A.* One in the ischiorectal fossa. *Metastatic A.* Secondary to an abscess elsewhere; caused by an infected embolus. *Psoas A.* One due to disease of the vertebrae. The pus descends in the sheath of the psoas muscle, forming a fluctuating tumour above or below Poupart's ligament. It is sometimes tuberculous in origin. *Residual A.* One developing in old inflammatory products. *Stitch A.* One formed around a stitch.

absolute values. In blood counts these are the actual numbers and not the percentage figures.

absorption (*ab-sorp'-shon*). Taking up by suction. Gauze and wool are absorbent dressings.

acanthosis (*ak-an-thō'-sis*). Any disease of the prickle-layer, the lowest stratum of the epidermis. *A. Nigricans.* General pigmentation of the skin with mole-like growths.

acapnia (*ā-kap'-ni-a*). A lessened amount of carbon dioxide in the blood often the result of hyperventilation.

acardia (*ā-kar'-di-ah*). Congenital absence of the heart.

Acarus (*ak'-a-rus*). The name of a group of animal parasites of the spider family, including ticks and mites. *A. Scabiei* is the parasite causing scabies.

acatalepsy (*ā-ka-ta-lep'-si*). Uncertainty, lack of understanding.

acataphasia (*a-kat-a-fā'-zi-a*). Difficulty in expressing ideas in logical sequence.

accessory nerves (*ak-se-so-ri*). Eleventh pair of cranial nerves.

accidental haemorrhage (*ak-si-den'-tal hem-o-rāj*). Bleeding from the pregnant uterus in the later months of pregnancy due to premature separation of normally situated placenta. It may be *concealed*, when the bleeding remains internal; or *external*, when the blood escapes by the vagina. *See* ANTEPARTUM HAEMORRHAGE.

accommodation (*ak-om-o-dā'-shon*). In ophthalmology the power to adjust the eye to obtain clear vision at different distances.

accouchement (*ak-koosh-mor*). Childbirth.

accretion (*ak-krē-shon*). Accumulation of foreign matter in an organ, *e.g.* the formation of renal calculi.

ACE 20

acephalic (*ā-ke-fa-lik*). Headless.

acetabulum (*a-se-tab'-ū-lum*). The cuplike socket in the hip or innominate bone into which the head of the femur fits.

acetate (*as'-et-āt*). A salt of acetic acid.

acetic acid (*a-sēt'-ik*). The acid of vinegar. It may be used in testing urine for albumin.

aceto-acetic acid (*as-ē-tō-a-sē-tik*). Produced at an intermediate stage of fatty acid oxidation. If metabolism is disturbed, as in diabetes mellitus, it is found in excess in the blood and the urine. *Syn*, diacetic acid.

acetonaemia (*a'-ē-tō-nē-me-ah*). The presence of acetone in the blood.

acetone (*as'-e-tōn*). A colourless volatile solvent. This substance is formed in the body when metabolism is upset, as in starvation, excessive vomiting, diabetes mellitus. It is excreted in the urine and the breath.

acetonuria (*as'-ē-tōn-ū'-ri-a*). The presence of acetone in the urine.

acetylcholine (*as'-ē-til-kō'-lēn*). A chemical substance liberated from parasympathetic nerve endings when they are stimulated. They are thus called cholinergic fibres.

acetylsalicylic acid (*as-ē'-til-sa-li-sil'-ik as-id*). Aspirin.

achalasia (*ak-al-ā'-ze-ah*). Failure of relaxation of a muscle sphincter. Applied particularly to the cardiac sphincter, often resulting in dilatation of the oesophagus.

Achilles tendon (*a-kil-lēz ten'-don*). The large tendon which attaches the calf muscles to the heel.

achillorrhaphy (*a-kil-o-ra-fi*). Surgery to rejoin the Achilles tendon after rupture.

achlorhydria (*ā-klor-hi'-dri-a*). Absence of hydrochloric acid in the gastric juice; may occur in pernicious anaemia and cancer of the stomach.

acholia (*ā-kō-li-a*). Absence of bile.

acholuria (*a-kol-ū'-ri-a*). The absence of bile pigment from the urine.

acholuric jaundice (*a-kol-ū'-rik*). *See* JAUNDICE.

achondroplasia (*a-kon'-drō-plā-zi-a*). A form of arrested development of the long bones, leading to dwarfism.

achromasia (*a-krō-mā'-zi-a*). (1) Absence of colour. (2) Loss of staining reaction in a cell.

achromatopsia (*a-krō-mat-op'-si-a*). Colour blindness.

achylia, achylosis (*a-ki'-li-a*). Absence of chyle. *A. gastrica*, atrophy of mucous membrane of the stomach resulting in reduction or absence of gastric juice.

acid (*as'-id*). A substance capable of uniting with alkalis to form salts. Acids turn blue litmus paper red and when in liquid form have a sour taste, *e.g.* vinegar and lemon juice both contain acids. (For individual acids *see under* special name.)

acidaemia (*a-sid-ē-mi-a*). The blood is abnormally acid and the pH below 7·3.

acid-base balance. The balance between the acidic and basic components which determine the pH of body fluids.

acid-fast. In bacteriology a term applied to certain bacteria which retain the red carbolfuchsin stain after the application of an acid solution. Other organisms are decolorized. Tubercle and leprosy bacilli are 'acid-fast'.

acidity (*as-id'-it-ē*). The strength of acid in a given substance, measured by its pH.

acidosis (*as-id-ō'-sis*). A condition in which the acid-base balance of the body fluids is disturbed, resulting in a fall in pH.

acid phosphatase (*fos-fa-tāz*). Enzyme produced by the prostate gland and secreted in seminal fluid. Serum acid phosphatase is raised in carcinoma of the prostate when there is bone involvement.

acinus (*a-sē-nus*), pl. **acini** (*a-sē-nē*). A minute grape-like structure whose cells secrete; as in the breast. Acini are also found in the lungs and other racemose glands. *Syn.* alveolus, pl. alveoli.

acne (*ak'-nē*). Inflammation of the sebaceous glands of the skin, causing the formation of little pustules, and of blackheads. Often found among adolescents.

acousma (*a-kūs-ma*). The hearing of imaginary sounds.

acoustic (*a-koo'-stik*). Relating to sound or hearing.

acquired (*ak-wī-rd*). Contracted after birth, not congenital.

acrid (*ak'-rid*). Pungent, corrosive.

acro- (*ak-rō*). Extremity of (prefix).

acrocephaly (*ak-rō-ke-fa-li*). Congenitally malformed cone-shaped head.

acrocyanosis (*ak-rō-sī-a-nō-sis*). Blueness of the extremities.

acrodynia (*ak-rō-din'-i-a*). See PINK DISEASE.

acromegaly (*ak-rō-meg'-a-lē*). A disease marked by enlargement of the face, hands and feet, and due to a pathological condition of the pituitary gland. The commonest form of gigantism.

acromion (*ā-krō'-mi-on*). The outward projection of the spine of the scapula. *See* SCAPULA.

acronyx (*ak'-rō-niks*). An ingrowing of the nail.

acroparaesthesia (*ak-rō-pa-res-thē-zi-a*). A tingling feeling in the hands with numbness caused by pressure on the brachial plexus.

acrophobia (*ak-rō-fō'-bi-a*). Morbid fear of being at a height.

acrylics (*a-kril-iks*). Plastic substances used for prostheses.

ACTH. Adrenocorticotrophic hormone, of the anterior lobe of the pituitary body, controlling the function of the adrenal cortex and the release of corticosteroids. It may be given by intramuscular or slow intravenous injection. ACTH gel is a long-acting form for intramuscular injection only.

actinism (*ak'-tin-izm*). Chemical changes produced by radiant energy, *e.g.* light rays.

actinodermatitis (*ak-ti-nō-der-ma-tī-tis*). Inflammation of the skin from ultra-violet or other rays.

Actinomyces (*ak-tī-nō-mī'-sez*). A pathogenic fungus causing actinomycosis.

actinomycosis (*ak-tīn-ō-mī-kō-sis*). Disease due to Actinomyces. There are usually chronic discharging abscesses.

actinotherapy (*ak-tin'-o-therapi*). Treatment by ultra-violet and infra-red radiations.

action potential (*ak-shon-po-ten-shal*). Electrical charges occurring when a nerve conducts an impulse.

action tremor. Tremor of the limbs or incoordination of movement as in ataxia.

activator (*ak-ti-vā'-tor*). A physical or chemical agent which initiates some reaction in which the activator itself does not take part.

active movements. A term used by physiotherapists to denote normal movement of a limb or part of the body.

active principle. The substance in a drug which gives it a medicinal character.

acuity (*a-kū-it-i*). Sharpness and clearness.

acupuncture (*ak-ū-pungk-chur*). (1) A treatment to relieve oedema. The oedematous tissue—usually of the legs—is stabbed all over with straight cutting needles. (2) A form of general treatment given by those who practise 'fringe' medicine.

acute (*ak-yoot'*). Rapid; severe. *A. abdomen*. A surgical emergency resulting from disease or damage of abdominal viscera.

acute yellow atrophy (*at'-ro-fi*). Severe damage to liver due to toxic agents.

acystia (*a-sis'-ti-a*). Absence of bladder.

adactylia (*ā-dak-til'-i-a*). Absence of fingers or toes.

Adam's apple. The laryngeal prominence formed by the thyroid cartilage.

adamantinoma (*a-da-man-ti-nō'-ma*). Epithelial tumour of jaw.

adaptation (*a-dap-tā'-shon*). (1) Adjustment by structural or functional change to new circumstances. (2) The process whereby the eye adjusts to sudden changes from light to dark and vice versa.

addiction (*ad-dik'-shon*). State of physical and mental dependence on a drug, usually alcohol or narcotics.

Addis count (*ad-dis kownt*). Number of red blood cells in the urine, per 24 hours.

Addison's anaemia. Pernicious anaemia.

Addison's disease. A disease of the suprarenal gland causing anaemia, vomiting, wasting, low blood pressure and a bronzed skin.

adducent muscle of eye (*a-dū-sent*). Internal rectus muscle.

adduct (*ad-dukt*). To draw towards the midline.

adduction (*ad-duk'-shon*). The act of moving a limb towards the midline of the body.

adductor (*ad-duk'-ter*). A muscle which draws towards the midline of the body, *e.g. A. muscles* of the thigh draw the legs together.

adendritic (*ā-den-dri'-tik*). A nerve cell without dendrons.

adenectomy (*ad-en-ek'-to-mē*). Excision of a gland.

adenine (*a-de-nēn*). An amino purine base important for the synthesis of nucleic acids.

adenitis (*ad-en-ī'-tis*). Inflammation of a gland.

adenocarcinoma (*ad-en-ō-kar-sin-ō'-ma*). A carcinomatous tumour of a gland.

adenoid (*ad'-en-oyd*). Lymphoid tissue, in the nasopharynx, which when swollen hinders breathing.

adenoidectomy (*ad-en-oyd-ek-to-mi*). Operation to remove adenoids.

adenoma (*ad-en-ō'-ma*). A benign tumour of glandular tissue.

adenomyoma (*ad-en-ō-mī-ō-ma*). A benign growth, esp. in uterus, of glandular and muscle tissue.

adenopathy (*ad-en-op'-ath-ē*). A disease of a gland, especially a lymphatic gland.

adenovirus (*a-de-nō-vīr'-*us). A group of viruses consisting partly of DNA. They attack lymphoid tissue.

adeps (*a-deps*). Lard. Once used as a basis for ointments, now replaced by more satisfactory bases. *A. lanae hydrosus*, lanolin.

adermin (*ad-er-min*). Pyridoxin or vitamin B_6, concerned with the metabolism of amino-acids.

adherent (*ad-hār'-ent*). Fixed firmly to.

adhesion (*ad-hē'-zhon*). A sticking together of two surfaces or parts. Bands of fibrous tissue, usually the result of inflammation.

adiaphoresis (*ā-dī-a-for-ē-sis*). Deficiency of perspiration.

adipose (*ad'-ip-ōz*). Fatty.

aditus (*ad'-it-us*). An entrance. A portal. *A. ad antrum* is the narrow passage between the mastoid antrum and the tympanic cavity of the ear.

adjustment (*ad-just-ment*). The change made by a person to adapt to circumstances.

adjuvant (*ad'-ju-vant*). A secondary ingredient in a prescription, aiding the chief drug.

Adler's theory. The theory that people develop neuroses to compensate for some inferiority.

adnexa (*ad-nek'-sa*). Appendages. Usually applied to the uterine appendages.

adolescence (*ad-ō-les'-sens*). The period between puberty and maturity.

adrenal (*ad-rē'-nal*). *See* SUPRARENAL GLAND.

adrenalectomy (*ad-rē-nal-ek'-to-mi*). The removal of one or both adrenal glands.

adrenaline (*ad-re'-na-lin*). Secretion of the suprarenal medulla. Used locally as a styptic as it constricts small blood vessels. Injected hypodermically it raises the blood pressure and is used for anaphylactic reactions. It relieves asthma.

adrenergic (*a-dren-er-jik*). Applied to automatic nerve fibres whose stimulation leads to the production of adrenaline and noradrenaline.

adrenocortical steroids (*ad-rē-nō-kor-ti-kal ste-royds*). Endocrine secretions of the adrenal cortex. *See* ALDOSTERONE, CORTISONE, DEOXYCORTICOSTERONE.

adrenocorticotrophic hormone (*ad-rē-nō-kor-ti-kō-tro-fik hor-mōn*). *See* ACTH.

adrenogenital syndrome (*ad-rē-nō-je-ni-tal sin'-drōm*).

Development of secondary male characteristics in the female or secondary female characteristics in the male. Usually due to hyperplasia or adenoma of the adrenal cortex.

adrenolytic (*ad-rē-no-li-tik*). A drug antagonistic to adrenaline.

adrenotropin (*a-drē-nō-trō-pin*). Also called adrenocorticotrophic hormone. An anterior pituitary hormone acting upon the adrenal gland.

adsorbent. Substance causing adsorption.

adsorption (*ad-sorp'-shon*). The property possessed by certain porous substances, *e.g.* charcoal, of taking up other substances.

adulteration (*a-dul-te-rā'-shon*). Fraudulent addition of unnecessary substances to foods or medicines.

advancement (*ad-vans-menĭ*). An operation for the cure of squint. The procedure consists in dividing one of the eye muscles at its insertion into the eyeball and reattaching it farther forward.

adventitia (*ad-ven-tish'-a*). Outer coat of a blood vessel.

adventitious (*ad-ven-tish-us*). Coming from without. Accidental.

Aëdes aegypti (*a-ē-dās ā-jĭp'-tē*). Species of mosquito transmitting yellow fever, etc.

aeration (*ā-rā-shon*). Charging with air or other gas.

aerobes (*ā-rōbs*). Term applied to bacteria needing oxygen for respiration, *cf.* anaerobes.

aerobic (*ā-rō'-bik*). Requiring free oxygen or air to support life.

aerocele (*ār-ō-sēl*). A diverticulum of larynx, trachea or bronchus.

aerogen (*ā-rō-jen*). Any gas-producing bacterium, *e.g. Clostridium welchii*, the cause of gas gangrene.

aerophagy (*ār-of'-a-ji*). Excessive air swallowing.

aerosol (*ā'-rō-sol*). Finely atomized solution used to sterilize the air, or may be used as an inhalation.

Aesculapius (*ē-skŭ-lā-pē-us*). A Greek god, the founder of the art of healing.

aesthesia (*es-thē'-zi-a*). Feeling.

aetas (*ā-tas*). Latin for age. Abbrev. *aet.*

aetiology (*ē-tē-ol'-o-ji*). The science of the causation of disease.

afebrile (*ā-feb'-ril*). Without fever.

affect (*af-ekt*). Term used in psychology for an emotion associated with ideas.

affective disorders. Group of psychiatric illnesses primarily due to reaction to internal or external stress. They include anxiety states, depression, mania and hypomania.

afferent (*af'-er-ent*). Leading to the centre, applied to the lymphatic vessels and to sensory nerves.

affiliation (*a-fil-ē-ā'-shon*). The fixing of paternity of an illegitimate child on the putative father.

affinity (*af-fin'-it-ē*). Attraction. In chemistry the property of an element which prefers to combine with some other particular element.

after-birth (*ahf'-ter-berth*). The placenta, cord, and membranes as expelled after labour.

after-care (*ahf'-ter-kār*). Care of the convalescent, including rehabilitation.

after-image. A retinal impression persisting although the stimulus of light has eased.

after-pains (*ahf'-ter pānz*). Pains from uterine contractions following labour.

Ag. Chemical symbol for silver.

agammaglobulinaemia (*ā-gama-glo-bū-lin-ē'-mi-a*). Absence of deficiency of gamma globulin in plasma proteins, leading to inadequate response to infection.

agar-agar (*ā-ga-ā-ga*). A gelatinous substance prepared from seaweed and used by bacteriologists for the culture of bacteria. Also prescribed as a laxative, as it absorbs water and increases bulk in the colon.

agenesis (*ā-je'-ne-sis*). Defective development of a structure.

agglutination (*a-gloo-ti-nā-shon*). The sticking together of cells, *e.g.* red blood cells, bacteria, due to an alteration of surface charge. Usually brought about by the effect of antibodies.

agglutinins (*ag-gloo'-tin-ins*). Antibodies such as those found in the blood serum of persons suffering from typhoid or paratyphoid fever. They have the property of causing bacteria to clump together or 'agglutinate'. See WIDAL REACTION.

agglutinogen (*ag-gloo-ti-nō-jen*). A factor stimulating the production of specific antibodies in the blood.

aggregate (*ag-re-gāt*). To group together.

aggressin (*ag-gre-sin*). A product of certain bacteria increasing their action on the host.

aggression (*ag-gre-shon*). A hostile attitude born of a feeling of inferiority or frustration.

aglutition (*ā-glū-ti-shun*). Inability to swallow.

agnosia (*ag-nō-zia*). A disturbance in recognizing sensory impression.

agonist (*a-go-nist*). Muscle which shortens when in action.

agoraphobia (*a'-gor-af-ō'-bi-a*). Neurotic fear of open spaces.

agranulocyte (*ā-gran-ū-lō-site*). The non-granular leucocytes *i.e.* monocytes and lymphocytes.

agranulocytosis (*ā-gran-ū-lō-sī-tō'-sis*). Absence or marked reduction in the blood of the polymorphonuclear cells. May be caused by drugs such as the sulphonamides or irradiation of the bone marrow.

agraphia (*ā-graf'-i-a*). Loss of the power to express words and ideas in writing.

ague (*ā-gū*). *See* MALARIA.

AID. Artificial insemination (donor other than husband).

AIH. Artificial insemination with semen from the husband.

air. *See* ATMOSPHERE. *A., tidal.* The air breathed in and out in ordinary breathing.

air embolism. Embolism caused by air entering the circulatory system.

air-encephalography (*ār-en-ke-fal-o'-gra-fi*). Radiography of the brain after air has been introduced into the subarachnoid space.

air hunger. Respiratory distress caused by lack of available oxygen especially in haemorrhage.

akinesis (*ā-ki-nē'-sis*). Loss or imperfection of movement.

Al. Chemical symbol for aluminium.

ala (*ā-la*). A wing. *A. nasi.* The outer side of the external nostril.

alastrim (*a-la'-strim*). Variola minor.

Albee's (*al-bēz*) **operation.** (1) The hip joint is ankylosed by a plastic operation. (2) A bone grafting operation to the spine performed in tuberculous disease of the spine. The graft is taken from the tibia.

Albers-Schönberg's disease (*al-bers shern-bārgs*). Marble bone disease.

albino (*al-bē-nō*). A male with white hair, fair skin, and pink eyes, due to pigmentary deficiency.

albumin (*al-bū'-min*). Serum protein with relatively low molecular weight (MW = 70,000) which is of great importance in controlling water exchanges between the blood and tissue fluids.

albuminuria (*al-bū-min-ū'-ri-a*). Albumin in the urine; occurs in diseases of the kidneys. Nowadays known as proteinuria.

albumose (*al-bū-mōs*). Inter-mediate product formed in digestion of protein.

alcohol (*al-ko-hol'*). The term usually refers to ethyl alcohol, the alcohol present in intoxicating drinks. *Absolute A.* May contain up to 1 per cent by weight of water. Rectified spirit is 90 per cent alcohol.

alcoholism (*al'-kō-hol-izm*). A morbid state produced by excessive use of alcoholic drinks.

aldosterone (*al-dos'-ter-ōn*). One of the adrenocortical hormones which regulates metabolism of electrolytes.

aleukaemia (*ā-lū-kē'-mi-a*). Deficiency of leucocytes in the blood.

alexia (*a-leks'-i-a*). Inability to understand the written or printed word, owing to a lesion of the brain.

Algae (*al-jē*). A group of plants including seaweed and some fresh-water plants. Used for purification of water by their filtering action.

algesia (*al-jē'-si-a*). Sensibility to pain. (-**algia** is a suffix meaning pain.)

alienation (*āl-yen-ā'-shon*). Insanity.

alignment (*a-līn'-ment*). Bringing into line.

alimentary (*al-i-men'-tar-'e*). Pertaining to the absorption of nourishment. The *alimentary canal* is the whole digestive tract, extending from the mouth to the anus.

alimentation (*a-lē-men-tā'-shon*). Nourishment.

aliquot (*a-li-qwot*). One of equal parts of a specimen, *e.g.* a sample of known volume taken from a specimen of known volume.

alkalaemia (*al-ka-lē-mi-a*). Abnormally alkaline blood with a pH above 7·5.

alkali (*al'-ka-lī*). A substance which combines with an acid to form a salt, and with a fat to form a soap. Turns red litmus paper to blue. Ammonia, soda and potash are examples of alkalis. *A. reserve.* The amount of buffer-alkalis available in the body to neutralize acids.

alkaline. Containing alkali. Blood, milk and saliva are normally slightly alkaline.

alkalinity (*al-ka-lin'-it-ē*). Proportion of alkali in a given substance.

alkaloid (*al'-ka-loyd*). An organic substance having some of the properties of an alkali, especially that of combining with an acid to form a salt. Morphine and quinine are alkaloids. Salts of these are morphine tartrate, morphine hydrochloride, quinine sulphate, etc.

alkalosis (*al-kal-ō'-sis*). Alkalaemia. An increase in the alkalinity of the blood due to excessive intake of alkali or accumulation of it, or to loss of acids in the body caused by sweating, vomiting, diarrhoea or deep breathing.

alkapton (*al-kap'-ton*). A nitrogenous substance derived from the decomposition of proteins.

alkapotonuria (*al-kap-ton-ūr-i-a*). The presence of alkapton in the urine due to a chemical disorder of metabolism.

alkylating agents (*al-ki-lā-ting-ā-jens*). Drugs such as nitrogen mustard interfering with the growth of malignant cells.

all or none law. Physiological law regarding irritable tissues, *e.g.* nerves, by which there are only two possible reactions to a stimulus, either no reaction or full response. There is no grading of response according to the strength of the stimulus.

allantois (*al-lan'-tō-is*). A diverticulum formed as an outgrowth of the yolk sac of the developing embryo, present as a vestigial structure in the umbilical cord. (*See* illustration.)

allelomorphs (*al-lē-lō-morfs*). Inborn characteristics determined by contrasting genes.

allergen (*al'-er-jen*). A substance that produces the allergic state.

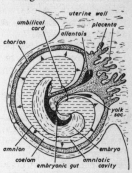

3 Diagram of early embryo showing the allantois

allergic state (*al'-ler-jik*). The patient is sensitive to a particular foreign protein which acts as a poison, producing certain reactions. Some of these proteins are derived from animal emanations, from pollens, or are found in the diet. Asthma, urticaria, hay fever are often allergic conditions. *Syn.* allergy.

allocheiria (*al-lō-ki-ri-a*). A sensation felt on the opposite side to that which is touched.

allograft (*a-lō-grahft*). Graft with material obtained from a donor.

alloy (*al'-oy*). A mixture of two or more metals obtained by fusing them together.

alopecia (*al-ō-pē'-si-a*). Absence of hair, baldness.

alpha cells. Cells of the Islets of Langerhans in the pancreas which secrete glucagon, an antagonist of insulin.

alpha rays (*al-fah räs*). Nuclear radiation consisting of two protons and two neutrons which is the helium nucleus. Will penetrate only a few mm into tissue.

alternating current (*orl'-ter-nā-tin ku-rent*). Electric current in which the direction periodically reverses.

alum. Ammonium or potassium aluminium sulphate. Astringent and haemostatic. Alum precipitated toxoid protects against diphtheria.

aluminium (*al-yū-min'-ium*). A white metal of low specific gravity. *A. hydroxide* used as an antacid for gastric ulcer. *A. silicate*. Kaolin used for poultices and also given by mouth as a gastric antacid.

alveoli (*al-vē'-ō-lī*). (Sing. is **alveolus**.) (1) The sockets of the teeth. (2) The air cells in the lungs. (3) The secreting units of the breasts.

alveolitis (*al-vē-ō-lī-tis*). Inflammation of an alveolus.

Alzheimer's disease (*alz'-hī-mer*). Degeneration of the brain cortex. Loss of memory, aphasia, and paralysis occur.

amalgam (*am-al-gam*). An alloy of mercury and other metals. *Dental A*, is of silver, tin and mercury. Used for filling teeth.

amastia (*ā-mas-ti-a*). Absence of breasts.

amaurosis (*am-aw-rō'-sis*). Blindness from disease or defect of the nervous system of the eye; occurs in uraemia.

amaurotic family idiocy (*a-maw-ro-tik*). This condition, also known as Tay-Sach's disease, occurs in infants. There is optic atrophy, rigidity of the limbs and coma.

ambidextrous (*am-bi-deks'-trus*). Equally skilful with each hand.

ambivalence (*am-bi-va-lens*). Contrary emotions, such as love and hate, are experienced towards the same object or person.

amblyopia (*am-bli-ō'-pi-a*). Indistinct vision; approaching blindness.

amblyoscope (*am-bli-o-skōp*). Instrument used in orthoptics for the correction of squint.

amboceptor (*am'-bo-sep'-tor*). Immune body.

ambulance (*am-bū-lanz*). A vehicle for the conveyance of sick and wounded.

ambulant (*am-bū-lant*). Able to walk.

ambulatory (*am'-bū-lā-to-rē*). Relating to walking; moving about. *A. treatment of fractures.* Enables the patient to remain up and about. The limb is immobilized in plaster of Paris.

amelioration (*a-mēl-i-or-ā'-shon*). General improvement in the condition of the patient.

amenorrhoea (*a-men-o-re'-a*). Absence of menstruation. In *primary A.*, menstruation has never been established. *Secondary A.* occurs after menstruation has commenced. There is amenorrhoea in pregnancy, and it may occur in certain endocrine disorders, anaemia, etc.

amentia (*a-men'-she-a*). Absence of intellect; idiocy.

ametria (*a-mē-triā*). Absence of uterus.

ametropia (*am-e-trō'-pi-a*). Defective vision due to abnormal form or refractive power of the eye.

amino-acids (*am'-īn-ō*). Nitrogen-containing organic acids of which proteins are built. Ten are considered to be essential to health and must be present in the food. They are leucine, phenylalanine, lysine, arginine, histidine, valine, tryptophane, isoleucine, methionine and threonine.

aminopterin (*a-min-op'-ter-in*). A folic acid antagonist.

amitosis (*a-mit-ō'-sis*). Simple cell division without chromosome formation.

ammonia (*am-mō'-ne-a*). A volatile alkali with a pungent odour.

amnesia (*am-nē'-si-a*). Loss of memory. *Anterograde A.* Inability to remember recent events. *Retrograde A.* Symptom of concussion. The patient cannot remember what happened immediately before the accident.

amniocentesis (*am-ni-ō-sen-tē-sis*). Aspiration of liquor amnii from the uterus for diagnostic purposes.

amniography (*am-ni-o-gra-fi*). Radiographic demonstration of amniotic sac by injection of radio-opaque dye.

amnion (*am'-nē-on*). The sac directly encircling the fetus in utero. (*See diagram of early embryo*, p. 29.)

amniotic fluid (*am-nē-o-tik floo-id*). *See* LIQUOR AMNII.

amoeba (*am-ē'-ba*). A microscopic unicellular animal, one variety of which causes amoebic dysentery.

amoebiasis (*am-ē-bī'-as-is*). Infection with pathogenic amoebae (plural of amoeba).

amoebicide (*am-ē-bi-s̆id*). Substance lethal to amoeba.

amorphous (*ā-mor-fus*). Formless.

ampère (*ahm-pār*). Unit measure of electric current.

amphiarthrosis (*am-fi-ar-thrō'-sis*). A slightly movable joint, *e.g.* the articulations of the spine.

amphoteric (*am-fo-ter'-ik*). Capable of acting both as acid and base.

ampoule (*am'-pūl*). A sealed phial containing some drug or solution sterilized ready for use.

ampulla (*am-pū-la*). Any flask-shaped dilatation. *A. of Vater. See* VATER'S AMPULLA.

amputation (*am-pū-tā'-shon*). The removal of a limb or organ.

amylase (*am'-il-āz*). An enzyme which has a digestive action on carbohydrates. It converts starch into maltose. It is found as ptyalin in the saliva and as amylopsin in the pancreas.

amyloid disease (*am'-il-oyd*), also called fatty or lardaceous (*lar-dās'-he-us*) disease. Wax-like material is laid down in the liver, kidneys, spleen and blood vessels. It usually occurs as a result of long-standing infection.

amylopsin (*am-il-op'-sin*). Amylase.

amylum. Starch.

amyotonia (*ā-mī-o-tōn'-i-a*). A form of muscular feebleness or paralysis, often congenital.

amyotrophic (*ā-mī-o-trō'-fik*). Pertaining to muscular atrophy.

ana. Used in prescriptions to mean so much of each. *Syn.* aa.

anabolic compound (*a-na-bo-lik kom-pownd*). Chemical substance which helps to repair body tissue.

anabolism (*an-ab'-o-lizm*). *See* METABOLISM.

anacrotism (*an-a'-krot-ism*). A small additional wave or notch found in the ascending limb of the tracing of the pulse curve.

anaemia (*a-nĕ-mi-a*). Diminished oxygen-carrying capacity of the blood, due to a reduction in the number of red cells or in their content of haemoglobin, or both. The cause may be inadequate production of red cells or excessive loss of blood. (For different types, *e.g.* Pernicious A., see under special name.) *See* BLOOD COUNT.

anaerobe (*an-ār-ōb*). Any micro-organism that can live and multiply in the absence of free oxygen, *e.g.* tetanus.

anaesthesia (*an-es-thē'-zi-a*). Absence of sensation; loss of feeling. *Basal A.* Partial general anaesthesia obtained by a drug such as morphine given before an inhalation anaesthesia. *Dissociated A.* Loss of sensation to pain and temperature, sense of touch being retained. *General A.* This gives loss of consciousness. *Glove A.* Hysterical loss of feeling in the area of the hand a glove covers. *Intravenous A.* A general anaesthesia produced by intravenous injection. *Local A.* Anaesthesia of a certain area only. *Nerve block A.* Local anaesthesia produced by injecting an anaesthetic into a sensory nerve. *Rectal A.* General anaesthesia by administering an anaesthetic rectally. *Refrigeration A.* Anaesthesia produced by intense cold. *Spinal A.* An anaesthetic is injected into the subarachnoid space of the spinal cord producing anaesthesia in the lower half of the body.

anaesthetic (*an-es-thet-ik*). An agent which produces insensibility. (As an adjective it means insensible to touch.)

anaesthetist (*an-ēs'-thet-ist*). The administrator of anaesthetics.

anal (*ā-nal*). Of the anus.

analeptic (*an-a-lep-tik*). A restorative. A drug which restores to consciousness, *e.g.* nikethamide.

analgesia (*an-al-jē'-zia*). Diminished sensibility to pain. A symptom in certain nervous diseases, *e.g.* syringomyelia.

analgesic (*an-al-jē-zik*). Relieving pain; remedy for pain.

analogous (*a-nal'-ō-jus*). Similar in certain respects.

analysis (*a-na'-li-sis*). In chemistry, the breaking down of a substance into its constituent parts. In psychiatric medicine, psycho-analysis.

analyst (*an'-al-ist*). The person who analyses.

anaphase (*an'-a-fāz*). A stage in mitosis.

anaphoresis (*an-a-for-ēs'-is*). Diminished activity of the sweat glands.

anaphylaxis (*a-na-fi-lak'-sis*). A state of shock induced by an antigen-antibody reaction occurring in cells which cause the release of substances acting on the vascular system.

anaplasia (*an-a-plā'-si-a*). The reversion of a special tissue or cells to a less differentiated type.

anastomosis (*an'-as-to-mō'-sis*). In anatomy the intercommunication of the terminal branches of two or more blood vessels. In surgery the establishment of some

artificial connection, as, for
instance, between two parts
of the intestine.

anatomy (*an-at'-o-mē*). The science of organic structure. *A.,
applied*. As applied to diagnosis and treatment.

anconeus (*an-kŏ'-nĕ-us*). A
small extensor muscle of the
forearm.

androgen (*an-drŏ-jen*). A hormone producing male sex
characteristics.

android pelvis (*an-droyd pelvis*). Shaped like a male pelvis. The narrow forepelvis,
shallow posterior segment
and straight lateral walls
make child-bearing difficult.

androsterone (*an-dro-ste-rŏn*).
A breakdown product of testosterone.

anencephalous (*an-en-kef'-al-
us*). Having no brain; occurs
in monsters; incompatible
with life.

anergic (*an-er'-jik*). Inactive.
Slack.

aneroid (*a-nār'-oyd*). Without
liquid. *A. barometer*. One
that measures air pressure by
its action on elastic lid of box
exhausted of air, not by
height of fluid column.

aneurine hydrochloride (*a-nū-
rin hī-drŏ-klo-rīd*). Vitamin
B₁. *See* VITAMINS.

aneurysm (*an'-ū-rizm*). A permanent dilatation of an
artery usually with rupture of

the internal and middle coats.
It may be *fusiform* or *sacculated* (*see diagrams*). The
thoracic aorta and the
innominate artery are those
usually affected, more rarely
the abdominal aorta.
Arteriovenous A. is a communication between an
artery and a vein, usually the
result of injury.

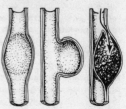

*4 Types of aneurysm: fusiform,
sacculated and dissecting*

aneurysm needle (*an'-ū-rizm*) A
blunt instrument which can
be passed under a vessel; the
eye is then threaded and the
needle withdrawn, leaving
the ligature beneath the
vessel ready to tie.

angiectasis (*an-ji-ek'-ta-sis*).
Dilatation of blood vessel.

angiitis (*an-ji-ī-tis*). Inflamation
of blood vessels.

angina (*an-jī'-na*). Suffocating
pain; thus any severe sore
throat associated with swelling of the walls of the air
passages may be termed
angina. Ludwig's angina,

Vincent's angina, are examples; but the commonest use of the term is in angina pectoris.

angina pectoris (*an-jī'-na pek'-tor-is*). A disease characterized by sense of suffocation, with pain in the chest due to insufficient blood supply to the heart, the arteries being diseased. It occurs on effort. Sublingual glyceryl trinitrate is helpful.

angiocardiogram (*an-jē-ō-kar'-dē-o-gram*). The x-ray film which shows up the heart and great vessels.

angiocardiography (*an-jē-ō-kar-dē-o'-graf-i*). To demonstrate the activity and function of the heart and great vessels by the injection of contrast medium.

angiogram (*an-jē-ō-gram*). X-ray film showing blood vessels.

angiography (*an-jē-og'-raf-ē*). An opaque liquid is injected to show the blood vessels on x-ray.

angioma (*an-jē-ō'-ma*). A tumour composed of blood vessels, often called a naevus.

angioneurotic (*an'-ji-ō-nū-rot'-ik*). Having to do with the nervous control of the blood vessels. Thus *angioneurotic oedema* is a persistent or intermittent swelling of parts such as the eyelid or lip. It may be an allergic symptom.

angioparalysis (*an-jē-ō-pa-ra'-li-sis*). Vasomotor paralysis.

angioplacentography (*an-ji-ō-pla-sen-to'-gra-fi*). Radiography of placental blood vessels by injection of radioopaque dye.

angioplasty (*an-jē-ō-plas'-ti*). Plastic surgery of the blood vessels.

angiosarcoma (*an-jē-ō-sar-kō'-ma*). A sarcoma composed of vascular tissue.

angiospasm (*an-jē-ō-spazm*). The blood vessels contract in spasms.

angiotensin (*an-ji-ō-ten-sin*). A polypeptide raising blood pressure and formed by the action of renin on plasma globulins.

Angström unit (*ang-strer-m*). Unit of measurement of wavelengths of light, equal to one ten thousand millionth of a metre.

anhidrosis (*an-hī-drō'-sis*). Deficiency of perspiration.

anhidrotics (*an-hid-rot'-iks*). Drugs which reduce the amount of perspiration, *e.g.* belladonna, hyoscyamus.

anhydrous (*an-hī'-drus*). Without water.

aniline (*a-nil-in*). Phenylamine. Used in preparing dyestuffs.

animalcule (*an-im-al'-kūl*). Microscopic animal.

anion (*an'-ī-on*). An ion which holds a negative charge of electricity and is repelled from the negative pole, or cathode, of a battery.

aniridia (*a-ni-ri-di-a*). Absence or defect of iris.

anisocoria (*an-is-o-ko'-ri-a*). Inequality of the pupils.

anisocytosis (*an-i-so-sī-tō'-sis*). Inequality of size of the red blood cells.

anisomelia (*an-is-o-me'-li-a*). Unequal limbs which should be a pair.

anisometropia (*a-ni-sō-me-trō-pi-a*). Refraction of the two eyes is different.

ankle (*ang'-kl*). The joint between the leg and the foot. The bones which articulate are the tibia and fibula above and the talus below.

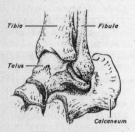

5 *The ankle joint*

ankyloblepharon (*an-ki-lō-blef'-a-ron*). Adhesion of the edges of the eyelids.

ankyloglossia (*an-ki-lō-glo'-si-a*). Inability to protrude the tongue fully and tendency for it to deviate to one side, usually the result of damage to the tongue muscles.

ankylosing spondylitis (*an-ki-lō-sing spon-di-lī-tis*). Disease of joints, of unknown aetiology, in which destruction of the joint space occurs and is followed by sclerosis and calcification. The sacro-iliac joints are predominantly affected.

ankylosis (*an-kilō'-sis*). Immobility in a joint, following inflammation or prolonged immobilization. *False A.* Fixation or stiffness produced by conditions around the joint, such as contraction of skin, *e.g.* after burns, or of tendons, by ossification of muscles, or by outgrowths of bone. *True A.* Fixation or stiffness produced by conditions in the joint such as injury or arthritis. *Fibrous A.* Fixation by fibrous tissue. *Bony A.* The articular surfaces of the bones are fused together.

Ankylostoma duodenale (*an-ki-lo-stō'-ma du-ō-den-ar'-li*). A minute parasitic hookworm which may inhabit the duodenum in large numbers and cause profound anaemia.

ankylostomiasis (*an-ki-lō-stō-*

mi'-a-sis). Hook-worm disease. Infection with the Ankylostoma duodenale.

annular (*an'-ū-lar*). Ring-shaped. *A. ligament.* The ligament around the wrist or ankle.

anode (*an'-ōd*). Electrode with positive charge.

anodyne (*an'-o-dīn*). A pain-relieving drug.

anomalous (*an-om'-al-us*). Irregular. Out of the ordinary.

anomia (*a-nō-mi-a*). Inability to name objects and recall names.

anonychia (*ā-nō-ni'-ki-a*). Without nail formation.

anoperineal (*ā-nō-pe-rin-ē-al*). Relating to anus and perineum.

Anopheles (*an-of'-el-ēz*). A genus of mosquitoes. They are carriers of the malarial parasite, their bite being the means of transmitting the disease to human beings.

anorchous (*an-or'-kus*). Having no testes, or the condition in which the testes have not descended into the scrotum.

anorectal (*ā-nō-rek-tal*). Of the anus and rectum.

anorexia (*an-o-rek'-sē-a*). Lack of appetite, abhorrence of food. *A. nervosa.* Patients may imagine that certain articles of diet are harmful to them. Their diet becomes

progressively limited resulting in extreme emaciation. Psychological treatment is indicated.

anosmia (*an-os'-mi-a*). Loss of sense of smell.

anovular (*a-no-vū-la*). Without ovulation, esp. of menstrual bleeding when ovulation has not occurred.

anovulation (*an-ov-ū-lā'-shon*). Cessation of ovulation.

anoxaemia (*an-ok-sē'-mi-a*). Insufficient oxygen in the blood.

anoxia (*a-nok-si-a*). Absence of oxygen. Often implies insufficient oxygen available for normal respiratory metabolism, *i.e.* hypoxia.

antacid (*ant-as'-id*). Any substance neutralizing an acid, *e.g.* sodium bicarbonate.

antagonist (*an-tag'-on-ist*). An organ such as a muscle that acts in opposition to another, or a drug neutralizing another drug.

antaphrodisiac (*ant'-af-ro-diz'-i-ak*). An agent which diminishes sexual desire.

ante (*an-tē*). Before.

anteflexion (*an-tē-flek'-shon*). A bending forward, as of the normal position of the uterus.

ante mortem (*an-tē maw-tem*). Before death.

antenatal (*an-tē-nā-tal*). Before birth.

antepartum (*an-tē-par'-tum*).

Before birth. *Antepartum haemorrhage* may be inevitable or accidental when it is due to partial separation of the placenta; incidental when it is due to diseases of the cervix.

anterior (*an-te'-ri-or*). In front of.

anterior chamber of eye. The space between cornea in front and the iris and lens behind, which contains the aqueous humour.

anterior commissure (*kom'-mis-sūr*). A bundle of nerve fibres crossing in the mid-line in front of the third ventricle and serving to connect certain parts of the two cerebral hemispheres.

anterior fontanelle. *See* FONTANELLE.

anterior poliomyelitis (*pol-i-ō'-mī-el-ī'-tis*). Inflammation of the anterior horns of the grey matter in the spinal cord. Infantile paralysis.

anterior root. Motor root, *syn.* ventral root. Nerve root emerging from the spinal cord carrying motor fibres.

anterograde (*an-ter-ō-grād*). Going forwards.

antero-inferior (*an-te-rō-in-fār'-i-or*). Lying in front and below.

antero-interior (*an-te-rō-in-tār'-i-or*). Lying to the front and internally.

anterolateral (*an-te-rō-la'-ter-al*). In front and to the side.

anteromedian (*an-te-rō-mē'-di-an*). Lying in front and near the mid-line.

anteroposterior (*an-te-rō-pō-stā'-ri-or*). From front to back.

anterosuperior (*an-te-rō-soo-pā'-ri-or*). In front and above.

anteversion (*an'-tē-ver'-shon*). The state of being inclined forward. It is the normal position of the uterus.

anthelmintic (*an-thel-min'-tik*). A remedy for intestinal worms, *e.g.* santonin, extract of filix mas, etc.

anthracosis (*an-thra-kō'-sis*). Disease caused by inhaling coal dust or soot into the lungs. Seen in miners.

anthrax (*an'-thrax*). An acute, infectious disease produced by the Anthrax bacillus. *Skin A.* and *Pulmonary A.* are the two main forms.

anthropoid (*an'-thro-poyd*). Manlike. *A. apes* include animals most closely related to man. *A. pelvis* has a narrowed transverse inlet which is long antero-posteriorly.

anthropology (*an-throp-ol'-o-ji*). The natural history of mankind.

anti (*an-ti*). Prefix meaning against.

antibiotic (*an-ti-bī-o'-tik*).

Opposed to life; drugs used in the treatment of bacterial infections.

antibodies (*an-ti-bo-dis*). Protein substances, usually circulating in the blood, which neutralize corresponding antigens.

anticholinergic (*an-ti-kō-li-ner-jik*). Term applied to drugs inhibiting the action of acetylcholine.

anticoagulant (*an-ti-kō-ag-ū-lant*). Substance which delays the clotting of blood.

anticonvulsant (*an-ti-kon-vul'-sant*). A drug used to prevent a convulsion.

antidepressants (*an-ti-de-pre-sants*). Drugs used to treat depression. They may be mono-amine oxidase inhibitors, the imipramine group of drugs or stimulants.

antidiuretic hormone (*an-ti-dī-ū-re-tik hor-mōn*). Posterior pituitary hormone regulating the amount of water passing from the uriniferous tubules into the renal substance.

antidote (*an'-ti-dōt*). The corrective to a poison.

antigen (*an'-ti-jen*). Substance capable of stimulating the formation of antibodies.

antihistamine (*an-ti-his'-ta-mēn*). Drug counteracting the effects of the liberation of histamine in the tissues, *e.g.*

Anthisan, Benadryl, Dramamine, Phenergan, etc.

anti-infective factor (*an-ti-in-fek-tif fak-tor*). Found in vitamin A.

antimetabolites (*an-ti-me-ta-bo-līts*). Chemical substances used to prevent cell division in malignant disease.

antimitotic (*an-ti-mī-to-tik*). Substance which prevents mitosis.

antimony (*an-ti'-mo-ni*). A metallic poison, like arsenic in its properties.

antimycotic (*an-ti-mi-ko-tik*). Substance used to treat fungus diseases.

antiperistalsis (*an-ti-pe-ri-stal'-sis*). Reverse peristalis, *i.e.* from below upward. *See* PERISTALSIS.

antiphlogistic (*an-ti-flo-jis'-tik*). Relieving inflammation.

antipruritic (*an-ti-proo-rit-ik*). Substance relieving itching.

antipyretic (*an-ti-pī-ret'-ik*). A drug which reduces the high temperatures of feverish conditions.

antirachitic factor (*an-ti-rak-it-ik fak-tor*). *Syn.* Vitamin D. Prevents rickets.

antiscorbutic (*an-ti-skor-bū'-tik*). *Syn.* Vitamin C or ascorbic acid. Prevents scurvy.

antiseptic (*an-ti-sep'-tik*). A substance opposing sepsis by arresting the growth and multiplication of micro-organisms. Iodine, phenol, biniodide of mercury, chlorine, formalin, lysol, quaternary ammonium compounds, chloroxylenols, hypochlorities are common antiseptics.

antiserum (*an-ti-sā-rum*). Serum, usually prepared from horses containing a high titre of antibody to a specific organism or toxin.

anti-siphonage (*an-ti-sī-fon-āj*). Preventing siphonage. *A. pipe.* Small pipes leading from the soil pipe which contain air. They are necessary when lavatories are placed one above another on different floors. They prevent the suction of water from the traps of the lavatories as the water from the upper floors rushes down.

antisocial (*an-ti-sō-shal*). Against the normally accepted behaviour in society.

antispasmodic (*an-ti-spaz-mo'-dik*). An agent relieving spasm.

antistatic (*an-ti-sta-tik*). Preventing a build-up of static electricity.

antithrombin (*an-ti-throm'-bin*). A substance in the blood having the power of

retarding or preventing coagulation.

antithyroid drugs (*an-ti-thī-royd*). Substances which restrict the secretion of thyroid hormones by interference in the intermediary metabolism of the gland.

antitoxin (*an-ti-tok'-sin*). A specific antibody produced in the blood in response to a toxin or poison. The antibody is capable of neutralizing that particular toxin.

antitragus (*an-ti-trā'-gus*). The prominence of the lower portion of the external ear.

antivenin (*an-ti-ven'-in*). An antidote injected in cases of poisoning by snake bite.

antrostomy (*an-trost'-o-mi*). Incision of an antrum.

antrum (*an'-trum*). A cave; applied to the maxillary sinus, called the antrum of Highmore, and the cavity in the mastoid bone communicating with the middle ear. *See* SINUS, MAXILLARY.

anuria (*an-ū'-ri-a*). Cessation of the production of urine; to be distinguished from retention of urine, due to inability to empty the bladder.

anus (*ā'-nus*). The rectal exit. *Imperforate A.* A congenital malformation where a child is born with no anal opening, or an anus is present but does not communicate with the bowel above. Treatment is operative and success depends on degree of development of lower bowel.

anxiety neurosis (*ang-zī-e-ti nū-rō'-sis*). A neurosis in which fear and apprehension mainly control the patient's behaviour and ideas.

aorta (*ā-or'-ta*). The large artery arising from the left ventricle of the heart and supplying blood to the whole body.

aortic incompetence (*ā-or'-tik in-kom'-pe-tens*). Blood from the aorta regurgitates back into the left ventricle, due to inefficiency of the valve.

aortic stenosis (*a-or-tik ste-nō-sis*). Narrowing of the aortic valve due to malformation or disease.

aortic valves. Three semi-lunar valves guarding the entrance from the left ventricle to the aorta and preventing the backward flow of the blood.

aortitis (*ā-or-tī'-tis*). Inflammation of the aorta.

apathy (*ap'-a-thi*). Listlessness. Lack of activity.

apepsia (*ā-pep'-si-a*). Failure of digestion due to deficiency of gastric juice.

aperient (*a-pār-i-ent*). A purgative medicine, *e.g.* cascara.

aperistalsis (*ā-per-i-stal'-sis*). Cessation of peristalsis.

apex (*ā-peks*). Top, extreme point, summit. *A. of the heart.* Narrow end of heart enclosing left ventricle. *A. beat.* The heart beat as felt at its most forcible point on the chest wall. This corresponds with the position of the apex of the left ventricle.

Apgar score (*ap-gah-skaw*). System for assessing vitality of new-born infant, esp. heart rate and respiratory effort.

aphagia (*a-fā'-ji-a*). Inability to swallow.

aphakia (*a-fā-ki-a*). Absence of lens of the eye.

aphasia (*a-fā'-zi-a*). Speechlessness; due to disease or injury of brain.

aphonia (*a-fō'-ni-a*). Loss of voice.

aphrodisiac (*af-rō-diz'-i-ak*). An agent which increases sexual power.

aphthae (*af'-thē*). Small white ulcers in the mouth.

aphthous stomatitis (*af-thus sto-ma-tī'-tis*). Inflammation of the mucous membrane of the mouth due to herpes simplex virus, *cf.* thrush.

apical (*ā'-pik-al*). Pertaining to the apex. *A. abscess.* Abscess of root of tooth.

apicectomy (*ā-pi-sek-to-mi*). Excision of the root-end of a tooth.

apicolysis (*ā-pi-ko-lī'-sis*). Stripping of the parietal pleura from the chest wall to collapse a tuberculous apex of lung.

aplasia (*ā-plā'-si-a*). Non-development of an organ or tissue.

aplastic anaemia (*ā-plas-tik a-nē-mi-a*). Anaemia resulting from destruction of bone marrow cells.

apnoea (*ap-nē'-a*). Suspended respiration.

apocrine glands (*a-po-krin glans*). Specialized sweat glands found in the axillae and genital regions.

aponeurosis (*ap-o-nū-rō'-sis*). A tendon-like fibrous tissue, which invests the muscles and transmits their movements to the structures upon which they act.

apophysis (*ap-off'-is-is*). A bony protuberance or outgrowth.

apoplexy (*ap'-o-plek-si*). A stroke. The effects of a cerebrovascular accident.

apothecary (*ap-oth'-e-ka-ri*). A druggist or pharmacist.

appendicectomy (*ap-pen-di-sek'-to-mi*). Removal of the vermiform appendix.

appendices epiploicae (*ep-pi-plō'-i-sē*). Small peritoneal bags of fat projecting from the peritoneal coat of the large intestine.

appendicitis (*ap-pen-di-sī'-tis*). Inflammation of the appendix.

appendix vermiformis (*ap-en-diks ver-mi-for'-mis*). A wormlike offshoot from the caecum, ending blindly, and 1 to 5in long.

apperception (*ap-er-sep-shon*). The conscious reception of a sensory impression.

applicator (*ap'-li-kā-tor*). An instrument for applying local remedies, *e.g.* radium.

apposition (*ap-o-zi'-shon*). The lying together or the fitting together of two structures.

apraxia (*a-prak'-si-a*). Inability to perform certain purposive movements. The lesion is in the cerebral cortex.

APT. Alum precipitated toxoid. A diphtheria prophylactic.

aptitude (*ap'-ti-tūd*). A facility or a particular bent for certain work or actions.

aptyalism (*ap-tī-a-lism*). Absence of salivation.

apyrexia (*ā-pī-rek'-si-a*). Without fever.

aqua (*a'-kwa*). Water: abbreviation is *aq.*

aqueduct (*ak'-wē-dukt*). Certain canals of the body, such as the A. of Sylvius which leads from the third to the fourth ventricle of the brain.

aqueous humour (*ā'-kwē-us hū'-mor*). Fluid in the eye between the cornea and the iris and the lens.

arachnodactyly (*a-rak-nō-dak-*

ti-li). Abnormally long and slender bones of the extremities.

arachnoid (*a-rak'-noyd*). Resembling a web. *A. membrane*, surrounds the brain and spinal cord. It is between the dura and pia mater.

Aran-Duchenne's disease (*a-ran-dū-shenz*). The commonest myopathy occurring in children. Also known as pseudo-hypertrophic muscular dystrophy.

arbor vitae (*ah-bor vē-tī*). Tree-like appearance seen in a section of the cerebellum and also applied to that seen in the interior folds of the cervix of the uterus.

arborization (*ah-bor-ī-zā-shon*). Branching of processes of nerve cells.

arboviruses (*ah-bo-vi'-ru-sez*). Insect-borne viruses causing diseases such as yellow fever.

arcus. An arch or ring. *A. Senilis*. An opaque circle round the edge of the cornea, occurring in the aged.

areola (*ā-re'-ō-la*). The pigmented skin round the nipple of the breast.

areolar tissue (*a-rē'-ō-la ti-shoo*). Filmy connective tissue of the body.

argentaffinoma (*ar-jen-ta-fi-nō-ma*). Also known as carcinoid tumour. Arises

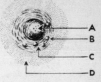

6 *Areola of breast: A = Nipple*
B = Montgomery's tubules
C = Primary areola
D = Secondary areola,
develops in the early weeks of
pregnancy

from so-called argentaffin cells in the gastro-intestinal tract.

argenti nitras (*ar-jen'-ti nī'-tras*). *See* NITRATE OF SILVER.

argentum. Silver.

arginine (*ah-ji-nēn*). One of the essential amino-acids formed from the digestion of dietary protein. It is present as a stage in urea formation.

argon (*ar'-gon*). An inert gaseous element in the atmosphere in very small quantities.

Argyll-Robertson (*ar-gīl-ro'-bert-son*) **pupil.** Pupil of eye which is small, reacting to accommodation but not to light. Seen in diseases of the nervous system, *e.g.* tabes dorsalis.

argyria (*ar-ji'-ri-a*). Discolouration of the skin from the continued use of preparations of silver.

arrector pili (*a-rek-tor pē-lē*). Muscle fibres around the hair follicles which on contraction produce 'goose-flesh'.

arrhenoblastoma (*a-rā-nō-blas-tō-ma*). A neoplasm of the ovary associated with masculinization.

arrhythmia (*a-rith'-mi-a*). Disturbance of rhythm (usually the heart's rhythm). *Sinus A.* Increased pulse rate during inspiration, decreased during expiration; common in infants.

artefact (*ar'-te-fakt*). A lesion produced by artificial means.

arterial (*ar-tār-i-al*). Pertaining to an artery. Thus *arterial tension* means the pressure of the blood circulating in a given artery.

arteriectomy (*ar-tar-i-ek-to-mi*). Excision of part of an artery.

arteriography (*ar-tār-i-og'-raf-i*). To demonstrate blood vessels following the injection of contrast medium opaque to x-rays.

arterioles (*ar-te-ri-ōls*). Small arteries with contractile muscular walls which control the supply of blood to the capillaries.

arteriopathy (*ar-tār-i-o-pa-thi*). Disease of the arteries.

arterioplasty (*ar-tār-i-ō-pla-sti*). Surgery to reform an artery, especially for aneurysm.

arteriorrhaphy (*ar-tār-i-ōr'-raf-i*). Suture of an artery.

arterio-sclerosis (*ar-tār'-i-ō-skler-ō'-sis*). Degeneration of an artery with hardening of its walls, seen chiefly in old age. The condition is accompanied by high blood pressure.

arteriotomy (*ar-tār-i-o-to-mi*). Incising an artery.

arteriovenous aneurysm (*ar-tār-ō-vē'-nus an'-ūr-ism*). See ANEURYSM.

arteritis (*ar-ter-ī'-tis*). Inflammation of the arteries.

artery (*ar'-te-ri*). A vessel carrying blood from the heart.

arthralgia (*ar-thral'-ji-a*). Pain in the joints.

arthrectomy (*ar-threk'-to-mi*). The removal by operation of the whole or part of a joint.

arthritis (*ar-thrī'-tis*). Inflammation of a joint. See RHEUMATOID A.

arthro (*ar-thrō*). Prefix referring to a joint.

arthroclasia (*ar-thrō-klā-si-a*). An operation for breaking up an ankylosed joint to produce free movement.

arthrodesis (*ar-thrō-dē'-sis*). Fixation of a joint by means of a surgical operation.

arthrodial (*ar-thrō'-di-al*). Term applied to a joint which glides.

arthrodynia (*ar-thrō-din'-i-a*). Pain in the joints.

arthrography (*ar-thro'-gra-fi*). Radiography of joint after the injection of radio-opaque fluid to outline the joint space.

arthropathy (*ar-thro-pa-thi*). Disease of the joints. Commonly used to imply secondary damage to joints as a result of other disease processes.

arthroplasty (*ar-thrō-plas'-ti*). The making of an artificial joint.

arthrotomy (*ar-throt'-o-mi*). Incision into a joint.

articular (*ar-tik'-ū-lar*). Relating to the joints; the articulation of a skeleton is the manner in which the bones are joined together.

articulation (*ar-tik-ū-lā-shon*). (1) A joint between two or more bones. (2) The enunciation of words.

artificial feeding (*ar-ti-fi-shal*). Feeding of an infant with food other than its mother's milk.

artificial insemination. Artificial introduction of spermatozoa into the vagina.

artificial kidney. Dialysing apparatus through which blood from the patient is pumped so that excretory products such as urea may be extracted in the event of the patient's own kidneys not functioning.

artificial pneumothorax. See PNEUMOTHORAX.

arytenoid (*ar-i-tē-noyd*). The term applied to two funnel-shaped cartilages of the larynx.

asbestos (*as-bes'-tos*). A mineral substance which is incombustible and which does not conduct heat.

asbestosis (*as-bes-tō-sis*). Disease of the lung caused by inhalation of asbestos dust.

ascariasis (*as-kar-ī-a-sis*). Infestation of the bowel by roundworms (ascarides).

ascaricide (*a-ska-ri-sīd*). Lethal to roundworms.

Ascaris (*as'-kar-is*). A genus of parasitic roundworm. *A. lumbricoides*, long roundworm.

Aschheim-Zondek test. See ZONDEK-ASCHHEIM TEST.

Aschoff nodules (*ash-off nodūls*). The focal lesions of acute rheumatism consisting of perivascular necrosis of collagen. These nodules tend to occur in the heart, muscles and connective tissues.

ascites (*as-sī'-tēz*). Fluid collection in the abdominal cavity.

ascitic fluid (*a-si-tik floo-id*). Fluid of ascites which can be aspirated.

ascorbic acid (*a-scaw-bik*). Vitamin C. See VITAMINS.

asepsis (*ā-sep'-sis*). The state of

being free from living pathogenic micro-organisms.

aseptic (*ā-sep'-tik*). Free from pathogenic micro-organisms. In aseptic surgery all instruments, dressings, etc., are sterilized before use.

asexual (*ā-sek-shal*). Having no sex. A method of reproduction in which there is no gamete formation.

Aspergillus (*as-per-gil-us*). The name of a group of fungi, some species of which are pathogenic, causing aspergillosis which may infect the ear, eye or lungs.

aspermia (*ā-sper-mi-a*). Inability to produce semen.

asphyxia (*as-fik'-si-a*). Suffocation.

aspiration (*as-pi-rā'-shon*). The operation of drawing off fluids from the body, for example, in a case of pleural effusion or an abscess. Suction is usually applied by means of a syringe or aspirator. Fluid may be removed from the pleural cavity by *siphonage*, or a two-way aspirating syringe is used.

aspirator (*as'-pi-rā-tor*). The apparatus used for aspiration.

assimilation (*as-im-il-ā'-shon*). The utilization of nourishment by the living tissues. *A. pelvis.* One in which the fifth lumbar vertebra is incorporated in the sacral body.

association (*as-sō-si-ā'-shon*). Co-ordination. 'Association of ideas,' *i.e.* a phrase used to denote the secondary thoughts that arise on the receipt of any individual mental impression.

asteatosis (*ā-ste-a-tō'-sis*). Deficient action of sebaceous glands.

astereognosis (*a-ster-e-og-nō'-sis*). Loss of power to recognize the shape of objects by touch.

asthenia (*as-the'-nē-a*). Failure of strength; debility.

asthenopia (*as-then-o'-pi-a*). Weakness of sight.

asthma (*as'-ma*). Paroxysms of difficult breathing, with sense of suffocation. There is difficulty in expiration due to bronchospasm. *Bronchial A.* is generally an allergic state.

astigmatism (*as-tig'-ma-tizm*). Inequality in the curvature of the cornea or lens, with consequent blurring and 'distortion of the images thrown upon the retina.

astragalus (*as-trag'-a-lus*). The ankle bone. *See* ANKLE.

astringent (*as-trinj'-ent*). A substance applied to produce local contraction of blood vessels and inhibit secretion, *e.g.* tannin, adrenaline.

astrocytoma (*as-tro-sī-tō-ma*). A tumour occurring in the central nervous system.

asymmetry (*ā-sim'-me-tri*). Lack of symmetry.

asymptomatic (*ā-simp-tō-ma-tik*). Without any symptoms.

asynclitism (*a-sin'-clit-ism*). Engagement in the pelvis of a diameter of the fetal head other than the biparietal. It may occur with a contracted pelvis.

atavism (*at'-a-vizm*). The recurrence of some hereditary peculiarity which has skipped one or more generations.

ataxia, ataxy (*at-ak'-si*). Literally, disorder; applied to any defective control of muscles and consequent irregularity of movements. *See also* LOCOMOTOR ATAXIA and FRIEDREICH'S ATAXIA.

atelectasis (*at-e-lek'-ta-sis*). Imperfect expansion of the lungs of the new-born. Term also used for collapse of part of the lung from some other cause.

atherogenic (*a-the-rō-je-nik*). Applied to factors which may cause atheroma.

atheroma (*ath-e-rō'-ma*). A degeneration of the walls of the arteries.

atherosclerosis (*a-the-rō-skle-rō-sis*). Fatty degeneration and hardening and narrowing of the arteries.

athetosis (*ath-e-tō'-sis*). A condition marked by continuous and purposeless movements, especially of the hands and fingers.

athlete's heart. Aortic incompetence from strain. *A. foot.* Infectious disease of the skin, between and behind the toes, due to parasitic fungi.

atlas (*at'-las*). First cervical vertebra.

atmosphere (*at'-mōs-fē-er*). The air surrounding the earth. 1 atmosphere of pressure = 101·3kPa (760mm Hg). As it is equal in all directions it is not felt. It is measured by means of a barometer and is sufficient to support a column of mercury 760mm high at sea level. The higher the altitude, the lower the pressure. Moist air is lighter than dry air, and so the barometer falls in damp weather.

atom (*a'-tom*). The structural unit of an element.

atomic weight (*ā-tom'-ik wāt*). The weight of an atom as compared with that of an atom of hydrogen.

atomizer (*at'-omi-i-zer*). A spray for providing a shower of very minute droplets.

atony (*at'-o-ni*). Wanting in muscular tone or vigour; weakness.

atresia (*at-trē'-si-a*). Absence of

a natural passage. Closure of a duct.

atria (*ā-tri-a*) (sing., **atrium**). The two thin-walled chambers of the heart into which the veins drain.

atrial fibrillation (*ā-tri-al fi-bri-lā-shon*). Cardiac arrhythmia caused by the independent contraction of muscle bundles in the atrial walls. There is no co-ordinated atrial contraction and the ventricular contractions are stimulated irregularly.

atrial septal defect (*ā-tri-al septal dē-fekt*). Defect in the development of the heart leaving a hole in the wall separating the right and left atrium.

atrio-ventricular bundle (bundle of His) (*ā-tri-ō ven-tri-kū-la*). A neuromuscular bundle of fibres connecting the atria with the ventricles of the heart, by means of which the impulse to contract is conducted. Degeneration of this bundle produces heart-block, a condition in which the ventricle contracts independently of the atrium. *See* STOKES-ADAMS' SYNDROME.

atrophy (*at'-ro-fi*). Wasting of a part, from disuse or lack of nutrition.

atropine (*at'-ro-pin*). The active principle of belladonna. It paralyses parasympathetic nerve endings, therefore inhibits glandular secretions, and peristalsis, increases the rate of the heart beat and dilates the pupil of the eye. It is used to inhibit bronchial secretion before an anaesthetic and 0·6mg atropine sulphate may be given subcutaneously together with 15mg morphine sulphate. To dilate the pupil of the eye, drops are instilled in a 1 per cent solution.

atropine methyl nitrate. Eumydrin.

atropinism (*at'-rō-pin-ism*), **atropism** (*at'-rō-pism*). Poisoning by atropine. *Symptoms*: Dryness of throat and mouth, restlessness and delirium, red erythematous rash.

attenuation (*at-ten-ū-ā-shon*). A weakening or dilution, term applied particularly to the production of vaccines.

atypical (*ā-ti-pi-kal*). Not typical, *e.g. A. pneumonia* which does not follow the usual pattern.

audiogram (*aw-di-ō-gram*). Chart showing how the ear responds to sounds of differing pitch.

audiometer (*aw-dē-om'-et-er*). An instrument for measuring the acuteness of hearing.

audiometry (*aw-di-o'-me-tri*). Measurement of hearing

ability. The results are usually plotted as an audiogram.

auditory (*aw-di-to-ri*). Pertaining to the sense of hearing.

Auerbach's plexus (*ow'-er-bax*). The collection of nerve fibres (terminations of vagus and sympathetic nerves) and ganglia situated in the intestinal wall. Function: regulates peristalsis.

aura (*aw-ra*). A sensation arising indigenously in the percipient. May precede epileptic fits.

aural (*aw'-ral*). Pertaining to the ear.

auricle (*aw'-ri-kl*). (1) The external ear. (2) One of the upper cavities of the heart now usually termed atrium. (3) An appendage to the atrium. *See* HEART.

auricular (*aw-rik'-ū-lar*). Pertaining to the ear or to the auricles of the heart.

auricular fibrillation (*aw-rik-ū-lar fibri-lā-shon*). *See* ATRIAL FIBRILLATION.

auriculo-ventricular bundle (bundle of His) (*aw-rik'-ū-lō ven-trik'-ū-lar*). *See* ATRIO-VENTRICULAR BUNDLE.

auriscope (*aw-ri-skōp*). An instrument for examining the drum of the ear. An otoscope.

aurist (*aw-rist*). A specialist in diseases of the ear.

auscultation (*aws'-kul-tā-shon*). Listening to sounds of the body for the purpose of diagnosis. Usually a tube is employed, *e.g.* stethoscope.

autistic (*aw-tis-tik*). Self-absorbed. A congenital mental condition preventing the child from making normal relationships or contact with his environment. The child may appear to be mentally retarded.

auto (*aw'-tō*). A prefix meaning self, of itself.

autoclave (*aw'-tō-klāv*). An apparatus for sterilizing by steam under pressure.

autodigestion (*aw-tō-di-jest'-chon*). Process of self-digestion of tissues.

auto-eroticism (*aw-tō-e-ro-ti-sism*). Sexual gratification obtained by a person stimulating himself.

autogenous (*aw-toj'-en-us*). Self-produced.

autograft (*aw-tō-grahft*). Graft taken from the patient's own body. *See* GRAFT.

autographism (*aw-tog'-raf-ism*). Same as dermographism.

auto-hypnosis (*aw-tō-hip'-nō-sis*). Self-induced hypnotism.

auto-immunity (*aw-tō-im-mū'-ni-ti*). State of sensitization to products of one's own organs, *e.g.* as in Hashimoto's disease.

AUT 50

auto-infection (*aw'-tō-in-fek-shon*). Self-infection.

auto-intoxication (*aw-tō-in-toks-i-kā'-shon*). Poisoning by toxins generated within the body.

autolysis (*aw-tol'-is-is*). The process of self-digestion occurring in tissues under pathological conditions and in the uterus during the puerperium.

automatism (*aw-tom'-at-ism*). A condition in which actions are performed without consciousness or regulated purpose; sometimes follows a major or minor epileptic fit.

autonomic nervous system (*aw-to-no-mik ner-vus sis-tem*). Motor supply to smooth muscle and glands. Divided into sympathetic and parasympathetic systems and characterized by synapsing in ganglia after fibres leave the central nervous system. Not directly under conscious control but there is considerable cortical representation.

autoplasty (*aw'-tō-plas-ti*). See AUTOGRAFT.

autopsy (*aw-top'-si*). A post-mortem examination.

auto-radiography (*aw-tō-rā-di-o-gra-fi*). Photography showing localization of radioactive substance in a tissue section.

auto-suggestion (*su-jes-chon*). Self-suggestion: used in the treatment of functional nervous disorders.

auto-transfusion (*aw-tō-trans-fū-zhon*). Transfusion of blood to a patient taken from another part of his body.

avascular (*ā-vas-kū-la*). Bloodless.

aversion (*a-ver-shon*). An intensive dislike. *A. therapy*. The patient is made to dislike the desired object, such as alcohol, by associating something unpleasant with it.

avian tuberculosis (*ā-vē-an*). Tuberculosis in birds. This is rarely transmitted to man.

avirulent (*ā-vi-rū-lent*). Not virulent.

avitaminosis (*ā-vi-tā-mi-nō'-sis*). Lacking in vitamins. Usually the particular vitamin deficiency is specified, *e.g.* avitaminosis A.

avulsion (*a-vul'-shon*). A tearing apart.

axilla (*aks-il'-la*). The armpit.

axillary artery (*ak-sil'-a-rī ar-te-ri*). The artery of the armpit, connecting the subclavian and brachial arteries.

axis (*ak'-sis*). The second cervical vertebra. Also a straight line through the centre of a body. The *axis of the pelvis* is a curved line which is everywhere at right angles to the planes of the pelvic cavity. *Axis traction* is force so applied to the fetus by forceps that its effect is always exerted along the axis of the pelvis. *Axis traction forceps* is a special pattern of forceps, invented originally by Tarnier, to allow an axis traction to be secured.

axon (*aks-ōn*). The long process of a nerve cell conducting impulses away from the cell body.

axonotmesis (*ak-son-ō-tmē-sis*). Damage causing the breakup of nerve fibres but the supporting tissue remains intact.

azoospermia (*ā'-zo-o-sper'-mi-a*). Absence of viable sperms in the semen causing male sterility.

azotaemia (*az-o-tē'-mi-a*). Excess urea in the blood.

azoturia (*az-o-tū'-ri-a*). An increase of urea in the urine.

azygos (*ā-zī'-gos*). Not paired but single.

B

Ba. Chemical symbol for barium.

Babinski's reflex (*bab-in-skēz rē-fleks*). Extensor plantar reflex. Extension instead of flexion of the great toe on stroking the sole of the foot. The sign is normal in infants and abnormal after about two years.

bacillaemia (*ba-si-lē-mi-a*). Bacilli in the blood.

bacillary dysentery (*ba-si-la-ri di-sen-te-ri*). Infection of the gut with Shigella bacilli.

bacilluria (*ba-sil-ū'-ri-a*). Bacilli in the urine.

bacillus (*ba-sil'-us*). See BACTERIA.

bacitracin (*ba-si-trā-sin*). Antibiotic from the Bacillus subtilis group. Sometimes used externally to treat skin infections.

bacteraemia (*bak-ter-ē-mi-a*). Bacteria in the blood.

bacteria (*bak-tār'-i-a*). Microscopic unicellular living organisms; some cause disease and are called pathogenic. The principal forms are: (1) *Cocci*, those which are rounded in shape. When these are disposed in pairs they are called *Diplococci*—these occur in pneumonia, some forms of meningitis, and gonorrhoea. When these occur in chains they are called *Streptococci*, when in clusters *Staphylococci*. (2) *Bacilli* are rod-shaped bacteria which include the Gram-positive organisms causing anthrax, tetanus and diphtheria; Gram-negative causing dysentery, typhoid and plague and the acid-fast organisms of tuberculosis and leprosy. (3) *Spirilla* are corkscrew-like germs, or spiral rods with several twists, occurring in relapsing fever, and syphilis. The majority of bacteria are stationary, but some have power of movement. Bacteria have power of multiplying by splitting across their centre, this is known as binary fission: others form spores, which are small, round, glistening bodies able to withstand great extremes of heat and cold.

bacterial (*bak-tār'-i-al*). Pertaining to bacteria.

bactericidal (*bak-tār-i-sī'-dal*). Capable of killing bacteria.

bacteriologist (*bak-tār-ē-ol'-ō-jist*). One who specializes in the study of bacteria.

bacteriology (*bak-tār-ē-ol'-o-ji*). The study of bacteria.

bacteriolysin (*bak-tār-ē-ō-lī'-sin*). A specific antibody developed in the blood to destroy bacteria.

bacteriolytic (*bak-tā-ri-ō-lit'-ik*). Capable of dissolving bacteria.

bacteriophage (*bak-tār-i-ō-fāj'*). Micro-organism, resembling a virus, capable of attacking other larger micro-organisms and destroying them by lysis.

bacteriostatic (*bak-tār-ē-o-sta-tik*). Preventing the growth of bacteria.

bacteriuria (*bak-tā-ri-ū-ri-a*). Bacteria in the urine.

Bainbridge reflex (*bān-brij rē-fleks*). Increased venous return causing increased heart rate and thought to be associated with inhibition of vagal impulses.

Baker's cysts (*sists*). Cysts originating from synovial pouches connected with joints.

baker's itch. An eczematous disease occurring on the hands of bakers from constant irritation.

balanitis (*bal-an-ī'-tis*). Inflammation of the glans penis.

Balkan beam (*bawl-kan bēm*). Frame fitted over a bed to carry a sling for an injured limb.

ballooning (*ba-lū-nin*). The distension of a cavity by air, or by its natural contents.

ballottement (*bal-lot'-mo*). The sensation of a return tap against the fingers when the hand is suddenly pressed on the pregnant uterus and temporarily displaces the contained fetus as it floats in the liquor amnii. Ballottement may be elicited externally, or per vaginam.

balneotherapy (*bal'-ne-ō-*

ther'-a-pi). The amelioration of disease or pain by baths.

bandage (*ban'-dā-je*). An appliance, generally of woven material, used to give support, apply pressure or secure a dressing.

Bandl's ring. *See* RETRACTION RING.

Bankart's operation (*bankartz*). Operation to repair the glenoid cavity after repeated dislocation of the shoulder joint.

Banti's syndrome (*ban-tiz sin'-arŏm*). Characterized by anaemia with recurrent bleeding from the alimentary tract, leucopaenia and splenomegaly due to portal hypertension.

Banting's diet. Taken to reduce superfluous fat. It has a high protein and low carbohydrate content.

Barbados leg (*bar-bā-dos*). Elephantiasis.

barber's rash. A pustular eczema occurring in the area of the moustache and whiskers. Sycosis Barbae.

barbiturate drugs (*bar-bit-ū-rāt*). Derivatives of barbituric acid, *e.g.* Nembutal, Evipan, Pentothal.

Barlow's disease (*bar-lōs disēz*). Infantile scurvy due to lack of vitamin C in the diet.

Barlow's sign (*bar-lōs sīn*). Testing the newborn infant's legs for congenital dislocation of hip. Many hips become stable within a week or two after birth and the sign can then not be elicited. Early splintage may occasionally be necessary to overcome potential dislocation of the hip.

baroreceptor nerves (*ba-rō-re-sep-tor nervs*). Found in the carotids and arch of the aorta. They stem from the vagus and glossopharyngeal nerves.

barrier nursing (*ba'-ri-er*). The nursing of a patient with an infectious disease in a general ward, or a ward with patients having a variety of infectious diseases. Adequate precautions are taken so that cross infection does not occur.

Bartholin's glands (*bah-tō-lins*). Two small glands, one each side of the vulva, may develop into an abscess or its duct may distend into a cyst.

bartholinitis (*bah-tō-lin-ī'-tis*). Inflammation of Bartholin's glands.

basal ganglia (*bā-zal gan'-gli-a*). Four deeply-placed masses of grey matter within the cerebral hemisphere, known as the caudate, lentiform and amygdaloid nuclei, and the claustrum. Disease of the basal ganglia gives rise to athetosis and Parkinsonism.

basal metabolism (*met-ab'-o-lizm*). The amount of energy consumed in essential physiological processes without taking into account any voluntary activity.

basal metabolic rate. The heat given out per unit of time by the individual under standard conditions, at absolute rest, at least twelve hours after a meal. It indicates the rate of combustion of the foodstuffs and of the tissues of the body. In cases of exophthalmic goitre the metabolic rate is high, while in cases of myxoedema it is lower than normal. For clinical purposes it is determined indirectly by the amount of oxygen taken in and carbon dioxide given out.

basal narcosis (*nar-kō'-sis*). Sleep produced by drugs given before an anaesthetic. *See* ANAESTHESIA.

base (*bāss*). (1) The bottom. (2) The chief substance of a mixture. (3) In chemistry, the substance which combines with an acid to form its salt.

Basedow's disease (*baz'-e-dow*). Exophthalmic goitre.

basement membrane. A very fine membrane separating the epithelium from the underlying structures.

basic (*bā-sik*). 1. Basal. 2. Alkaline.

basila (*ba-si-lah*). Pertaining to the base.

basilic (*ba-zil'-ik*). The name of a vein on the inner side of the arm. *Median b. vein.* Short trunk opening into the b. vein, and usually the one chosen for intravenous injection or for withdrawing blood from the arm.

basophil(e) (*bās'ō-fil*). One of three types of glandular leucocyte readily stained with basic dyes in which the cation is the active part. Nucleic acids are basophilic.

basophilia (*bās-ō-fi-li-a*). (1) Abnormality of red blood cells found in lead poisoning in which there is punctate basophilic staining of the cytoplasm. (2) Increase in number of basophils in blood.

bath. Any liquid or gas used to bathe the body. A *water b.* may be cold, 32–70° F (0–21° C) used to stimulate body tissues; a warm bath is 90–104° F (32–40° C) and a hot bath is 98–108° F (37–42° C) and may be analgesic, sedative and diaphoretic. *Medicated bs.* These may contain sodium bicarbonate, saline, wax, etc. Starch, oatmeal and bran were formerly much used for emollient purposes.

Bassini's herniorrhaphy (*ba-si'-nis her-ni-or'-ra-fi*). Method of reconstruction of the inguinal canal in repair of hernia.

battered baby (*ba-terd bā-bi*). A young child physically injured by his parent or his guardian. *B.b.* syndrome. A recognized pattern of physical maltreatment of a young child by his parents. The parents are themselves psychologically disordered.

Battle's incision (*in-si-zhon*). Same as Lennander's.

battledore placenta (*pla-sen'-ta*). A placenta in which the umbilical cord is inserted into the edge instead of the centre.

Bazin's (*bā-zinz*) **disease.** Erythema induratum of tuberculous origin. Reddish or purple nodules appear on the legs which may ulcerate.

BCG. Bacille Calmette-Guérin. A vaccine used for inoculation against tuberculosis.

bearing down. Popular term for the expulsive contractions during the second stage of labour when the cervix uteri is fully dilated.

beat (*bēt*). Applied to the beating of the heart and the pulsation of the blood.

bed bug. Insect, Cimex lectularius, living in furniture.

bedsore. A sore on the buttocks, heels, ankles, shoulders or elbows, caused by constant pressure on these points when lying. This may arise in long illnesses if pressure is not relieved, and is specially likely to occur in cases of spinal injury if the patient is not frequently turned. Now usually called pressure sore.

Beer's knife. A knife with a triangular blade used in operations on the eye.

behaviour (*bē-hā-via*). Conduct; or response to certain stimuli.

behaviourism (*bē-hā-vūr-ism*). A psychological approach made through the study of the individual's behaviour pattern.

bejel (*be-jel*). Skin disease caused by a treponema.

Belcroy feeder. Small feeding bottle with teat and rubber bulb to help the flow of milk. Used for premature and weak infants.

Bell's paralysis. Peripheral paralysis or palsy of facial nerve.

belle indifference (*bel in-dif-er-enz*). An hysterical manifestation. Lack of emotional response in an obviously distressing situation.

Bellocq's cannula or sound. Hollow sound with curved

spring used to draw in a plug in acute nose bleeding.

Bence-Jones protein. A protein found in the urine in disease of the bone marrow, *e.g.* myelomatosis.

bends. Decompression sickness. *See* CAISSON DISEASE.

Benedict's solution. May be used in testing urine for sugar.

benign (*be-nīn*). Non-malignant. Not cancerous.

Bennett's fracture (*ben-netz frak-tūr*). Fracture of the base of the first metacarpal due to a blow on the base of the thumb.

benzene (*ben-zēn*). Hydrocarbon from coal tar.

benzyl benzoate (*ben-zō-āt*). Used in the treatment of scabies.

beriberi (*ber-i-ber'-i*). An acute neuritis, due to lack of vitamin B$_1$ (thiamine). Common in some parts of the tropics, associated with anaemia and dropsy. *See* VITAMINS.

Berkefeld filter (*berk-felt fil-ter*). A tubular filter, made of diatomaceous earth, which can be fitted to a tap.

beryllium window (*be-ri'-li-um win'-dō*). Apparatus designed to allow minimum penetration of the beam in X-ray therapy.

Besnier's prurigo (*bes-nē-ās proo-rī'-go*). Eczema affect-

ing nape of neck, behind the heels, etc. Occurs in children.

beta cells (*bē-ta sels*). The type of cell making up the major part of an island of Langerhans and producing insulin.

beta rays (*bē-ta rās*). Electrons emitted by radio-active substances. They will penetrate to about 1cm in tissue.

Betz cells (*bets sels*). Large cells in the deeper layers of the cerebral cortex.

bezoars (*be-zō-ars*). Masses of foreign material present in the gastro-intestinal tract.

Bi. Symbol for bismuth.

bi. Prefix meaning two or twice.

bicarbonate (*bī-kar-bon-āt*). Any salt containing two equivalents of carbonic acid and one of a base.

bicephalus (*bī-kef'-al-us*). A monster with two heads.

biceps (*bī'-seps*). The two-headed muscle in front of the humerus.

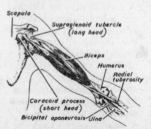

7 The biceps muscle

biconcave (*bī-kon-kāv*). Hollow or concave on both sides, usually of a lens.

biconvex (*bī-kon-veks*). Bulging or convex on both sides, usually of a lens.

bicornuate (*bī-korn-ū-āt*). Having two horns. *B. uterus* A congenital abnormality due to incomplete development—the uterus may be double or a single organ possessing two horns. Pregnancy may take place in one half and be normal. Very rarely twins may develop—one in each horn.

bicuspid (*bī-kus'-pid*). Having two points or cusps. The two teeth immediately behind the canines in each jaw are bicuspids. Bicuspid or mitral valve, the valve between the left atrium and left ventricle of the heart.

Bielchowski's disease (*bēl-chow-skis di-sēz*). Early juvenile cerebro-macular degeneration, characterized by mental deterioration and blindness.

bifid. (*bī-fid*). Cleft.

bifocal (*bī-fō'-kal*). With a double focus. *B. spectacles* can be used for near and distant vision.

bifurcate (*bi-fer'-kāt*). Forked.

bigeminal (*bī-je-mi-nal*). Occurring in two pairs.

bilateral (*bī-lat'-er-al*). Two sided. Pertaining to both sides.

bile (*bīl*). Gall. The secretion of the liver; greenish, bitter, and viscid. Alkaline. Specific gravity 1010 to 1040. It consists of water, inorganic salts, bile salts, bile pigments. It emulsifies fats and stimulates peristalsis.

bile pigments (*pig-ments*). Bilirubin, red, and biliverdin, green. These pigments are derived from haemoglobin and appear in the faeces as stercobilin, and in the urine as urobilin. In cases of jaundice the unaltered pigments bilirubin and biliverdin appear in the urine. *See* BILIURIA.

Bilharzia (*bil-har'-zi-a*). The same as Schistosoma. A parasitic worm infesting the portal vein and lymph spaces. The worm's eggs are the main cause of the symptoms in those affected; they are spiny, and therefore cause bleeding wherever they lodge. They are found in enormous numbers in the bladder and rectum.

biliary ducts (*bil'-ya-rē dukts*). Canals in the liver which convey the bile to the duodenum. *See* Fig. 8.

bilious (*bil'-yus*). Connected with bile. Term often used to denote nausea.

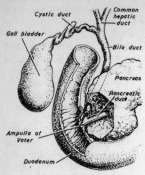

Cystic duct
Common hepatic duct
Gall bladder
Bile duct
Pancreas
Pancreatic duct
Ampulla of Vater
Duodenum

8 The bile ducts

bilirubin (*bil-i-rū'-bin*). *See* BILE PIGMENTS.

biliuria (*bil-i-ūr'-i-a*). Presence of bile in the urine. Choluria.

biliverdin (*bil-i-ver'-din*). *See* BILE PIGMENTS.

Billroth's operation. A type of partial gastrectomy.

bimanual (*bī-man'-ū-al*). With two hands. By the use of both hands.

binary fission (*bi-na-ri fish-on*). Division of a cell into two equal daughter cells.

binaural (*bi-naw'-ral*). Pertaining to both ears.

biniodide of mercury (*bīn-ī'-ō-dīd*). A very poisonous antiseptic, similar in composition and properties to perchloride of mercury, but less irritating and less potent. *See* CORROSIVE SUBLIMATE.

binocular (*bī-nok'-ū-la*). Relating to both eyes.

binovular (*bī-nov-ū-la*). Produced by two ova. Binovular twins develop from two separate ova fertilized at the same time.

bio-assay (*bī-ō-a-sā*). Quantitative estimation of biologically active substances such as hormones.

biochemistry (*bī'-ō-kem-is-tri*). The chemistry of cell life.

biogenesis (*bī-ō-jen'-es-is*). Hypothesis that living matter always arises from living matter.

biology (*bī-ol-o-ji*). The science of life and living organisms.

biopsy (*bī-op'-si*). Examination of tissue from the living body.

bios. The Greek word for life; hence the derivation of such words as 'biology', 'biogenesis'.

biotin (*bī-o-tin*). Vitamin H.

Biot's respiration (*bē'ō*). Seen most commonly in meningitis. There are pauses in the respiration, but no waxing or waning as in Cheyne-Stokes respiration.

biparous (*bīp-ar-us*). Bearing twins.

bipolar version. *See* VERSION.

birth (*berth*). The act of being born. *B. mark*, congenital naevus. *B. paralysis*, paralysis due to injury at birth.

59 **BLE**

bisexual (*bī-sek-shal*). Being of both sexes. Hermaphrodite.

bismuth (*biz'-muth*). A metal, the salts of which are used in medicine as a stomachic, sedative and tonic. Causes black stools. Is opaque to x-rays. When applied externally, soothing and astringent.

bistoury (*bis-tō-ri*). A surgical knife.

bitemporal hemianopia (*bī-tem-po-ral he-mi-a-nō-pi-a*). Loss of vision in the outer part of the visual field of each eye.

Bitot's spots (*bi-toz*). Shiny spots on the conjunctiva associated with vitamin A deficiency.

biurate crystals (*bī-ū'-rāt*). Found in the articular cartilage of joints in gout.

bivalve. Having two valves.

blackhead. See COMEDONES.

black stools (*blak stools*). Sign of bleeding from the intestine. May also occur in patients taking large quantities of iron tablets.

blackwater fever. A form of malaria in which there is rapid haemolysis of red blood cells so that the blood supply to vital organs such as the brain is impaired. There is high fever, haemoglobinuria and jaundice.

bladder. A hollow organ for the reception of fluid. *Urinary B.* receives the urine from the kidneys. See GALL BLADDER.

Blalock's operation (*blā-lok*). The subclavian artery is anastomosed to the pulmonary artery. Performed in cases of congenital pulmonary stenosis. See FALLOT'S TETRALOGY.

bland. Mild, non-irritating.

blastoderm (*blas-tō-derm*). Germinal layers of the developing fertilised ovum of three types, ectoderm, mesoderm, endoderm.

blastoma (*blas-tō'-ma*). A granular growth due to a micro-organism.

blastomycosis (*blas-tō-mī-kō'-sis*). A skin disease caused by the invasion of a yeast-like organism.

blastula (*bla-stū-la*). The fertilized ovum after the morula stage. It is hollow and filled with fluid.

bleaching powder (*blē-ching*). Chlorinated lime. A disinfectant and decolorizer.

bleb (*bleb*). See BLISTER.

bleeder. See HAEMOPHILIA.

bleeding time. The duration of bleeding following puncture of the skin as of the ear lobe.

blennophthalmia (*blen-of-thal'-mi-a*). Catarrh of the conjunctiva.

blennorrhoea (*blen-nor-re'-a*). (1) Discharge of mucus from the urethra or vagina. (2) Purulent conjunctivitis.

blepharadenitis (*blef-ar-ad-en-i'-tis*). Inflammation of the Meibomian glands. Terms commencing 'blephar' refer to the eyelids.

blepharitis (*blef-a-rī'-tis*). Inflammation of the eyelids.

blepharoptosis (*blef-ar-op-tō'-sis*). See PTOSIS.

blepharospasm (*blef-a-rō-spa-zm*). Spasmodic closure of the eye. Commonly due to the presence of a foreign body in the eye or to ulceration of the cornea.

blindness (*blind*). Lack of sight. *Colour B.*, an inability to distinguish certain colours. *Cortical B.*, blindness due to a lesion of the visual centre in the brain. *Night B.*, or nyctalopia, vision subnormal at night, thought to be due to a deficiency of vitamin A in the diet. *Snow B.*, dimness of vision with pain and lacrimation due to the glare of sunlight upon snow. *Word B.*, inability to recognize familiar written words owing to a lesion of the brain.

blind spot. Point where the optic nerve enters the retina.

blister. A collection of serum between the layers of the skin. A bleb, a vesicle.

blood (*blud*). The red fluid which circulates through the heart, arteries, capillaries and veins. Blood consists of a pale yellowish albuminous fluid, called plasma, in which are carried numerous minute cells. There are the red blood cells, or erythrocytes, which hold the haemoglobin, carry oxygen and give to blood its red colour; and the white blood cells or leucocytes. The leucocytes are of various kinds, named as follows: polymorphonuclears or granulocytes, of three kinds, neutrophils, eosinophils, basophils; lymphocytes, small and large, and monocytes. In blood diseases abnormal forms appear, and the total number and the ratio to each other of these various kinds differ. The blood also contains minute discs called platelets.

The functions of the blood are to carry to the tissues the water and nourishment which they require, to take off the waste products of their growth and activities, and to distribute heat equably through the body. In addition, the blood carries the antitoxins and other substances which defend the system against bacterial invasion, and certain other substances which are necessary for the general functions of the body or the individual functions of the various organs.

When blood is shed fibrinogen, a soluble protein in the plasma, is converted to an insoluble thread-like form, fibrin, which constitutes the clot. The change is affected by an enzyme, thrombin, which is not active in circulating blood, in which it exists as prothrombin. Prothrombin is converted to thrombin at the time of shedding blood by the action of a second enzyme, thrombokinase which is set free by the breaking-up of platelets. The process also requires the presence of calcium ions for its completion. (*See also* BLOOD COUNT.)

blood-brain barrier. Hypothetical barrier separating the blood from the parenchyma of the central nervous system.

blood casts (*karsts*). Small shreds of coagulated blood found in the urine in certain cases of disease or injury of the kidney.

blood count (*kownt*). Examination and enumeration microscopically of the various cells in the blood. A normal blood count would be, in an average healthy man between 20 and 40 years:

Red cells—4,000,000 to 5,000,000 per cubic millimetre; *White cells*—7,000 to 10,000. If the different forms of white cells are estimated, it is called a *differential white blood count* and the percentages are as follows: *polymorphonuclears*—60 to 70 per cent; *eosinophils*—2 to 3 per cent; *large and small lymphocytes*—20 to 25 per cent; *other rarer forms*—4 to 8 per cent. *See* HAEMOGLOBIN, COLOUR INDEX, EOSINOPHILIA, LEUCOCYTOSIS.

blood grouping. For a blood transfusion it is essential that the blood of the donor be compatible with that of the patient. Blood grouping is decided according to the presence or absence of certain agglutinogens in the cells, two in number, A and B. The international nomenclature of the different groups is as follows: AB, A, B, O. Group AB are those who may receive blood from any other group, and are called universal recipients. Group A may receive blood from Groups A and O. Group B may receive blood from Groups B and O. Group O may receive only from Group O. From the above it will be seen that Group O can give blood to all other groups, and therefore is a universal donor. Before transfusion a direct match is always made between the red cells of the donor and the serum of the recipient. Any clumping together or agglutination of the cells which can be seen even with the naked eye means incompatibility. *The Rhesus (Rh.) Factor.* It has been recently shown that 85 per cent of human beings of most races possess this agglutinogen in their red cells, and so are termed 'Rh positive'. The remaining 15 per cent, 'Rh negative', are liable to form an anti-body (agglutinin) against the agglutinogen, if it is introduced into their circulation. It may occur in an 'Rh negative' woman if she becomes pregnant with a fetus whose blood cells are 'Rh positive' or if an 'Rh negative' person is transfused with 'Rh positive' blood.

blood-letting. Bleeding, phlebotomy, venesection. The withdrawal of blood for therapeutic purposes from a vein.

blood plasma (*plaz-ma*). The fluid part of blood in which the cells are suspended.

blood pressure (*pre'-sher*). The pressure exerted by the blood in the vessels in which it is contained. It is taken in the brachial artery and estimated in terms of the number of millimetres pressure of mercury required, on the upper arm, just to obliterate the pulse at the wrist. This figure is the *systolic b. pressure.* The average systolic pressure in a young adult is 100–120. The *diastolic b. pressure* is the pressure in the artery during the resting phase of the cardiac cycle, *i.e.* the lowest pressure. The average diastolic pressure is 70 to 90 in a young adult. It rises with age. High blood pressure is present in arteriosclerosis, and some kinds of kidney and heart disease.

blood sedimentation rate (*sed-i-men-tā-shon rāt*). 0·4ml of a 3·8 per cent sol. of sodium citrate is drawn into a syringe. Blood is then taken into the syringe from a vein until the total quantity reaches 2ml mark. The blood and citrate are thoroughly mixed and then sucked into a standard pipette to make a column 200mm high. The pipette is placed vertically and the column of fluid examined exactly one hour later. It is found that the red cells have sedimented leaving a clear supernatant fluid. In health the length of clear fluid on top varies from 1 to 5mm. In active tuberculosis or other toxaemic states it may be 20 to 100mm or more.

blood serum (*sē-rum*). *See* SERUM.

blood sugar (*shoo'-ga*). The amount of sugar normally in the blood is about 0·08 to 0·12 per cent or 80 to 120mg per 100ml of blood. This figure rises slightly after a meal, but not to more than about 180mg. Above this figure, sugar leaks through into the urine. The blood sugar is raised in diabetes mellitus.

blood transfusion (*tranz-fū-zhon*). The transference of blood from a healthy individual to one suffering from a grave degree of anaemia due to either haemorrhage or disease. The donor must not have suffered from certain specified diseases and his blood must belong to the same or to a compatible group. *See* BLOOD GROUPING. Clotting is prevented by the addition of 3·8 per cent sodium citrate solution. The blood is taken from the median basilic or other suitable vein of the arm; the quantity is usually 500ml. This is allowed to flow from the needle in the

arm, along a piece of short tubing into a vacuum bottle containing citrate solution; all needles and tubing have previously been run through with citrate solution. The blood is injected into the patient by (1) the closed method, through a thick hollow needle or fine polythene tubing into the vein. (2) The vein of the patient is cut down upon, isolated and lifted; an incision is made into it, a small cannula slipped into the opening and tied there. The blood is then slowly run in from a giving set through a drip cannula. After the cannula in the arm is withdrawn, the vein is tied above and below and the skin incision closed.

blood urea (*ū-re-a*). Normally about 30mg per 100ml of blood, or 0·03 per cent, rising to a higher figure with increasing age. An abnormal amount of urea present usually shows deficient kidney action.

blood volume (*blud vo-lūm*). The calculated amount of blood in the whole body. About 5 litres in the normal adult.

bloodless operation. An operation unaccompanied by loss of blood. In the case of operation on a limb the blood is expelled from the part operated upon by raising the limb and applying a tourniquet or by applying an elastic bandage.

blue baby. A cyanosed infant, due to congenital cardiac defects called the tetralogy of Fallot.

blue line on gums. This is seen near the margin in cases of lead poisoning and aids diagnosis. The line is interrupted where there are no teeth.

blue stone. Copper sulphate.

BMR. Abbreviation for basal metabolic rate. *See* BASAL METABOLISM.

BNA. Abbreviation for *Basle Nomina Anatomica.* Naming of anatomical terms agreed in Switzerland in 1895.

Bodecker index (*bö'-dek-er in-deks*). The ratio between the number of tooth surfaces (five to a tooth) which are carious and the total number of surfaces of the teeth which could be affected.

Boeck's disease (*berks*). *See* SARCOIDOSIS.

Böhler's iron (*ber-lerz-ī-on*). An iron heel incorporated in plaster of Paris when applied to the leg, to permit walking.

boil (*boyl*). Furuncle. A staphylococcal infection of the skin, causing inflammation round a hair follicle.

bolus (*bō'-lus*). A large round mass such as that of food before it is swallowed.

bomb. An apparatus containing radium so that its rays may be applied to any desired part of the body.

bone. Hard material forming the skeleton. It is made mainly of collagen impregnated with mineral substance, chiefly phosphate and calcium and contains bone cells or osteocytes. The hard, outer part is compact tissue and the inner is cancellous tissue.

bone graft. A portion of bone is transplanted to remedy a defect.

bone marrow. Fatty substance contained within the marrow cavity of bones. In the flat bones, and with children in the long bones as well, the fat is replaced by active blood-forming tissue, which is responsible for production of the granular leucocytes, the red cells and platelets.

boracic acid (*bo-ras'-ik as-id*). Boric acid. A mild antiseptic used for irrigation of eyes, usual strength, half saturated solution.

borax (*bor'-aks*). Sodium biborate. A weak antiseptic. With glycerin and honey it is used as a soothing drug in inflammation of the mouth.

borborygmus (*bor-bo-rig'-mus*). Rumbling of intestinal flatus.

boric acid. Boracic acid.

Bornholm disease (*bawn-hōm*). Epidemic diaphragmatic pleurodynia.

boss (*bos*). A projection.

Botallo's foramen (*bot-al-ōs faw-rā-men*). The foramen ovale in the atrial septum of the fetal heart.

botulism (*bot-ū-lizm*). Food poisoning by Bacillus botulinus. Usually fatal.

bougie (*boo'-jē*). A slender solid instrument which is flexible and yielding, used for dilating contracted passages.

bouillon (*bū-i-yo*). (1) A broth or soup. (2) A liquid nutritive medium for culture purposes.

bovine (*bō-vīn*). Pertaining to or derived from the ox or cow.

bowel (*bow'-el*). The intestine. The gut. It consists of the small and large intestine. The small intestine is about 20ft long and is divided into: (1) *Duodenum*, 12in long; (2) *Jejunum*, about 8ft long; (3) *Ileum*, about 12ft long. The large intestine is about 5ft long and consists of (1) the *Caecum* with the *Vermiform Appendix*; (2) *Ascending Colon*, running up the right side; (3) *Transverse Colon*, running from right to left; (4) *Descending Colon*, running down left side; (5) *Sigmoid* or *Pelvic Colon*, passing to (6) *Rectum* which opens externally via (7) the *Anal Canal*.

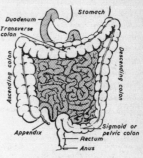

9 The bowel

bow-leg (*bō*). Genu varum.

Bowman's capusules (*bō-manz cap-sūlz*). *See* MALPIGHIAN CORPUSCLES.

Boyle's law. At any given temperature, the volume of a given mass of gas varies inversely to the pressure it bears.

Bozeman's catheter (*bō'-z-mans kath'-e-ter*). An intrauterine catheter grooved for ensuring the unobstructed return of fluid.

B.P. British Pharmacopoeia. *See* FORMULARY.

B.P.C. British Pharmaceutical Codex.

brachial (*brā'-ke-al*). Pertaining to the arm. *B. artery*, the main artery of the arm; it is a continuation of the axillary artery. *B. neuralgia. Syn.* B. neuritis. Pain in arm due to pressure on the brachial plexus. *B. plexus*, the plexus of nerves supplying the arm, forearm, and hand.

brachium (*brā'-ki-um*). The arm.

bradycardia (*brad-i-kar'-di-a*). Abnormally slow pulse. Occurs in heart block and head injuries.

brain (*brān*). The main integrating mass of nervous tissue situated in the skull. It may be divided into cerebral hemispheres, cerebellum and brain stem.

branchial (*bran'-ki-al*). Pertaining to the gills. Thus *branchial cysts* are sometimes found in certain regions of the neck as vestiges of the gill stage of fetal development.

Braun's splint. A combined splint and extension apparatus for the lower limb.

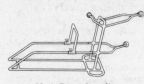

12 A Braun's splint

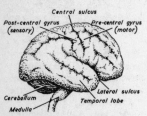

10 Lateral view of the brain

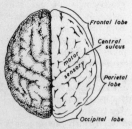

11 The brain from above

breast (*brest*). (1) The milk-secreting gland. (2) The anterior surface of the thorax. *See* MAMMAE.

breath (*breth*). Air taken into and expelled from the lungs. *B. holding.* A behaviour disorder of infants and children. *B. sounds*, the sounds heard by auscultation of the chest during respiration.

breech (*brēch*). The buttocks. *B. presentation*, presentation of buttocks of fetus.

bregma. *See* FONTANELLE.

Bright's disease (*brītz*). Disease of the kidney, characterized by proteinuria, casts, and oedema. Nephritis.

brilliant green (*bril'-yant grēn*). Antiseptic dye used as a lotion, 1 in 1000, and as ointment 2 per cent.

broad ligaments (*brawd*). The folds of peritoneum with the contained lymphatics, blood-vessels, Fallopian tubes, etc., which pass outwards on each side of the uterus.

Broadbent's sign. Retraction of the lower left part of the chest wall when the pericardium is adherent.

Broca's area (*brŏ'-ka*). The motor speech area normally on the left side of the brain in right-handed people.

Brodie's abscess. Chronic abscess of bone. The tibia is most commonly affected.

bromidrosis (*bro-mi-drŏ'-sis*). Offensive sweating, most common in the feet.

bromism (*brŏ'-mizm*). Poisoning by bromides. Symptoms: red, papular rash, conjunctivitis.

bronchi (*bron'-ki*). The two tubes into which the trachea divides, opposite the upper border of the fifth dorsal vertebra.

bronchial tubes (*bron'-ki-al*). The smaller tubes into which the bronchi divide in the lung.

bronchiectasis (*bron'-ki-ek'-tas-sis*). A disease of the bronchial tubes in which they become dilated and usually secrete offensive pus in large quantities. Treatment, postural drainage, antibiotics, lobectomy, pneumonectomy.

bronchiole (*bron'-ki-ōl*). A minute bronchial tube.

bronchiolitis (*bron-kē-o-li'-tis*). Inflammation of the bronchioles.

bronchitis (*bron-kī'-tis*). Inflammation of the bronchial tubes.

bronchocele (*bron'-kō-sēl*). A diverticulum of a bronchus.

bronchogenic (*bron-kō-jen-ik*). Originating from a bronchus.

bronchography (*bron-ko-gra-fi*). Instillation of radio-opaque dye in the bronchi, so that they are apparent on x-ray.

broncholith (*bron-kō-lith*). A bronchial calculus.

bronchomycosis (*bron-kō-mi-kō-sis*). Infection of the bronchi by fungus infection of lungs.

bronchophony (*bron-kof'-o-ni*). Resonance of patient's voice as heard on auscultating the bronchi.

broncho-pleural fistula (*bron-kō-plor-al fis-tū-la*). An opening between a bronchus and the pleural cavity found in disease.

broncho-pneumonia (*bron-kō-nū-mō'-ni-a*). Pneumonia,

beginning in the bronchioles, affecting scattered lobules of the lung and also the finest or capillary bronchioles.

bronchoscope (*bron'-ko-skōp*). An instrument for seeing into the main bronchi.

bronchoscopy (*bron-kos'-kō-pi*). Examination of the bronchi with a bronchoscope.

bronchospirometry (*bron-kō-spī-ro-me-tri*). The measurement of the capacity of a lung or one of its lobes.

brow. The forehead. *B. presentation.* An unfavourable but unusual presentation in labour at the uterine orifice. The mento-vertical diameter, which is 13·0cm, presents.

Brownian movement (*brow'-nian*). Oscillatory movement seen under the microscope in fine particles suspended in a liquid.

Brucella abortus bovinus (*broo-sel-la ab-or-tus bō-vī-nus*). The bacterium from an infected cow causing undulant fever.

Brucella melitensis (*broo-sel-la me-li-ten'-sis*). Bacterium from an infected goat whose milk causes Malta fever in man.

Brucellosis (*broo-sel-ō-sis*). Infection with an organism of the Brucella group.

bruise (*brooz*). A contusion.

The skin is not broken but is discoloured due to bleeding in the underlying tissues.

bruit (*broo-ē'*). The French for 'sound', used with regard to sounds heard in auscultation.

Brunhilde virus (*broon-hil-de vī-rus*). A strain of poliomyelitis virus.

Brunner's glands (*broo'-ner*). Glands of the duodenum.

bubo (*bū'-bō*). Inflammatory swelling of glands, particularly of groin.

bubonic plague (*bū-bon'-ik plāg*). Oriental plague, which in some forms is characterized by the development of buboes.

buccal (*buk-kal*). Pertaining to the mouth.

buccinator (*buk'-sin-ā-tor*). The muscle of the cheek; one of the muscles of mastication.

Buerger's disease (*ber-gerz di-sēz*). Thromboangiitis obliterans. Rare disease of blood vessels resulting in reduction of blood supply to extremities.

buffer. A substance allowing only slight changes of pH when an acid or alkali is added to it, *e.g.* sodium bicarbonate in blood and tissue fluids.

bulb. A rounded expansion of an organ.

bulbar palsy (*bul'-ba pawl'-zi*).

Paralysis due to disease of medulla oblongata.

bulimia (*bū-lim'-i-a*). Morbid hunger.

bullae (*bul'-lē*). Large blisters.

Buller's shield. Used to protect the sound eye from discharge poured from the infected one in contagious ophthalmia. It consists of sticking plaster and a watch glass.

bundle of His. *See* ATRIOVENTRICULAR BUNDLE.

bunion (*bun'-yon*). Inflammation of a bursa situated over the metatarsophalangeal joint of the great toe.

burette (*būr'-ret*). A graduated tube for measuring a reagent.

burns. Burns are of different degrees according to the depth of tissue involved. Those of the first degree show redness, of the second degree, blistering; third-degree burns involve the entire thickness of the skin, fourth-degree burns show charring of muscle and bone. The first-aid treatment is to exclude air by applying a dressing soaked in a solution of soda bicarb. or saline, and to treat the shock.

burr hole (*ber hōl*). Circular hole cut in the cranium to allow access to the brain.

bursa (*ber'-sa*). A small sac interposed between movable parts. *B. mucosa.* A sac lined

with synovial membrane secreting synovial fluid.

bursitis (*ber-sī'-tis*). Inflammation of a bursa.

buttock (*bu-tok*). Breech. Nates.

byssinosis (*bis-sin-ō'-sis*). A type of pneumoconiosis caused by inhalation of cotton dust.

C

C. (1) Chemical symbol for carbon. (2) Centigrade. (3) Celsius. (4) Calorie.

Ca. Chemical symbol for calcium.

cacao butter (*kak-a'-o*). Cocoa butter. *Syn.* theobroma.

cachet (*kash'-ā*). Capsule in which powders of disagreeable taste are enclosed.

cachexia (*ka-chek'-si-a*). A chronic state of malnutrition and debility produced by absorption of toxins.

cadaver (*kad-av-er*). A corpse.

caeco-sigmoidostomy (*sē'-kō-sig-mōy-dos'-to-mi*). Operation for establishing direct communication between the caecum and sigmoid colon.

caecostomy (*sē-kos'-to-mi*). Operation to provide an opening into the caecum through the abdominal wall.

caecum (*sē'-kum*). The blind intestine, a cul-de-sac at the commencement of the large intestine. *See* BOWEL and APPENDIX VERMIFORMIS.

caesarean section (*se-za'-rē-an sek'-shon*). Delivery of the fetus through an incision in the abdominal and uterine walls.

Caesium 137 (*sē-si-um*). Radioactive isotope used in radiotherapy in place of radium.

caffeine (*kaf'-fēn*). The alkaloid of coffee and tea; a cerebral stimulant and diuretic.

caisson disease (*kā'-son*). Also known as 'the bends'. The effect on those working under a heavier atmospheric pressure than normal, *e.g.* in deep mines or under water. Return to normal pressure should be effected gradually or nitrogren bubbles form in the blood and tissues.

calamine (*kal'-a-mīn*). Zinc carbonate used as an astringent.

calcaneus (*kal-kā'-ne-us*). The os calcis or heel bone.

calcareous (*kal-kā'-re-us*). Containing compounds of calcium.

calciferol (*kal-sif'-er-ol*). The official name for vitamin D.

calcification (*kal-si-fi-kā'-shon*). The deposit of lime-salts: occurs normally in bone tissue, and may occur in other tissues, if diseased, *e.g.* calcified fibroid of uterus.

calcitonin (*kal-si-tō-nin*). Hormone lowering plasma content of phosphorus and calcium.

calcium carbonate, c. lactate, c. gluconate. Salts of calcium. The carbonate is used as an antacid in gastric conditions. The other salts are prescribed in cases of calcium deficiency, *e.g.* rickets, tetany and for chilblains.

calculus (*kal'-kū-lus*). A concretion found in the various reservoirs of the body, *e.g.* pelvis of the kidney, bladder, gall bladder. Operations for the removal or crushing of the stone are lithotomy, lithotrity, and litholapaxy.

Caldwell-Luc operation (*kawl-dwel-look*). Operation to drain the maxillary sinus.

calibrate (*kal-ē-brāt*). To graduate an instrument for measuring by a given standard.

calipers or callipers (*kāl'-i-perz*). (1) Surgical instruments for measuring the chest, the pelvis, etc. (2) *Ice-tong caliper*, a two-pointed instrument used for fixing a bone by actual penetration of some part of it, as in the treatment of fractures. (3) *Walking caliper*, an instrument fixed at the lower end to a boot. At the upper end is a padded ring which fits round the groin and under the ischial tuberosity. This takes the weight off an injured leg on walking.

callosity (*ka-lo'-sit-i*). A thickened horny layer of epidermis formed on palmar and plantar surfaces subject to much friction.

callous (*kal'-lus*). Hard, insensible, thickened.

callus (*kal'-lus*). A new bony deposit around a fracture. Some of this is absorbed, the remainder develops into new bone which repairs the fracture.

calor. Heat.

calorie (*kal'-or-ē*). Scientific term for the standard unit of heat. 1 Calorie is the amount of heat required to raise 1 kilogram of water through 1 degree Celsius. The amount of heat produced in the body by the combustion of food can be estimated. 1 gram carbohydrate, 1 gram protein each yield 4·1 C. 1 gram fat yields 9·3 C. It is essential that a diet should yield an adequate number of calories per day, and that the three types of foodstuffs should be proportionally distributed. A man weighing 11 stone doing an average day's work requires about 3,300 Calories per day. *Small c.*, the amount of heat necessary to raise 1 gram of water through 1° Celsius. 1,000 small calories=1 kilocalarie (kcal)=4·2 kilojoule (kJ).

calorific (*kal-or-if-ik*). Producing heat.

calorimeter (*kal-or-im'-e-ter*). An apparatus for determining the amount of heat yielded by a substance.

calvarium (*kal-va'-ri-um*). The upper half of the skull. The cranial vault.

calyx (*kā-liks*). A cup-shaped organ or cavity such as those of the recesses of the pelvis of the kidney.

camphor (*kam'-for*). Substance with aromatic odour, given internally as a carminative, with syrup as an expectorant and applied externally as an analgesic in liniments.

canal of Nuck. A narrow passage along which the round ligament passes to the region of the pubes, it is sometimes the seat of inguinal hernia and occasionally of cysts.

canaliculus (*kan-al'-ik-ū-lus*). A small canal or groove, *e.g.* (1) the hairlike passage leading from the edge of the eyelid to the lacrimal sac. (2) One of the minute spaces in a cancellous bone. *See* BONE.

cancer (*kan'-ser*). A general term used to describe various types of malignant disease.

cancerophobia (*kan-ser-o-fō'-bi-a*). Excessive fear of cancer.

cancroid (*kan'-kroyd*). Like a cancer.

cancrum oris (*kan'-krum o'-ris*). Ulceration of the mouth: nothing to do with cancer.

Candida (*kan'-di-da*). A genus of fungi which may cause thrush.

canine teeth (*kā'-nin*). The four eye-teeth, next to the incisors. *See* TEETH.

canker (*kang'-ker*). Ulceration.

cannabis indica (*kan'-na-bis in'-dik-a*). Indian hemp, hashish; a soporific and cerebral stimulant. One of the drugs controlled by the Misuse of Drugs Act.

cannula (*kan'-nū-la*). Surgical name for a metal tube used to withdraw fluid from a cavity. *See* TROCAR.

canthus (*kan'-thus*). The angle of the eyelids, outer or inner.

capelline (*kap'-e-lin*). Bandage for the head.

capillaries (*kap-il'-ar-ēz*). The network of microscopic vessels which communicate with the arterioles and the venules. The walls are formed of a single layer of endothelium.

capillarity (*ka-pi-la-ri-ti*). Effect of surface tension causing liquid to rise up inside a small tube.

capillurgy (*kap'-il-er-ji*). The art of destroying superfluous hair.

capitate (*ka'-pi-tāt*). Like a head. One of the carpal or wrist bones.

capitulum (*kap-it'-ul-um*). The round eminence on the lower end of the humerus which articulates with the radius.

capsular ligament (*kap'-sū-la lig'-a-ment*). A ligament surrounding a movable joint.

capsule (*kap'-sūl*). A sheath enclosing a part or organism.

capsulotomy (*cap-sūl-ot'-o-mi*). An incision of the capsule of the lens of the eye.

caput succedaneum (*suk-sē-dā-ne-um*). Swelling on infant's scalp, due to pressure during labour.

carbohydrate (*kar-bō-hī'-drāt*). Organic compounds composed of carbon, oxygen, and hydrogen only. Sugar and starch are examples of carbohydrate foods.

carbolfuchsin (*kar-bol-fūk'-sin*). A solution of fuchsin and carbolic acid in alcohol and water, used as a stain in pathological and bacteriological work.

carbolic acid (*kar-bol'-ik as-id*). Phenol. A powerful antiseptic obtained from coal tar. Highly poisonous. Used in a solution of 2·5% to 5% as a disinfectant.

carbon (*kar'-bon*). Non-metallic element occurring as diamond, graphite, and charcoal, the latter only being used in medicine.

carbonate (*kar'bon-āt*). Compound of carbonic acid and a base.

carbon dioxide (*dī-oks'-īd*). CO_2. A gas which is a product of combustion. It is formed in the system by the metabolic process of the body, and excreted through the lungs. It is a respiratory stimulant and is administered diluted with oxygen when respiration is depressed. At extremely low temperatures this gas forms a liquid, and lower still a substance resembling snow. The latter is often used for destroying naevi and similar superficial growths on the skin.

carbon monoxide poisoning. Poisoning by inhalation of carbon monoxide, *e.g.* from coal gas or motor vehicle exhaust. *Symptoms* begin as giddiness and singing of ears, then lividity of face and body; later, owing to combination of the gas with the blood, the patient may have a rosy tinge; loss of muscular power; violent action of heart and lungs; fixed dilated pupils, convulsions, coma or asphyxia. *Treatment:* fresh air,

oxygen and artificial respiration if necessary.

carboxyhaemoglobin (*kar-bok-si-hēm-o-glō'-bin*). A compound of carbon monoxide and haemoglobin formed in coal-gas poisoning.

carbuncle (*kar'-bunk-l*). Severe staphylococcal inflammation of an area of skin and subcutaneous tissue. There is necrosis and liquefaction of the subcutaneous tissue and several points of discharge.

carcinogenic (*kar-sin-ō-jen-ik*). Term applied to substances producing or predisposing to cancer.

carcinoma (*kar-si-nō'-ma*). A type of cancer growing from epithelial tissue. One mode of spread is by way of the lymph channels, and therefore glands near, and at a distance, are involved.

carcinomatosis (*kar-sin-ō-ma-tō-sis*). Disseminated malignant disease.

cardia (*kar'-dē-a*). (1) The heart. (2) The aperture between the oesophagus and the stomach.

cardiac (*kar'dē-ak*). Relating to the heart. *C. catheterization.* Investigation to diagnose certain heart conditions. A catheter is introduced through a vein in the arm into the chambers of the heart from which pressure recordings can be obtained. *C. massage.* Squeezing the heart rhythmically to simulate the normal heart beat in an attempt to restart the circulation, having first gained access to the heart through an incision in the chest. *External C. massage.* Pressure on the chest with patient lying flat on back. The heart is rhythmically pressed between the front and back of the thoracic cage.

cardiac cycle. The changes in the heart to produce one heart beat.

cardinal (*kar'-din-al*). Chief or principal. *C. ligaments.* Fan-shaped muscular expansions from the cervix and vagina to the pelvic wall.

cardiogram (*kar'-di-ō-gram*). The tracing obtained by the use of the cardiograph.

cardiograph (*kar'-di-ō-graf*). An instrument which records the movements of the heart.

cardiology (*kar-dē-ol'-o-ji*). The study of the heart and circulatory disorders.

cardiomyotomy (*kar-dē-ō-mī-ot'-om-i*). Operation to relieve muscular spasm at the lower end of the oesophagus.

cardiopathy (*kar-dē-o-pa-thi*). Disease of the heart.

cardiospasm (*kar-dē-ō-spazm*). Cardiac achalasia. *See* ACHALASIA.

cardiovascular (*vas-kū'-la*). Pertaining to the heart and circulatory system.

carditis (*kar-dī'-tis*). Inflammation of the heart muscle.

caries (*kā-rēz*). Decay of teeth.

carina (*ka-rē-na*). A keel-shaped structure, esp. the base of the trachea where it is joined by the bronchi.

carminative (*kar'-min-a-tiv*). A remedy for flatulence, *e.g.* oil of peppermint.

carneous (*kar'-nē-us*). Flesh-like.

carneous mole (*mōl*). *See* MOLE.

carotene (*kar-o-tēn*). A yellow pigment occurring in some plants. It is a precursor of vitamin A.

carotid (*kar-rot'-id*). Name given to the two great arteries of the neck, and to structures connected with them.

carpal tunnel syndrome (*karpal tu-nel sin'-drōm*). Numbness and tingling in the hand as a result of compression of the median nerve at the wrist.

carpometacarpal (*kar-pō-me-ta-kar-pal*). Relating to a carpus and metacarpus.

carpopedal spasm (*kar-pō-pe-dal*). Cramp in hands and feet, due to deficiency of ionized calcium in the blood.

carpus (*kar'-pus*). The wrist.

carrier (*ka'-ri-er*). An individual who harbours in his body the micro-organisms of disease, and thus acts as a carrier of infection, *e.g.* typhoid carrier, diphtheria carrier. The typhoid bacillus can be harboured for years.

cartilage (*kar'-ti-lāj*). Gristle; a transparent substance of the body, very elastic and softer than bone.

caruncle (*ka-run-kl*). Small pedunculated granulomatous mass. *Lacrimal C.* The small red globe at inner corner of the eye.

cascara sagrada (*kas-kar'a sa-gra'-da*). A bark with laxative effects. It may be given as a tablet or in the form of an elixir.

caseation (*kā-sē-ā'-shon*). Conversion into cheesy material, as in breaking down of tuberculous glands.

casein (*kā-sēn*). An albuminous component of milk.

caseinogen (*kā-zin-ō-jen*). When acted upon by rennin this protein of milk yields casein.

Casilan (*ka-si-lan*). A proprietary protein powder containing all the essential aminoacids.

Castle's factors. Two factors, one in gastric juice, the other in certain foods, providing the anti-anaemic factor.

castor oil (*kas'-ter oyl*). *Oleum ricini.* A purge of unpleasant taste which can be mitigated by adding lemon. In the duodenum in the presence of bile, it is converted into glycerol and ricinoleic acid; the latter is an irritant.

castration (*kas-trā'-shon*). Removal of the testicles or ovaries.

casts. Pieces of material taking shape of cavity from which they have been expelled, *e.g.* blood or epithelial debris found in the urine in kidney disease, membranous casts from large bowel in mucous colitis.

CAT. Computerized axial tomography. The technique of examining body sections in the axial plane using very sophisticated equipment.

catabolism (*kat-ab'-ol-izm*). *Syn.* KATABOLISM.

cataclysm (*kat'-a-klizm*). Sudden shock; a deluge.

catacrotic (*kat'-a-krot'-ik*). Waverings in the downward mark of the sphygmograph.

catalepsy (*kat'-a-lep-si*). A period of trance, during which the limbs remain in any position in which they are placed.

catalyst (*ka'-ta-list*). Substance which facilitates a chemical reaction without itself being altered, *e.g.* enzyme.

catamenia (*ka-ta-mē-ni-a*). The menses.

cataphoresis (*kat-a-for-ē'-sis*). Introduction of drugs through the unbroken skin, especially by means of an electric current.

cataplasm (*kat'-a-plazm*). A poultice.

cataplexy (*ka'-ta-plek-si*). A rigid muscular condition produced by fear or shock.

cataract (*kat'-a-rakt*). Opacity of the lens of the eye, causing blindness. The commonest cause is old age. *Treatment*, extraction of the lens.

catarrh (*ka-tar'*). Inflammation of the mucous membrane, generally applied to the nose and throat, but also to internal organs, *e.g.* the bile ducts.

catatonia (*ka-ta-tō-ni-a*). A schizophrenic condition.

catgut. Material prepared from sheep's intestine and used for absorbable ligatures.

catharsis (*ka-thar'-sis*). Emotional relief brought about by the conscious realization of suppressed desires.

cathartic (*ka-thar'-tik*). A drastic purge.

catheter (*ka-the-ter*). Instrument used for the passage of fluids; usually from the bladder where there is urethral obstruction. *Nasal c.* (Ryle's tube). Used for the administration of fluid feeds. The tube passes through the nose down the throat into the stomach. *Eustachian c.* A special tube used to inflate the pharyngo-tympanic tube (Eustachian tube). *See also* CARDIAC.

cathode (*kath'-ōd*). The negative pole in an electric circuit.

cation (*kat-ī-on*). An ion which holds a positive charge of electricity and is attracted to the cathode when a current is passed through a solution which contains it.

cauda equina (*kaw'-da ek-wī'-na*). The bundle of sacral and lumbar nerves at the base of the spinal cord.

caudal analgesia (*kaw-dal an-al-jē'-si-a*). Regional anaesthesia of the rectum and perineum produced by injecting local anaesthetics into the sacral canal through the sacral hiatus.

caul (*kawl*). Fetal membranes about the face and head of some infants at birth.

cauliflower growth (*ko-li-flah*). Term applied to the shape of a tumour growing from a surface.

causalgia (*kaw-sal-ji-a*). Pain referred to in the distribution of a cutaneous nerve which persists long after an injury to that nerve. Often follows herpes zoster (shingles). The cause is not known.

caustic (*kaws'-tik*). A substance, usually a strong alkali or acid, which destroys cells and causes chemical burns. Silver nitrate, fused into a pointed cone and trichloroacetic acid, used as crystals, are common examples.

cautery (*kaw'-ter-i*). Application of heated metal to living tissue in order to destroy it or to arrest haemorrhage. Diathermy is used during operations to arrest bleeding and to destroy tissue when excising malignant growths.

cavernous respiration (*ka'-vern-us res-pī-rā'-shon*). A hollow sound, heard on auscultation, when there is a cavity in the lung.

cavernous sinus (*sī-nus*). A blood sinus on the body of the sphenoid bone.

cavernous tumour. An angioma.

cavitation (*ka-vi-tā-shon*). Process whereby cavities are formed.

cavity of pelvis. The space between the pelvic inlet and outlet.

cell (*sell*). (1) A minute mass of protoplasm. The structural unit of any living organism. An animal cell is usually of microscopic dimensions. It contains a nucleus which appears essential (*a*) for the chemical changes that go on in the cell; (*b*) for multiplica-tion of cells by division of the nucleus and cell substance into two parts (fission). (2) A small jar containing chemicals which can generate electricity when the two terminals are connected by a conducting material such as a wire.

cellulitis (*sel-lū-lī'-tis*). Inflammation of cellular tissue. *Pelvic C.*, *see* PARAMETRITIS.

cellulose (*sel-u-lōz'*). The woody, fibrous part of plants. It has no food value but forms bulk in the colon and so stimulates peristalsis. In the form of wood wool, cellulose is used as an absorbent dressing.

censorship (*sen-so-ship*). Freudian term for the barrier preventing repressed memories, ideas and impulses from easily coming into consciousness.

Centigrade (*sen'-ti-grād*). The scale of thermometers for scientific purposes now known as the Celsius scale. The freezing-point is 0 deg., normal body temp. 37 deg., boiling point 100 deg. *See* p. 13 for conversion of Fahrenheit into Celsius.

centimetre (*sen'-ti-mē-ter*). Metric unit of length, one hundredth part of a metre, about two-fifths of an inch.

Central Midwives Board. The

statutory authority which controls and regulates the practice of obstetrics by those who are not qualified medical practitioners.

central nervous system (*sen-tral ner′-vus sis-tem*). Abbreviation CNS. Generally term incorporating the brain and spinal cord, as opposed to the *peripheral nervôus system*, which includes the nerves and sensory receptors outside the brain and spinal cord.

centrifugal nerve fibres (*sen-tri-fū-gal*). Those which conduct impulses leaving the central nervous system—otherwise called efferent.

centrifuge (*sen′-tri-fūj*). An instrument for separating substances of different specific gravity by rotation.

centriole (*sen-tri-ōl*). Small granule situated just outside the nuclear membrane and found in many resting cells. Just before mitosis this granule divides and at mitosis the two resulting centrioles move apart and form the poles of the spindle.

centripetal nerve fibres (*sen-tri′-pē-tal*). Usually called *afferent* nerves; those which conduct impulses entering the central nervous system.

centromere (*sen-tro-mār*). A structure formed during nuclear division; a spindle-attachment. The region of the chromosome which attaches it to the spindle which is composed of long protein molecules passing between chromosomes and the centriole when the cell is dividing.

centrosome (*sen-trō-sōm*). Region of differentiated cytoplasm in which the centriole is situated.

cephalhaematoma (*kef-al-hē-ma-tō′-ma*). A subperiosteal haemorrhage on head of an infant, usually due to pressure during a long labour. It is gradually absorbed.

cephalic version (*kef-al′-ik ver′-shon*). The production artificially of a cephalic presentation, from a breech presentation or transverse lie. *See also* VERSION.

cephalocele (*kef′-al-ō-sēl*). Hernia of the brain.

cephalometry (*ke-fa-lō-me-tri*). Estimation of the size of the head of a fetus, usually by radiographic means.

cerebellum (*ser-ē-bel′-lum*). Outgrowth from the hindbrain overlying the medulla oblongata. Concerned with the co-ordination of movement. *See* BRAIN.

cerebral haemorrhage (*se′-re-bral hem′-o-räj*). Rupture of an artery of the brain, due to either high blood pressure or disease of artery. Escape of blood causes destruction of brain tissue, and paralysis occurs of that side of the body which is opposite to the injured side of the brain. If the haemorrhage has occurred on the left side of the brain, the speech is affected.

cerebral palsy (*pawl'-zē*). A condition in which the control of the motor system is affected due to a lesion in the brain resulting from a birth injury or pre-natal defect. The popular term is 'spastic'.

cerebral thrombosis (*se-re-bral throm-bō-sis*). Thrombus formation in vessels supplying the brain generally resulting in cerebrovascular accident.

cerebration (*ser'-e-brā-shon*). Activity of the brain. Thinking.

cerebrospinal fever. Epidemic meningitis of the brain and spinal cord, caused by the meningococcus. The fever is often accompanied by a rash; hence the popular name 'spotted fever'.

cerebrospinal fluid. The clear watery fluid which lies in the subarachnoid space, surrounding the brain and spinal cord. It also fills the cavities

or ventricles of the brain. Its function is to protect the brain and spinal cord.

cerebrovascular accident (*se-rē-brō-vas'-kū-ler ak'-si-dent*). General term referring to cerebral embolism, thrombosis or haemorrhage.

cerebrum (*ser'-e-brum*). The larger part of the brain occupying the cranium. *See* BRAIN.

cerumen (*se-rū'-men*). Waxy secretion of the external auditory meatus.

cervical (*ser-vī'-kal*). Pertaining to the neck or cervix of the uterus. *C. rib.* Outgrowth from the seventh cervical vertebra, passing out and down to join rib below. It may press on nerve trunks of the arm giving rise to tingling and pins and needles in hand and fingers. *C. spondylosis.* Degenerative changes in the intervertebral discs of the cervical spine with associated secondary osteo-arthritic changes in the intervertebral joints of the neck.

cervicectomy (*ser-vi-sek'-to-mi*). Excision of the cervix uteri.

cervicitis (*ser'-vi-sī-tis*). Inflammation of the cervix of the uterus.

cervix (*ser'-viks*). A neck. *C. uteri.* The neck of the uterus. The lowest third of the uterus, about one inch in length. It is traversed by a canal which opens into the vagina.

Cestoda (*ses-tōd'-er*). Tapeworms. *See* TAENIA.

Cetavlon (*set-av'-lon*). Official name Cetrimide, B.P., abbreviation CTAB, a detergent with antiseptic action, used as a 1% solution.

cetrimide (*set-ri-mīd*). Quaternary ammonium compound used to cleanse skin, etc.

chalazion (*kal-ā-zi-on*). Meibomian cyst. A small retention cyst in the eyelid, due to blocking of a meibomian follicle.

chancre (*shang'-ker*). Syphilitic ulcer of the first stage; occurs at the site of infection. Contagious.

chancroid (*shang-kroyd'*). *See* SOFT SORE.

change of life. Popular term for the menopause.

character (*ka-rak-ter*). Applied to a person's mental features and according to which his actions are made relatively stable and predictable.

charcoal (*tshar'-kol*). Prescribed as a powder, lozenges or biscuits to absorb gases in the gastro-intestinal tract and thus relieve flatulence.

Charcot-Marie-Tooth disease (*shar-kō-ma-rē-tooth di-sēz*). Peroneal muscular atrophy.
A familial condition of unknown cause in which there is atrophy of the spinal nerves and neuritis affecting the peroneal nerves with resultant wasting of the muscles of the feet and lower legs. The hands may also be affected.

Charcot's joint (*shar-kō'*). Painless destructive changes in a joint due to loss of sensation.

cheilitis (*kī-lī'-tis*). Inflammation of the lip.

cheiloplasty (*kī'-lo-plas-ti*). Plastic operation on the lips.

cheilorrhaphy (*kī-lo-ra-fi*). Operation to repair a hare lip.

cheiloschisis (*kī-lō-ski-sis*). Hare lip.

cheilosis (*kī-lō-sis*). Condition affecting the lips and angles of the mouth which can be caused by riboflavin deficiency.

cheiropompholyx (*kī'-rō-pom'-fo-liks*). A disease characterized by the appearance of small vesicles on the hands.

chelating agents (*kē-lā-ting ā-jents*). Substances which inactivate certain metals and are thus used in the treatment of poisoning by them.

chemoreceptor (*ke-mō-rē-sep'-tor*). Nerve ending capable of reacting to chemical stimuli, *e.g.* taste and smell.

chemosis (*kē-mō'-sis*). Oedema of the conjunctiva.

chemotaxis (*kem-o-tak'-sis*). The attraction or repulsion of living cells for various chemical substances.

chemotherapy (*ke-mō-the-ra-pi*). Healing by chemical means, administration of drugs. A term which was commonly applied to the use of sulphonamide drugs. Nowadays used to define treatment of malignant disease by cytotoxic drugs.

Cheyne-Stokes breathing. Irregular respiration, at first shallow, then increasing in depth till a maximum is reached, when it decreases again until imperceptible and a pause ensues, during which breathing is absent. Usually a bad sign, and due to a poor supply of oxygen to that part of the brain containing the respiratory centre.

chiasm (*ki'-asm*). A crossing.

chiasma opticum (*ki'-as-ma op'-ti-kum*). The meeting and crossing of the optic nerves.

chicken-pox (*chi'-ken poks*). A virus disease. Varicella. Rash appears on the chest on the first day; the disease runs its course in a fortnight. Incubation period ten to sixteen days. Quarantine period for contacts, twenty days.

chilblain (*chil-blān*). Pernio.

Inflammation of the skin due to cellular damage as a result of local deficiency in the circulation.

chiropodist (*ki-rop'-ō-dist*). One skilled in the treatment of the feet.

chirurgical (*ki-rur'-ji-kal*). Surgical.

chloasma (*klō-az'-ma*). Pigmentation of the skin. *C. gravidarum*, the brown discolouration of pregnancy.

chlorhexidine (*klor-hex-i-dēn*). Antiseptic derived from coal tar.

chlorine (*klo'-rēn*). A yellow gaseous element. A disinfectant used in swimming baths and in minute quantities to disinfect drinking water. Poisonous.

chlorocresol (*klo-rō-krē-sol*). A powerful bactericide.

chloroma (*klo-rō'-ma*). A green-coloured sarcoma especially affecting the bones of the skull.

chlorophyll (*klo'-ro-fil*). The green colouring matter in the leaves of plants by which photosynthesis takes place. This is the assimilation of carbon dioxide under the influence of light.

cholaemia (*ko-lē'-mi-a*). The presence of bile pigment in the blood.

cholagogue (*kol'-a-gog*). A medicine which increases the flow of bile into the intestine, *e.g.* directly, bile salts; indirectly, calomel.

cholangiogram (*kō-lan-jē-o-gram*). X-ray showing the biliary system.

cholangitis (*kōl-an-jī'-tis*). Inflammation of the biliary system.

cholecystectomy (*ko'-lē-sis-īek'-to-mi*). Removal of the gall bladder.

cholecystenterostomy (*ko'-lē-sis-ten-ter-os'-to-mi*). Operation for forming an artificial communication between the gall bladder and the intestine.

cholecystitis (*ko'-lē-sis-ti'-tis*). Inflammation of the gall bladder.

cholecystogastrostomy (*ko'-lē-sis-tō'-gas-tros'-to-mi*). An operation for forming an artificial communication between the gall bladder and the stomach.

cholecystography (*ko'-lē-sis-tog'-ra-fi*). X-ray examination of the gall bladder, after it has been rendered opaque to x-rays by drugs such as pheniodol. Low fat meal 15 hours before, then no further food allowed but water as desired. The first skiagram taken is twelve hours later, and two further ones at intervals of 2½ to 3 hours. Sometimes a meal rich in fat is ordered before taking the later pictures, in order that the emptying power of the gall bladder may be observed.

cholecystolithiasis (*kō-lē-sis-tō-li-thī-a-sis*). A stone or stones in the gall bladder.

cholecystostomy (*ko'-lē-sis-tos'-to-mi*). Operation for making the gall bladder open to the exterior.

choledocholithotomy (*kol-ē-dok-o-li-thot'-o-mi*). Incision of the common bile duct for the removal of gall-stone.

choledochotomy (*ko'-lē-dok-ot'-om-i*). Incision of the common bile duct.

cholelithiasis (*ko-lē-li-thī'-a-sis*). Formation of gall-stones.

cholemesis (*kō-lem'-e-sis*). Vomiting of bile.

cholera (*kol'-e-ra*). An epidemic tropical disease spread by infected water. *Symptoms:* Cramp, vomiting, and rice-water stools caused by cholera vibrio.

cholesteatoma (*kol-es-tē-a-tō'-ma*). Small tumour containing fat-like material which occasionally is found in the external auditory meatus.

cholesterol (*ko-les'-ter-ol*). A sterol widespread in animal tissues, first isolated from bile. One of the substances which on precipitation gives rise to gall-stones.

choline (*kō-lēn*). An organic base which is a constituent of some important substances, *e.g.* phospholipids, acetylcholine. It is used in fat metabolism.

cholinergic (*ko-lin-er-jik*). *See* ACETYLCHOLINE.

cholinesterase (*kō-li-li-nes-te-rāz*). Specific for acetylcholinesterase: an enzyme found at motor end plates and other sites, which breaks down and inactivates acetylcholine. Non-specific or pseudocholinesterases are found in the blood.

choluria (*ko-lū'-ri-a*). Bile in the urine.

chondralgia (*kon-dral'-ji-a*). Pain in a cartilage.

chondrin (*kon'-drin*). Cartilaginous tissue.

chondritis (*kon-drī-tis*). Inflammation of cartilage.

chondroblast (*kon-drō-blahst*). The embryonic cell forming cartilage.

chondroma (*kondrō'-ma*). A benign tumour of cartilage cells.

chordae tendineae (*kor-dē ten-di-ni-ē*). Thin musculotendinous bands extending between the walls of the ventricles of the heart and the tricuspid and mitral valves.

chordee (*kor-dē'*). Painful erection of penis, common in gonorrhoea.

chorditis (*kor-dī'tis*). Inflammation of the vocal cords.

chordotomy (*kor-do-to-mē*). Division of an antero-lateral column of the spinal cord.

chorea (*ko-rē'-a*). Involuntary twitchings of the muscles, and incoordination of movement. In children it is rheumatic in origin and known as St. Vitus's Dance. The adult form, due to cerebral degeneration, is known as Huntington's Chorea.

chorion (*ko'-ri-on*). Layer enclosing embryonic structures and enveloping the fetus. *See* ALLANTOIS.

chorion epithelioma (*ko'-ri-on epi-thē-li-ō'-ma*). A malignant growth of the uterus after abortion or delivery. Especially to be dreaded after hydatidiform mole. *See* MOLE.

chorionic villi (*kor-i-ō'-nik*). Vascular processes developing on the external surface of the chorion.

choroid (*ko'-royd*). The posterior five-sixths of the middle coat of the eye, containing blood vessels and pigment. It lies between the retina and the sclera.

choroid plexus (*ko-royd plek-sus*). Specialized vascular epithelium which produces the cerebrospinal fluid. One choroid plexus is situated in each of the four ventricles of the brain.

choroiditis (*kor'-oyd-ī'-tis*). Inflammation of the choroid.

choroidocyclitis (*kor-oyd-ō-sī-klī-tis*). Inflammation of the choroid and ciliary body.

Christmas disease (*kris'-mas*). Rare defect of blood coagulation.

chromatography (*krō-ma-to-gra-fi*). A method of separating different substances in solution and used in chemical analysis.

chromatosis (*krō-ma-tō-sis*). Pigmentation of the skin, *e.g.* as in Addison's disease.

chromic acid (*krō'-mik as-id*). Red crystals used as a caustic.

chromocyte (*krō'-mo-sīt*). Any coloured cell.

chromophil adenoma (*krō-mo-fil a-de-nō-ma*). Tumour of the pituitary gland found in acromegaly.

chromophobe adenoma (*krō-mō-fōb a-de-nō-ma*). Pituitary tumour causing hypopituitarism.

chromosomes (*krōm-o-sōmz'*). When a cell divides, the genetic material present in the nucleus becomes segregated into thread-shaped bodies which are visible under the microscope. These are known as chromosomes and consist of connected strands of DNA molecules known as genes. In man there are 46 chromosomes per cell: 22 pairs of *autosomes* and two pairs of *sex chromosomes*; females have two X chromosomes, males one X and one Y. The Y chromosome is shorter than the X chromosome.

chronic (*kron'-ik*). A disease from which complete cure is never obtained and which tends to worsen.

Chvostek's sign (*shfos-teks*). A spasm of the facial muscles produced by tapping the facial nerve. This sign is present in tetany.

chyle (*kīl*). The milk-like fluid which is lymph draining from the villi of the small intestine.

chyluria (*kī-lū'-ri-a*). Passing of chyle in the urine.

chyme (*chīm*). Food which has been digested in the stomach.

cicatricial (*sik'-a-trish-al*). Pertaining to a scar, or cicatrix.

cicatrix (*sik'-a-triks*). The scar of a healed wound or ulcer.

cilia (*sil'-i-a*). (1) Eyelashes. (2) Hairlike processes of certain cells. *See* CILIATED EPITHELIUM.

ciliary body (*sil'-i-a-ri*). Consists of the ciliary muscle and processes, forming part of the middle coat of the eye, and which changes the size of the pupil.

ciliated epithelium (*sil'-i-a-ted*).

Epithelium with hair-like processes on the surface which waft in one direction only. It lines the respiratory tract and the Fallopian tubes.

Cimex lectularius (*sē-meks lek-tū-lā-rē-us*). The common bed bug.

cinchonism (*sin'-ko-nizm*). Intolerance to quinine, indicated by buzzing in the ears, nausea, vomiting.

circa (*ser'-ka*). About.

circinate (*ser-kin-āt*). Ring-shaped.

Circle of Willis (*wi'-lis*). Circular intercommunication of arteries supplying the brain.

circulation (*ser-kū-lā'-shon*). *See* HEART. *Systemic or general circulation.* Arterial blood received into the left atrium passes through the mitral valve to the left ventricle. It then passes into the aorta and through its smaller branches to the capillaries—into smaller veins, then larger, until on reaching the superior and inferior venae cavae it passes into the right atrium. *Pulmonary circulation.* The venous blood which is received into the right atrium passes through the tricuspid valve into the right ventricle. From there into the pulmonary artery, which divides into two branches, one going to each lung. The artery divides in the lung into capillaries, and here, by means of the haemoglobin in the red cells, takes up oxygen from the inspired air. Oxygenated blood returns to the heart by the four pulmonary veins, two from each lung entering the left atrium. *Portal circulation.* Veins from the pancreas, spleen, stomach, intestines, unite behind the pancreas and form the portal tube or vein. This takes blood, rich in the products of digestion, to the liver where it divides into smaller vessels and capillaries. Blood leaves the liver by the hepatic veins which enter the inferior vena cava.

circumcision (*ser-kum-si'-zhon*). Surgical removal of the foreskin.

circumduction (*duk'-shon*). Circular movement of a limb.

circumflex nerve. This arises from the brachial plexus to supply the deltoid and teres minor muscles.

circumoral (*sir-kum-or'-al*). Around the mouth. *Circumoral pallor*, especially seen in scarlet fever, when the white area around the mouth is in great contrast to the colour of the rest of the face.

circumvallate (*ser-kum-val-lāt*). Surrounded by a wall.

cirrhosis (*sir-rō'-sis*). Chronic diffuse damage to an organ, usually applied to the liver.

cirsoid (*sir'-soyd*). Resembling a varix.

cisterna magna (*sis-ter'-na mag'-na*). A subarachnoid space at the back of the hind-brain between cerebellum and medulla oblongata. Contains CSF.

cisternal puncture (*sis-ter'-nal*). A puncture made with a hollow needle at the nape of the neck into a space called the cisterna magna which contains cerebrospinal fluid. Used when the fluid cannot be obtained by lumbar puncture.

citrate (*sit'-rāt*). Compound of citric acid and a base. Sodium citrate renders milk more digestible. A citrate solution added to shed blood delays clotting.

citric acid (*sit'-rik as-id*). Acid prepared from lemon juice. Antiscorbutic. Makes an astringent mouthwash.

Cl. Symbol for Chlorine.

clamps (*klamps*). Instruments used to compress vessels or to secure a grip on a structure.

claudication (*klaw-dik-ā'-shon*). Limping. *Intermittent C.* Limping with severe pain on walking which disappears with rest; due to insufficient blood supply to the limb.

claustrophobia (*klaw-'strō-fō'-bi-a*). Fear of a confined space, such as a room. Opposite of agoraphobia.

clavicle (*klav'-e-kl*). The collar bone, going from each shoulder to the breast-bone across the front of the chest.

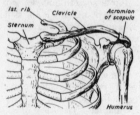

13 The shoulder girdle showing the clavicle

clavus (*klā-vus*). A corn.

claw foot (*klor*). The foot is shaped like a claw and has a very pronounced arch.

claw hand. Claw-shaped hand due to flexor spasm followed by contracture of the muscles flexing the fingers. Often caused by ulnar nerve damage.

cleft palate (*pal'-et*). Failure of fusion of the lip and palate during development; the line of cleavage is shown in the diagram. The cleft is variable in extent; the deformity can be remedied by plastic surgery.

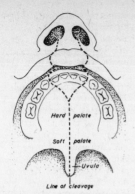

Hard palate

Soft palate

Uvula

Line of cleavage

14 A cleft palate

cleidocranial dysostosis (*klī-dō-krā-ni-al di-so-stō'-sis*). Rare hereditary condition in which there is a failure of development of membranous bone; consequently there may be partial or total absence of the clavicles and imperfect ossification of the skull in the region of the fontanelle. The striking feature is the ability to approximate the shoulders in front of the chest.

cleidotomy (*klī-dot'-o-mē*). Cutting the collar bone.

climacteric (*klī-mak'-ter-ik*). Termination of reproductive period. The menopause.

climatology (*klī-ma-tol'-o-ji*). The study of climates as affecting the treatment of disease.

clinic (*klin'-ik*). An institution to treat patients.

clinical (*klin'-ik-al*). Relating to the observation and treatment of a patient.

clinical thermometer (*thermom'-et-er*). *See* THERMOMETER.

Clinitest (*kli-ni-test*). Proprietary tablets containing reagent for testing urine for sugar.

clitoris (*kli'-tor-is*). A small organ of erectile tissue, found in the female in front of the urethra. The seat of sexual excitement.

cloaca (*klo-ā-ka*). Aperture through which both urine and faèces are discharged.

clonic (*klon'-ik*). Spasmodic contractions, short and irregular. They occur in the second stage of an epileptic convulsion and in certain other fits.

clonus (*klō-nus*). Reflex spasms with contractions and relaxations of muscles.

Clostridium (*klos-tri-di-um*). Large spore-bearing anaerobic bacilli. The genus includes *Cl. botulinum*, *Cl. tetani* and the gas gangrene group.

clotting time (*klo'-ting tīm*). Time taken for blood to clot when bleeding has occurred. Normal time is 4 to 13 minutes at 37° C.

clove hitch (*klōv hit'-ch*).

Useful knot for a temporary sling.

clubbing (*klu-bing*). The appearance of fingers and sometimes toes when the normal angle at the base of the nail is lost. It results from hyperplasia of connective tissue. Clubbing is associated with longstanding respiratory or cardiovascular disease.

clubfoot (*klub-foot*). *See* TALIPES.

clumping. Packing together of cells, usually red blood cells, due to loss of membrane charge resulting from reaction with antibody. *See* AGGLUTININS.

Clutton's joints (*klut'-tons joyntz*). Swelling of the knee joints found in congenital syphilis.

CMB. Abbreviation for Central Midwives Board.

CNS. *See* CENTRAL NERVOUS SYSTEM.

coagulase test (*kō-a-gū-lās test*). Test used for identification of pathogenic staphylococci which depends on the demonstration of the enzyme coagulase which breaks down fibrinogen and clots plasma.

coagulation (*kō-ag-ū-lā'-shon*). Thickening of a fluid into curds or clots. Almost always applied to blood. *See* BLOOD and BLOOD TRANSFUSION.

coal-tar (*kōl-tah*). A viscid liquid, from dry distillation of bituminous coal.

coalesce (*kō-a-les*). To converge or come together as may occur with spots in a skin rash.

coarctation (*kō-ark-tā'-shon*). The compression of the walls of a vessel. When this occurs in the aorta it is narrowed where it is joined by the ductus arteriosus.

cobalt (*kō'-bawlt*). Trace element. Its absence from the diet of young animals may lead to anaemia. *C. bomb.* Source of irradiation in deep X-ray therapy using Co^{60}.

cocaine (*ko-kān'*). A powerful local anaesthetic, much used in ophthalmology. It enlarges the pupil of the eye. Included in the Misuse of Drugs Act.

cocainism (*ko-kān'-izm*). Chronic poisoning from indulgence in the drug.

coccus (*kok'-us*). Any spheroidal-shaped micro-organism. *See* BACTERIA.

coccydynia (*kok-si-din'-i-a*). Pain in the coccyx.

coccyx (*kok'-siks*). The tail-like termination of the spine.

cochlea (*kok'-le-a*). The spiral cavity of the internal ear, containing the nerve endings of the eighth cranial or auditory nerve.

cock-up splints (*kok'-up*) for hand and wrist. Usually made of metal.

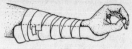

15 A cock-up splint

cod-liver oil (*kod-li-ver oyl'*). *Oleum Morrhuae*; contains vitamin D. Used in the prevention and treatment of rickets.

coeliac (*sēl'-i-ak*). Related to the abdominal cavity.

coeliac disease (*sēl'-i-ak dizēz*). A condition commencing in early childhood, associated with deficient absorption of fat from the intestines, resulting in the passage of loose, bulky, pale, offensive stools, abdominal enlargement, wasting and retarded development.

coelioscopy (*sē-lē-os'-ko-pē*). Also known as peritoneoscopy. Examination of the abdominal contents as follows: a small incision is made through the abdominal wall under a local anaesthetic. Air is passed into the peritoneal cavity and the contents viewed by means of a laparoscope. This method may be used when an exploratory laparotomy is unjustifiable.

coffee ground vomit. Vomit which contains partly digested blood.

cognition. Awareness. Part of a mental process. There is cognition when there is perception or memory of a material thing or idea.

coitus (*kō-it'-us*). Sexual intercourse.

colchicum (*kol-chi-kum*). Drug used in the treatment of gout.

colectomy (*ko-lek'-to-mē*). The operation of removing the colon.

colic (*kol'-ik*). Severe abdominal pain due to muscular spasm of a hollow viscus frequently caused by obstruction. *Biliary colic.* Intense pain due to lodging of a gallstone in the cystic or common bile duct. Sudden relief when it passes into duodenum. *Intestinal colic.* Severe pain in the abdomen due to irritation of the gut as in food poisoning. *Renal colic.* Same when due to a stone in the pelvis of kidney blocking up upper end of ureter. *Uterine colic.* Spasmodic contractions of the uterus as it endeavours to expel its contents.

colicystitis (*ko-li-sist-ī'-tis*). Cystitis from the colon bacillus.

coliform (*ko'-li-form*). Resembling *bacillus coli communis*.

colitis (*ko-lī'-tis*). Inflammation of the colon. *Acute, ulcerative* c., due to an infection, *e.g.* Dysentery. *Chronic ulcerative c.,* cause unknown. *Mucous c.,* thought to be of nervous origin and associated with constipation.

collagen (*kol'-a-jen*). A protein constituent of fibrous tissue.

collagen diseases. A group of diseases in which there is inflammation of the small blood vessels, *e.g.* disseminated lupus erythematosus, polyarteritis nodosa, dermatomyositis.

collapse (*kol-laps'*). Severe sudden prostration. *Symptoms: see* SHOCK. *Massive c.,* of one or more lobes of the lung, may result from a chest wound. *C. of the lungs.* Lack of air in previously expanded air tissue.

collar bone (*ko'-la*). Clavicle.

collateral. Accessory or subordinate but from same source. *C. circulation.* Blood flowing in accessory vessels, generally when main vessels are blocked.

Colles' fracture (*kol'-es*). Transverse fracture of the radius just above the wrist with displacement of the hand backwards and outwards.

Colles' law (*kol'-es*). A woman may breast-feed her baby, and this child being syphilitic may affect others and yet apparently not the mother. The explanation is—the mother is already affected, not yet showing any signs of the disease, but her Wassermann will be positive, and later in life she will show some signs of late tertiary syphilis, *e.g.* gummata, GPI or tabes.

collodion (*kol-lō'-di-on*). Pyroxylin dissolved in alcohol and ether; used in surgery to form a false skin for clean wounds. Highly inflammable.

colloid (*kol'-oyd*). A substance which will not pass through an animal membrane, *e.g.* starch. Various metals can be reduced into a peculiar semi-gelatinous or colloidal state in which they are said to be very active therapeutically: *e.g.* gold, silver, copper, manganese, antimony, etc.

collutorium (*kol-ū-to'-ri-um*). A mouthwash; a gargle.

collyrium (*kol-lir'-i-um*). An eyewash.

coloboma (*kol-ob-ō'-ma*). A fissure or gap in the eyeball or in one of its component parts, *e.g.* coloboma iridis.

colocynth (*kol'-ō-sinth*). A very powerful purge, dose 120 to 300mg. Seldom used.

colon (*kō'-lon*). The part of the

large intestine between the caecum and the rectum. *See* BOWEL.

colon bacillus (*bas'-il-us*). *Bacillus coli communis*: a microbe present in vast numbers in the intestine, and the cause of serious diseases if it gets a foothold anywhere else in the body. *See* BACILLURIA.

colony (*ko'-lo-ni*). A collection of bacteria growing in culture medium.

colorimeter (*kol-or-im'-et-er*). An instrument for estimating the depth of colour of a fluid.

colostomy (*ko-lost'-o-mi*). Operation to make an artificial opening so that the colon opens out into the anterior abdominal wall.

colostrum (*ko-los'-trum*). A milky fluid flowing from the breasts the first two or three days after confinement, before the true milk comes.

colotomy (*kol-ot'-o-mi*). An incision into the colon.

colour blindness (*ku'-ler blindnes*). Inability to distinguish certain colours, known sometimes as Daltonism.

colour index (*in'-deks*). Is a measure of the amount of haemoglobin contained in each red cell, compared to the normal amount. It is calculated thus:

$$\text{Normal} \quad \frac{\text{Haemoglobin percentage}}{\text{Red cell percentage}} \quad \frac{100}{100} = 1$$

colpitis (*kol-pī'-tis*). Inflammation of the vagina.

colpocele (*kol'-po-sēl*). A tumour or hernia in the vagina.

colpohysterectomy (*kol-pō-his-ter-ek'-to-mi*). Removal of the uterus through the vagina.

colpoperineorrhaphy (*kol'-po-per-i-nē-ŏr'-af-i*). Operation for repairing a torn vagina and perineum.

colporrhaphy (*kol-por'-af-i*). Operation for repairing a torn vagina or for preventing prolapse of the vaginal walls. *Anterior colporrhaphy.* Repairing the anterior vaginal wall and preventing recurrence of a cystocele. *Posterior colporrhaphy.* Repairing the posterior vaginal wall and preventing the recurrence of a rectocele.

colpotomy (*kol-pot'-o-mi*). Incision of the vagina.

coma (*kō-ma*). Insensibility, stupor, sleep.

comatose (*kō'-ma-tōs*). In a state of coma.

comedones (*ko-me-dōns*). Accumulations of sebaceous secretions in the hair follicles, commonly called blackheads.

comma bacillus (*ko'-ma*). The

bacillus which produces cholera.

commensal (*komen-sal*). Refers to members of different species living in close association but without influencing each other, *cf.* symbiosis.

comminuted fracture (*kom'-me-nūt-ed frak'-tūr*). See FRACTURE.

commissure (*kom-mis-sūr*). A connecting structure. Bundle of nerve fibres connecting the right and left side of the brain and spinal cord. In gynaecology the anterior and posterior commissures of the vulva are used to denote its two ends. The anterior commissure passes immediately above the clitoris, the posterior constitutes the anterior edge of the perineum.

communicable disease (*ko-mū-ni-kabl di-sēz*). A disease caused by micro-organisms transmitted indirectly or directly from one person or animal to another. How the disease spreads and its clinical and social aspects all provide fields for study.

commutator (*ko-mū-tā-ter*). A mechanical device for reversing the direction of an electric current.

compact tissue (*kom'-pakt ti-sū*). The hard, external portion of a bone. *See* BONE.

compatibility (*kom-pa'-ti-bil-iti*). Able to be mixed together without ill result: thus *compatible blood* is used for transfusion since it can be mixed with that of the recipient. *Compatible drugs* are those which can be mixed without producing undesirable chemical interactions. *See* BLOOD GROUPING and BLOOD TRANSFUSION.

compensation (*kom-pen-sā'-shon*). Psychiatric term for tendency to exaggerate features of behaviour opposite to those which seem to the patient to be unsatisfactory. In *Cardiac c.* the heart muscle hypertrophies to compensate for valvular defects.

Complan (*kom-plan*). A powdered food of which each 100g contains 31g protein, 16g fat and 44g carbohydrate, vitamins and essential minerals. Used in tube feeding and as a complete or supplementary food.

complement (*kom'-ple-ment*). A protein present in the blood which forms an essential component of certain antibody-antigen reactions.

complement fixation test. The disappearance of complement from the serum is used to detect antigen-antibody reactions. This complement 'fixation' forms the basis of certain serological tests such as the Wassermann reaction.

complemental air (*kom-ple-ment'-al*). The additional air drawn into the lungs on deep inspiration.

complex (*kom'-pleks*). A group of ideas with an emotional background. Partially or entirely repressed in the unconscious mind, it may be the underlying cause of mental abnormality.

complicated fracture (*kom'-plē-kā-ted frak'-tūr*). See FRACTURE.

complication of disease (*kom-pli-kā'-shon*). A disease occurring in the course of some other disease and more or less dependent upon it.

compos mentis (*kom-pos men'-tis*). Of sound mind.

compound (*kom-pownd*). Chemical substance made up of more than one element and having special properties.

compound fracture. See FRACTURE.

comprehension (*kom-prē-hen-shon*). The understanding of ideas and the relationship between them.

compress (*kom'-press*). (1) A tightly folded pad of lint, gauze, or other material used to secure local pressure. (2) A sterile dressing applied

over an area which has been prepared for a surgical operation.

compression (*kom-presh'-on*). The state of being compressed. *Cerebral c.*, increased intracranial pressure from a tumour, etc.

compulsive (*kom-pul-siv*). Applied to some action which a person feels he must perform, however irrational. It may be done to work out some anxiety.

computerized axial tomography. See CAT.

concave (*kon-kāv*). With outline curved like interior of a circle.

concavity (*kon-kav'-i-ti*). A depression.

concentration (*kon-sen-trā-shon*). The amount of dissolved substance in a solution.

concentric (*kon-sen-trik*). With a common centre.

conception (*kon-sep'-shon*). (1) The impregnation of the ovum. (2) An idea.

concha auris (*kong'-ka aw'-ris*). Deepest hollow of pinna of the outer ear.

concretion (*kon-krē'-shon*). A calculus. An abnormal deposit in the body such as stone in the gall bladder.

concussion (*kon-kush'-on*). Interruption of function of the brain as the result of compression wave set up by a blow to the head. The wave of compression transmitted through the cerebrospinal fluid and the brain substance obliterates momentarily the blood capillaries supplying the brain. Recovery may take many hours.

condensation (*kon-den-sā-shon*). The transformation of a gas to a liquid, or a liquid to a solid.

condenser (*kon-den'-ser*). (1) Apparatus to cool and thus cause condensation of gas. (2) Apparatus used to store charges of electricity. It consists of metal plates separated by non-conducting material. (3) Means of focussing light in optical apparatus.

conditioned reflex (*kon-dish-ond rē-fleks*). Reflex action produced by association of ideas.

condom (*kon-dom*). Rubber sheath for the penis preventing conception.

conduction (*kon-duk'-shon*). Passage of a physical disturbance through matter. Biologically, the passage of a nerve impulse.

conductor (*kon-dukt'-or*). An instrument used to direct surgical knives, called also a director. In electricity, a substance which allows the passage of electric currents.

condyle (*kon'-dīl*). A round projection at the ends of some bones. *See* HUMERUS.

condyloma (*kon-dē-lō'-ma*). Wartlike growth about the anus or pudendum.

cones, retinal (*kōns*). Together with rods form the vision receptor layer of the retina.

confabulation (*kon-fab-ū-lā'-shon*). The narration of fictitious occurrences.

confection (*kon-fek'-shon*). Medication with sweet covering.

confinement (*kon-fin'-ment*). Childbirth.

conflict (*kon-flikt'*). In psychology a mental disturbance denoting antagonism between contradictory desires.

confluent smallpox (*kon-flū-ent'*). A severe form of smallpox in which the individual papules coalesce.

confusion (*kon-fū-zhon*). Inability to think clearly.

congenital (*kon-jen'-i-tal*). Existing at birth.

congenital heart disease. Heart disease present from birth. Due to developmental abnormalities of the cardiovascular system.

congestion (*kon-jest'-chon*). Hyperaemia. Accumulation of blood in a part of the body, as in the lungs or brain. *Congestion of the lungs*, pneumonia.

Congo red (*kon'-gō*). A red dye turned blue by acid substances.

conisation (*ko-nī-zā-shon*). Part of the cervix is removed, by excision or diathermy.

conjugate (*kon'-jū-gāt*). (1) United in pairs or couples; fused. (2) An important diameter of the pelvis, measured from the most prominent part of the upper half of the sacrum to the nearest point on the back of the symphysis pubis. This is the *true* conjugate, which should measure not less than 10·8cm and is sometimes as large as 11·4cm or 12·0cm. If less than 10·8cm, the pelvis is a deformed one. The *diagonal* conjugate is measured from the lower edge of the symphysis to the sacrum, and can be determined clinically, whereas the true conjugate cannot. The diagonal conjugate is about 1·3cm to 1·9cm longer than the true conjugate. The *external* conjugate is measured from the spine of the last lumbar vertebra to the front of the symphysis pubis (this can only be done with calipers), and is normally about 20cm.

conjunctiva (*kon-junk-tī'-va*). Mucous membrane covering the anterior eyeball.

conjunctivitis (*kon-junk-ti-vi'-tis*). Inflammation of the conjunctiva.

connective tissue (*kon-nek'-tiv tish'-ū*). Supporting or packing material consisting of a fibrous gel made up of collagen and elastin fibres.

Conn's syndrome (*kons sin-drōm*). A condition caused by the oversecretion of aldosterone.

consanguinity (*kon-san-gwin'-i-ti*). Blood relationship.

conservative (*kon-ser'-va-tiv*). Aiming at preservation or repair, *e.g.* conservative treatment of a tooth.

consolidation (*kon-sol-i-dā-shon*). Becoming solid, as with a lung in pneumonia.

constipation (*kon-sti-pā-shon*). Infrequent bowel action, leading to the rectum being filled with hard faeces.

constitutional (*kon-sti-tū'-shon-al*). Affecting the whole body, not local.

constrict (*kon-strikt*). Contract or draw together.

consumption (kon-sum-shon). Using up. Popular term for pulmonary tuberculosis.

contact (*kon'-takt*). One who has been exposed to an infectious disease. *C. lens,* plastic lens worn directly on the cornea.

contagious (*kon-tā'-jus*). Communicable disease which is transmitted by contact, *i.e.* not communicable through atmosphere.

contraception (*kon-tra-sep'-shon*). Preventing conception.

contraceptives, oral. Drugs, usually combined oestrogens and progestogens, which inhibit ovulation. They prevent blastocyst implantation and make cervical mucus unfavourable to sperm migration.

contracted pelvis (*kon-trak'-ted pel'-vis*). A pelvis is contracted if any of its diameters is shorter than normal (*see* CONJUGATE and DIAMETERS). The commonest form of contraction is the *simple flat* pelvis, in which the true conjugate is the only diameter materially shortened. Other common forms are the *generally contracted* or *small round* pelvis; and the *generally contracted flat* pelvis. The obliquely distorted, the triradiate, the osteomalacic, the spondylolisthetic and others are rare. A contracted pelvis may lead to difficulty during delivery.

contraction (*kon-trak'-shon*). Shortening. A drawing together.

contraction ring. *See* RETRACTION RING.

contracture (*kon-trak-tūr*). Permanent contraction of structure due to the formation of fibrous tissue which is inelastic. *Dupuytren's c.* Localized thickening of palmar fascia which involves the overlying skin of the palm. There is a strong tendency for this to contract, drawing the affected fingers into rigid flexion.

contra-indication (*kon-tra-in-di-kā'-shon*). Sign that a particular treatment is unsuitable.

contralateral (*kon-tra-la'-teral*). On the opposite side.

contre-coup (*kon-tr-koo*). Injury through transmission of force of the blow, remote from original point of contact.

Controlled Drugs. *See* MISUSE OF DRUGS ACT.

contusion (*kon-tū'-zhon*). A bruise.

convalescence (*kon-val-es-enz*). Period of regaining full health after an illness.

convection (*kon-vek'-shon*). The heat of liquids and gases transmitted by a circulation of heated particles.

conversion (*kon-ver'-shon*). In psychology when an emotion becomes transformed into a physical manifestation.

convex (*kon-veks*). With outline curved like exterior of circle.

convolutions (*kon-vo-lū'-*

shons). The folds and twists of the brain or the intestines. *See* BOWEL and BRAIN.

convulsions (*kon-vul'-shons*). Violent spasms of alternate muscular contraction and relaxation, due to disturbance of cerebral function. A fit.

convulsive therapy (*kon-vul-sif the-ru-pē*). Electroplexy. Shock treatment given by electrical apparatus to psychiatric patients. *See* ELECTROCONVULSIVE THERAPY.

Coombs' test (*kooms*). Coombs' reagent detects the presence of any antibody coating the red cell, i.e. in a newborn baby with haemolytic disease and following a mis-matched blood transfusion.

copper sulphate (*sul'-fāt*). Blue stone, blue vitriol.

copulation (*kop-ū-lā-shon*). Sexual intercourse.

cor pulmonale (*kor-pul-mon-ah-le*). Congestive cardiac failure resulting from chronic respiratory disease.

coracoid (*kor'-a-koyd*). A process of bone on the scapula which resembles a crow's beak. *See* SCAPULA.

cord (*kawd*). Any string-like body such as the spinal cord or umbilical cord.

cordotomy. *See* CHORDOTOMY.

corium or **dermis** (*ko'-re-um*). Internal layer of the skin. The true skin.

corn (*kawn*). A local thickening of the skin due to pressure such as found on the feet.

cornea (*kor'-ne-a*). Transparent epidermis and connective tissue which forms the front surface of the eye.

corneal graft (*kor-nē-al grah-ft*). Healthy cornea is given by grafting to replace a diseased cornea.

cornu (*kaw-nū*). Horn-like.

corona dentis. Crown of a tooth.

coronal suture (*ko-rō'-nal sū-tūr*). The suture which joins the parietal and frontal bones of the skull.

coronary (*ko-ron'-a-ri*). Encircling as a vessel. *C. arteries* supply the heart muscle; narrowing and spasm of these produce angina pectoris. There are also coronary arteries in the stomach. *C. sinus*, a passage for the venous blood into the right atrium.

coronoid (*ko-ro-noyd*). Like a crow's beak as with certain bony processes.

corpora quadrigemina (*kor'-por-ah kwod-ri-jem'-in-ah*). Four rounded bodies consisting chiefly of grey matter in the midbrain.

corpulency (*kaw'-pū-len-si*). Undue fatness. Obesity.

corpus callosum (*kal-ō-sum*). The band of nervous tissue which connects the two hemispheres of the cerebrum.

corpus luteum (*loo-tē-um*). A temporary organ secreting the hormone progesterone which favours the establishment and continuity of a pregnancy. It is formed under the influence of luteinizing hormone of the pituitary, by growth of the wall of a Graafian follicle after ovulation. If ovulation does not result in fertilization, the corpus luteum degenerates, but if fertilization occurs, the corpus luteum persists.

corpus striatum (*strī-ā-tum*). Basal ganglion in the midbrain.

corpuscle (*kor'-pusl*). Usually refers to a cell esp. red or white blood cells.

corrective (*kor-rek'-tiv*). A drug which modifies the action of another drug.

Corrigan's pulse (*ko'-rig-anz puls*). Known also as water-hammer pulse, occurs in aortic regurgitation. The artery distends forcibly and then appears to empty suddenly and completely.

corrosive (*kor-rŏ'-siv*). Eating into, consuming.

corrosive sublimate (*sub'-li-māt*). Perchloride of mercury. Powerful, very poisonous antiseptic. For douches is used in strengths of 1 in 1,000 to 1 in 10,000. Itself colourless, it is generally coloured blue to distinguish it.

cortex (*kaw'-teks*). The outer layer of an organ.

Corti's organ (*kaw-tēz aw'-gan*). The collection of nerve endings of the auditory nerve in the cochlea.

corticosteroids (*kor-ti-kō-steroyds*). Steroidal hormones from the adrenal cortex.

corticotrophin (*kor-ti-kō-trō'-fin*). ACTH. Hormone from the anterior pituitary gland stimulating the adrenal cortex.

cortisone (*kaw'-ti-z'on*). One of the hormones of the adrenal cortex. Used in the treatment of a variety of diseases because of its anti-inflammatory and anti-allergic action.

Corynebacterium diphtheriae (*ko-rin-e-bak-tār-ium dif-thā-ri-ā*). The bacillus causing diphtheria.

coryza *ko-rī'-za*). Cold in the head, nasal catarrh.

cosmetic (*kos-me-tik*). Improving the appearance. *C. operation*. Operation designed to improve the appearance of disfigured or unsightly part.

costal (*ko'-stal*). Relating to the ribs.

costive (*ko'-stiv*). Constipated.

cotyledon (*kot-i-lē'-don*). One

of the constituent portions of the placenta.

counter-extension (*kown'-ter eks-ten'-shon*). Extension by means of holding back the upper part of a limb while the lower is pulled down.

counter-irritation (*kown'-ter-i-ri-tā-shon*). The application of an irritant stimulus to the skin in order to divert attention from sensory information coming from another site, *e.g.* application of hot water bottle to relieve abdominal pain.

coupling (*ku'-pling*). Abnormal heart beat which occurs in overdose of digitalis. The normal heart beat is followed by an extra ventricular contraction (ventricular extrasystole). The latter may be too weak to transmit a pulse.

Cowper's glands (*koo'-perz*). Two small glands near the bulb of the urethra in the male.

cowpox. *See* VACCINIA.

coxa (*kok'-sa*). The hip joint.

coxalgia (*koks-al-ji-a*). Pain in the hip joint.

coxa valga (*koks'-a val'-ga*). Deformity of the hip joint in which the angle made by the neck and shaft of the femur is greater than normal. *C. vara.* In this case the angle is less than normal.

Coxsackie virus (*kok-sa-ki*

virus). Group of viruses which may cause epidemic myalgia (Bornholm disease) and benign lymphocytic meningitis, and possibly other relatively mild diseases.

crab louse (*krab' lows*). The phthirus pubis which infests the pubic region.

cracked nipple (*krakt*). Fissure in mother's nipple due to overfull breasts and aggressive sucking by infant. If untreated leads to mastitis.

cramp (*kramp*). Sudden painful tonic contraction of the muscles.

craniometry (*krā-nē-o'-me-tri*). Measurement of skulls.

craniotabes (*krā-ni-ō-tā'-bēz*). Thinning of the bones of the vault of the skull; occurs in rickets.

craniotomy (*krā-ni-ot'-o-mi*). Operation in which the skull is opened.

cranium (*krā'-nē-um*). The skull.

creatine (*krē'-at-in*). A nitrogenous constituent of muscle. *Blood c.* is raised in hyperthyroidism.

creatinine (*krē-at'-in-in*). A substance formed from creatine and excreted in the urine. *Blood c.* may rise in kidney disease.

Crede's method (*kred'-āz method*). Expelling the

placenta by means of compression of the fundus of uterus.

crepitation, crepitus (*krep-i-tā'-shon*). The grating of ends of a fractured bone.

cresol (*krē'-sol*). An antiseptic, similar to phenol, and obtained from coal-tar.

cretinism (*kret'-in-izm*). Congenital deficient thyroid secretion, causing impaired mentality, small stature, coarseness of skin and hair and deposition of fat on the body. Treated early with thyroid extract, great improvement may result.

cribriform (*kri'-bri-form*). Perforated like a sieve.

cricoid cartilage (*kri'-koyd kar'-ti-lāj*). A ring-shaped cartilage below the thyroid.

crisis (*krī'-sis*). The deciding point of a disease, from which the patient either begins to recover or sinks rapidly; often marked by a long sleep, profuse perspiration, or other phenomena.

Crohn's disease (*krōns*). Chronic form of enteritis affecting the terminal part of the ileum. *Syn.* regional ileitis.

crossed laterality (*krost la-te-ral'-iti*). Combination of either right-handedness with left eyedness or left-handedness with right eyedness.

cross-infection. Hazard in hospitals where for various reasons, infection is transferred from one patient to another. Particularly dangerous in surgical and obstetric wards where wound infection is a problem despite stringent efforts to minimize the spread of bacteria.

cross-resistance. Microorganisms which are resistant to one antibiotic, tend to have resistance to other antibiotics of the same type.

croup (*kroop*). Dyspnoea and stridor due to obstruction of the larynx. It may be due to inflammation, or spasm of the muscles.

crucial (*kroo'-shul*). Critical or decisive.

cruciate (*kroo-shē-āt*). Cross-shaped.

crural (*krū'-ral*). Relating to the thigh.

crus (*kroos*). Latin for leg. A limb-like structure.

crush syndrome (*krush sin'-drōm*). As the result of extensive crushing of muscles, toxic substances pass into the circulation which cause the medullary circulation of the kidney to be opened up so that blood is diverted from the glomeruli in the renal cortex. This results in oliguria.

crutch paralysis (*kru'-tch*

paral'-is-sis). Caused by pressure on the axillary nerves and vessels by a crutch.

cryosurgery (*krī-ō-ser-je-ri*). Surgery which entails the use of freezing as for replacement of detached retina, removal of lens in cataract operation.

cryptomenorrhoea (*krip-to-men'-o-re-a*). Apparent amenorrhoea due to obstruction to the flow of menstrual blood.

cryptorchid (*krip-tor'-kid*). A male in whom one or both testicles have failed to reach the scrotum.

crypts of Lieberkühn (*kripts of lē-ber-koon*). Glands found in the mucous membrane of the small intestine. They secrete a mixture of digestive enzymes collectively termed intestinal juice.

crystalline lens (*kris-ta-lin*). Lens of the eye.

crystalloids (*kris'-tal-loyds*). Substances which will pass through an animal membrane. They easily crystallize and are readily soluble, *e.g.* salt, sugar.

crystalluria (*kris-ta-lū-ri-a*). Crystals which are found in the urine esp. when patient's intake of water is too small when sulpha drugs are prescribed.

cubit (*kū'-bit*), **cubitus.** (1) The forearm. (2) The elbow.

cuirass respirator (*kyor-as*). Respirator, fitting over patient's chest and abdomen like a breastplate, used in ventilatory failure. Rarely seen today.

culdoscope (*kul-dos-kōp*). Instrument passed through the posterior vaginal wall to view the pelvic cavity.

culture (*kul'-cher*). The artificial cultivation of tissues, cells or viruses.

culture media (*mē'-dia*). Substances used for cultivating bacteria, *e.g.* gelatin, broth.

cumulative action (*kū'-mulativ*). A term applied to the prolonged use of certain drugs which are excreted slowly. After several doses have been given, symptoms of poisoning may arise, *e.g.* mercury, digitalis.

cuneiform (*kū-nē-form*). Wedge-shaped. Three of the tarsal bones.

curare (*kū'-rah'-rē*). A poison derived from a South American plant. It paralyses motor nerves. Used by anaesthetists to produce muscular relaxation, thus reducing the amount of anaesthetic required.

curettage (*kū-re-tahj*). The operation of scraping with a curette; most commonly the uterus is the seat of operation.

curette (*kū-ret'*). A spoon-shaped instrument. *C., suction.* Hollow tube of metal, glass or plastic, connected to a vacuum pump and used to terminate pregnancy in the early stages.

curie (*kū'-rē*). Unit of radioactivity.

Cushing's disease (*ku'-shings di-zēz*). Adenoma of the pituitary with hypersecretion of ACTH resulting in adrenal cortical overactivity.

Cushing's syndrome (*ku'-shings sin'-drōm*). Syndrome due to oversecretion of adreno-cortical hormones and characterized by moonface, redistribution of body fat, polycythaemia, hirsutism, acne, amenorrhoea, osteoporosis, glycosuria, hypertension, purpura, muscular weakness and occasionally mental derangement.

cusp (*kusp*). Projection, esp. on crown of tooth; also applied to part of heart valve.

cutaneous (*kū-tā'-ne-us*). Pertaining to the skin.

cuticle (*kū-ti-kl*). The external or scurf skin.

cutis (*kū'-tis*). True skin or derma.

cyanocobalamin (*sī-an-ō-kō-bal-a-min*). Vitamin B_{12}, the antipernicious anaemia principle of liver extract.

cyanosis (*sī-an-ō'-sis*). Blue appearance; due to deficient oxygenation of the blood. It occurs in heart failure, diseases of the respiratory tract, and congenital heart disease. *See* BLUE BABY.

cycle (*sī-kl*). Repeated series of events, *e.g.* cardiac cycle, menstrual cycle.

cyclical vomiting (*sik'-li-kal*). Recurrent attacks of vomiting occurring in childhood, usually with headache, and signs of acidosis.

cyclitis (*sīk-lī'-tis*). Inflammation of ciliary body of the eye.

cyclodialysis (*sī-klō-dī-a-li-sis*). Ophthalmic operation to drain the anterior chamber of the eye.

cycloplegia (*sī-klō-plē'-ji-a*). Paralysis of the ciliary muscle of the eye.

cyclopropane (*sī-klō'-prō-pān*). A gas that is used to produce general anaesthesia. It must be used in a closed circuit. Used for operations on the chest as it causes the minimum respiratory movement.

cyclothymia (*sī-klō-thī'-mia*). A mental state in which depression alternates with exuberance.

cyclotomy (*sī-klot-o-mē*). Incision through the ciliary body of the eye.

cyesis (*sī-ē-sis*). Pregnancy.

cyst (*sist*). A tumour containing fluid in a membranous sac. *Daughter c.* One developed from the walls of a large one.

cystadenoma (*sis-tad-e-nō'-ma*). Benign growth containing cysts.

cystectomy (*sis-tek'-to-mi*). Removal of the urinary bladder.

cystic disease of the lung. Congenital disease in which the pancreas is first affected and then the lung.

cystic duct (*sis'-tik*). The duct leading from the gall bladder to the common bile duct.

cysticercosis (*sis-ti-ser-kō'-sis*). Normally the cysticercus stage of the tapeworm occurs in the pig. Occasionally it develops in the muscle or nervous system of man producing serious symptoms, *e.g.* epilepsy.

cystine (*sis'-tin*). A sulphur-containing amino-acid.

cystitis (*sis-ti'-tis*). Inflammation of the urinary bladder.

cystitome (*sis-ti-tōm*). Knife used by ophthalmic surgeon in operation for cataract.

cystobubonocele (*sis-to-bū-bo'-n'o-s'el*). Hernia involving the bladder.

cystocele (*sis'-tō-sēl*). Hernia of the bladder into the vagina.

cystogram (*sis-tō-gram*). X-ray of urinary bladder.

cystolithiasis (*sis-to-li-thi'-a-sis*). Stone in the bladder.

cystometry (*sis-to-me-tri*). Measurement of tone of the bladder.

cystoscope (*sis'-to-skōp*). An instrument for examining the bladder.

cystostomy (*sis-tos'-to-mi*). Operation of producing an opening from the bladder to the exterior.

cystotomy (*sīs-tot'-o-mi*). Incision of the bladder or division of the anterior capsule of the lens of the eye.

Cytamen (*sī-ta-men*). Cyanocobalamin.

cytology (*sī-tol'-o-ji*). The study of cells. *Exfoliative c.* The study of shed cells used in the diagnosis of pre-malignant disease.

cytolysis (*sī-tol'-is-is*). Cell disintegration.

cytometer (*sī-tom'-et-er*). An instrument for counting cells, usually of the blood.

cytoplasm (*sī-to-pla-sm*). Protoplasm.

cytotoxic (*sī-tō-tōk-sik*). Substance which damages cells. *C. drugs.* Used in malignant disease to destroy cancer cells.

cytotoxin (*sī-tō-tok-sin*). Antibody inhibiting a cell's normal activity.

D

Dacron (*dak-ron*). Man-made fibre used in vascular surgery.

dacryadenitis (*dak-ri-ad-en-ī'-tis*). Inflammation of the lacrimal gland.

dacryocystitis (*dak'-ri-ō-sis-tī'-tis*). Inflammation of the tear sac.

dacryocystorhinostomy (*dak-ri-ō-sis-tō-rī-nos'-to-mi*). Operation to establish a communication between the tear (lacrimal) sac and the nose.

dacryolith (*dak'-ri-ō-lith*). Stone in the lacrimal duct.

dacryoma (*dak-ri-ō-mah*). Benign tumour arising from lacrimal epithelium.

dactyl (*dak-til'*). A digit of the hand or foot.

dactylion (*dak-til-i'-on*). Webbed fingers or toes.

dactylitis (*dak-ti-lī'-tis*). Inflammation of the fingers or toes. Generally used of the bones only.

dactylology (*dak-ti-lol'-o-jē*). Talking by the fingers; deaf and dumb language.

Dakin's solution (*dā'-kinz*). An antiseptic solution containing sodium hypochlorite and boric acid used to irrigate wounds.

Daltonism (*dal'-tōn-izm*). Colour blindness.

dandruff (*dan'-druf*). A scaly condition of the scalp.

dandy fever. *See* DENGUE.

day hospital. Hospital for patients, esp. the elderly and psychiatric patients, who go home at night.

Darwinism (*dar'-win-izm*). The theory of descent by evolution as taught by Charles Darwin in the nineteenth century.

DDA. Dangerous Drugs Act. Now replaced by the Misuse of Drugs Act 1971, and special drugs known as Controlled Drugs.

DDT. A synthetic insecticide.

deaf mute (*def mūt*). An individual who is both deaf and dumb.

deafness (*def-nes*). Lack of hearing. *Word d.* Agnosia.

deamination (*dē-am-in-ā-shon*). The breaking down of aminoacids in the liver.

debility (*de-bil'-i-ti*). Weakness, loss of power.

debridement (*dā-brēd'-mo*). Thorough cleansing of a wound and excision of the edges.

decalcification (*dē'-kal-si-fi-kā'-shon*). Loss or removal of calcium salts from bone.

decapitation (*dē'-kap-e-tā'-shon*). The operation of severing the fetal head from the body, very occasionally necessary in cases of obstructed labour.

decapsulation (*dē-kap-sū-lā'-shon*). Removal of the capsule of an organ, *e.g.* of the kidney.

decidua (*de-sid'-ū-a*). The thickened lining of the uterus formed to receive the fertilized ovum. As the ovum grows larger, the decidua covering it is called the *decidua reflexa*; the part where it is attached to the uterine wall and which later becomes the placenta, the *decidua basalis*; while that lining the rest of the uterine cavity is the *decidua vera*.

deciduoma malignum (*de-sid-ū-ō-ma ma-lig'-num*). *See* CHORION EPITHELIOMA.

decompensation (*dē-kom-pen-sā'-shon*). Failure of compensation, as of the heart.

decomposition (*dē-kom-pō-zish'-on*). (1) Putrefaction. (2) Breakdown of substances by hydrolytic enzymes.

decompression (*dē-kom-presh'-on*). An operation performed to relieve internal pressure, *e.g.* trephining of the skull. *D. sickness*. Caisson disease.

decortication (*dē-kor-ti-kā'-shon*). Removal of the cortex or external covering from an organ, *e.g.* of the cerebrum or

of the kidney. *D.*, *pulmonary*, pleurectomy: removal of one or more ribs and the visceral layer of the pleura.

decubitus (*de-kū'-bit-us*). The recumbent or horizontal position.

decussation (*dē-kus-ā'-shon*). (1) An interlacing or crossing of fellow parts. (2) The point at which the crossing occurs. *D. of the pyramids*. The crossing of the motor fibres from one side of the medulla to the other.

defaecation (*dē-fē-kā'-shon*). The act of evacuating the bowels.

defibrillator (*dē-fi-bri-lā-tor*). Apparatus which applies electrical impulses to the heart. Designed to stop fibrillation and restore the normal cardiac cycle.

deficiency diseases (*de-fish'-en-sē*). Due to an inadequate supply of vitamins in the diet, *e.g.* rickets, scurvy, beriberi.

deformed pelvis (*dē-fawm'd*). *See* CONTRACTED PELVIS.

degeneration (*dē-je-ner-ā'-shon*). Deterioration in structure or function of tissue. When the structural changes are marked, descriptive terms are sometimes used, *e.g.* colloid, fatty, hyaline, etc.

deglutition (*deg-lū-tish'-on*). Act of swallowing.

dehydration (*dē-hī-drā'-shon*). Loss of water.

déjà vu phenomenon (*dā-ja vū fe-no-me-non*). Illusion of familiarity when experiencing something new.

Delhi boil (*del'-ē*). A form of boil prevailing in the East. Cutaneous leishmaniasis.

delinquent (*de-lin-kwent*). One who acts against the accepted moral code.

deliquescent (*de-li-kwe-sent*). Able to absorb moisture and become fluid.

delirium (*de-lir'-i-um*). Extravagant talking, raving, and physical agitation generally due to high fever.

delirium tremens (*de-lir'-i-um tre'-menz*). An acute psychosis usually associated with chronic alcoholism. The patient is disorientated, has hallucinations and is excited. There is a coarse tremor of the fingers, tongue and facial muscles.

delivery (*de-li'-ver-i*). Parturition. Childbirth.

deltoid (*del'-toyd*). The muscle which covers the prominence of the shoulder.

delusion (*de-lū'-zhon*). A false idea, entirely without foundation in the facts of the environment.

demarcation (*de-mar-kā'-shon*). The marking of a boundary. *Line of d.*, red

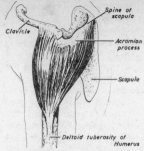

16 The deltoid muscle

line which forms between dead and living tissue in gangrene.

dementia (*de-men'-she-a*). Feebleness of the mental faculties, inconsequent ideas. A form of insanity. An acquired condition. *D. praecox*, schizophrenia.

demographic (*de-mō-gra-fik*). Relating to vital statistics and social science.

demulcents (*de-mul'-sents*) Agents which protect sensitive surfaces from irritation.

dendron, dendrite (*den'drīt*). A protoplasmic filament of a nerve cell through which synapse occurs.

denervated (*de-ner-vā-ted*). Deprived of nerve supply.

dengue (*deng'-ge*). A virus disease of the tropics, transmitted by mosquitoes and characterised by fever, headache, pains in the limbs, and a rash.

Denis Browne splints. A number of splints designed to correct congenital deformity, as that of the hip, bear this surgeon's name. His padded metal splints to correct congenital talipes equinovarus are widely used.

dens. A tooth.

density (*den'-si-ti*). Compactness. The weight of matter contained in a unit of volume.

dental (*den'-tal*). Pertaining to the teeth.

dentine (*den'-tēn*). The substance which forms the body of a tooth. *See* TEETH.

dentition (*den-tish'-on*). Teething. *See* TEETH.

denture (*den'-tūr*). A set of artificial teeth.

deodorant, deodorizer (*dē-ō'-dor-ī-zer*). Destroyer of smells; the chief deodorants are chloride of lime, sulphurous acid, nitrous acid, chlorophyll, iodoform, scents, and fumigating pastilles. They are all more or less disinfectants.

deoxidation (*dē-ok-si-dā'-shon*). The removal of oxygen from a substance.

deoxycorticosterone (*dē-ok-si-kaw-ti-kos'-te-rōn*). A constituent of suprarenal cortex extract, prescribed in Addison's disease.

deoxyribonucleic acid (*dē-ok-si-rī-bo-nū-klā-ik a-sid*). DNA. A complex chemical found in the cell nucleus and containing the genetic information.

depersonalization (*dē-per-son-al-ī-zā-shon*). A neurotic state when the person feels that he has no reality in existence but is only an onlooker at his own behaviour and actions.

depilatory (*dē-pil'-a-to-ri*). An agent for removing superfluous hairs from the body.

depletion (*dē-plē'-shon*). Act of emptying; bleeding; purging.

deposit (*de-poz'-it*). A sediment.

depressant (*de-pres'-ant*). An agent reducing functional activity.

depression (*dē-pre'-shon*). A feeling of gloom due to disappointment, loss or failure. In *reactive depression*, due to stress, the patient does not lose touch with reality. *Endogenous depression* is a psychotic state and there is usually a predisposition to it in the person's make-up. He then loses all touch with reality and needs expert help. *Involutional depression* occasionally occurs at the menopause.

depressor (*de-pres'-or*). (1) Down-drawing muscle.

(2) An instrument for depressing a part.

Derbyshire neck (*dah-bi-shu nek*). Term used to describe a swollen neck due to goitre. Once common in Derby.

derealization (*dē-rē-al-ī-zā-shon*). A feeling that the world is unreal and strange.

derma, dermis (*der'-ma*). The cutis or true skin.

dermalgia (*der-mal'-jia*). Pain of the skin.

dermatitis (*der-ma-ti'-tis*). Inflammation of the skin. The numerous causes may be of external or internal origin. Some common external irritants are dyes, metals, disinfectants, flowers.

dermatology (*der-ma-tol'-oji*). The science of the skin and its diseases.

dermatome (*der-ma-tōm*). Instrument for cutting a skin graft.

dermatomycosis (*der-mat-o-mī-kō'-sis*). A skin disease caused by a fungus.

dermatomyositis (*der-mat-o-mī-ō-sī'-tis*). One of the collagen diseases characterized by inflammation and breakdown of skin and progressive weakness of muscles.

dermatophyte (*der-ma-tō-fīt*). Group of fungi on skin and mucous membranes.

dermatosis (*der-ma-tō'-sis*). Any skin disease.

dermis (*der'-mis*). The true skin which lies below the epidermis.

dermographism (*der-mo'-graf'-izm*). The production of wheals on the skin, resembling urticaria, on gently stroking the skin.

dermoid cyst (*der-moyd sist'*). A cyst containing epithelial substances, especially hair, teeth, and sebaceous material.

Descemet's membrane (*des-e-mă*). Lining membrane behind the cornea of the eye.

desensitization (*de-sen-si-tī-zā'-shon*). To remove sensitivity to a substance. A method of treatment used for the allergic state.

desiccation (*des-ik-ā'-shon*). The act of drying.

desmoid (*des'-moyd*). Like a bundle. Fibrous tissue.

desquamation (*des-kwa-mā'-shon*). Peeling off of the skin, *e.g.* after scarlet fever.

detergent (*de-ter'-jent*). Substance which effectively lowers the surface tension of a fluid and thereby disperses fat. Used for cleansing purposes.

deterioration (*dē-tār-i-or-ā'-shon*). A worsening condition.

detoxicated (*dē-toks-i-kā'-ted*). With toxic properties removed.

detritus (*de-trē'-tus*). Debris. Accumulation of disintegrated material.

detrusor (*dē-trū-sor*). An expelling muscle.

Dettol (*de'-tol*). Official name: Liq. Chloroxylenol. An antiseptic lotion.

dexter (*dek'-ster*). Right. Upon the right side.

dextran (*deks'-tran*). A blood-plasma substitute. Used as 6% solution.

dextrin (*deks'-trin*). An intermediate product in the conversion of starch into sugar.

dextrocardia (*dek-stro-kar'-dia*). Congenital transposition of the heart from the left to the right side of chest.

dextrose (*deks-'trōs*). Grape sugar. Glucose. For rectal or intravenous injection, 5 per cent solution, *i.e.* 5g in 100ml aqueous solution is the usual strength.

dhobie itch (*dō'-bē*). Ringworm, mainly in the inguino-crural region. Also called tinea cruris.

diabetes insipidus (*dī-a-bē'-tēz*). Syndrome cause by deficient secretion of antidiuretic hormone (ADH) by the pituitary gland and characterized by the passage of enormous quantities of pale urine of low specific gravity, containing no sugar.

diabetes mellitus. A disease marked by an excessive flow of urine containing sugar, and thirst. It is due to failure of the pancreas to manufacture insulin; this being necessary for the metabolism of carbohydrates. The nurse will have to measure and test urine. The specific gravity may be as high as 1030 to 1045. The treatment is dietetic with the administration of the prescribed amount of insulin, or oral hypoglycaemic drugs *e.g.* chlorpropamide.

diacetic acid (*dī-as-ē'-tik*). Aceto-acetic acid. This is a substance occasionally present in the urine: especially in serious cases of diabetes.

diagnosis (*dī-ag-no'-sis*). The decision as to the nature of an illness, arrived at by studying the case.

dialysis (*di-al'-is-is*). The separation of certain substances from a mixture by passing the latter through a membrane. Usually applied to dialysis of blood to remove toxic waste in cases of renal insufficiency (kidney machine). *See* HAEMODIALYSIS.

diameters of pelvis (*dī-am'-eterz*). Besides the three conjugate diameters (described under CONJUGATE), the most important pelvic measurements are as follows: *The right and left oblique*, from the right and left sacro-iliac joints to the left and right pectineal eminences respectively; these should measure 12–13cm. The *transverse*, which at the brim measure 12cm and at the outlet about 10cm. *The distance between the anterior superior spines* of the ilia should be not less than 25cm, and *between the iliac crests* at least 2·5cm more than this.

diameters of skull. The important diameters of the fetal skull at term are as follows: Sub - occipito - bregmatic, 9cm; cervico-bregmatic, 9cm; fronto-mental, 8cm; occipito-mental, 13cm; supra - occipito - mental, 14cm; occipito-frontal, 11cm; sub-occipito-frontal, 10cm; biparietal, 9cm; bitemporal, 8cm (Jellett).

diamorphine (*dī-ah-mor'-fin*). An alkaloid obtained by the action of acetic anhydride on morphine. It allays cough, induces sleep and does not leave the depressing after-effects of morphia, but its narcotic action is less. (*Syn.* Heroin.) Addiction is a constant risk.

diapedesis (*dī-a-ped-ē'-sis*). The passage of leucocytes through the walls of blood-vessels. It occurs in inflammation.

diaphoresis (*dī-a-fo-rē'-sis*). Perspiration.

diaphoretics (*dī-a-for-et'-iks*). Agents which increase perspiration, *e.g.* pilocarpine.

diaphragm (*dī-a-fram*). The muscular septum separating the chest from the abdomen.

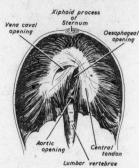

17 The undersurface (abdominal) of the diaphragm

diaphragmatic hernia (*dī-a-frag-ma-tik her-ni-a*). Herniation of abdominal viscera through the diaphragm into the chest. Usually due to a congenital defect of the diaphragm. Hiatus hernia is an acquired form in adults.

diaphysis (*dī-af'-fe-sis*). The middle part of long bones; the shaft, *cf.* epiphysis.

diarrhoea (*dī-ar-rē'-a*). Frequent loose stools.

diarthrosis (*dī-ar-thrō'-sis*). A freely movable joint permitting movement in any direction.

diastase (*dī'-as-tās*). An enzyme which converts starch into sugar with intermediate dextrins.

diastasis (*dī-as'-tā-sis*). Forcible separation of bones without fracture; dislocation.

diastole (*dī-as'-tō-lē*). That part of cardiac cycle when the ventricles fill with blood, *cf.* systole.

diastolic (*dī-as-tol'-ik*). Connected with diastole. Thus a *diastolic murmur* is one produced during the relaxation or diastole, of the heart.

diathermy (*dī-ath-er'-mi*). The passage of high frequency electric current through a tissue. Because of the electrical resistance of the tissue, heat is generated. This is diffuse when large electrodes are used, as in physiotherapy. Tissues may be cauterized by using a small electrode. Diathermy is used so that tissues are destroyed, *e.g.* as in removal of superficial new growths. It is also used as a cautery to arrest bleeding.

diathesis (*dī-ath'-e-sis*). Constitutional disposition to a particular disease.

dichotomy (*dīu-kot'-o-mi*). Division into two parts.

dicrotic pulse (*dī-krot'-ik*). Having two beats. Usually applies to secondary pulse wave due to the closure of semilunar valves since, when this is marked as in conditions associated with vaso-dilatation, *e.g.* high fever, it gives the impression of a double pulse.

didactyle (*dī-dak'-tīl*). Having only two fingers, or two toes.

didymitis (*did-i-mī'-tis*). Inflammation of the testicle.

dielectric (*dī-e-lek'-trik*). The non-conducting material separating the conducting surface in an electrical condenser.

diet (*dī-et*). A pattern of food intake developed according to physiological need, availability and individual preference.

dietetics (*dī-e-tet'-iks*). The study of food values.

Dietl's crises (*dē'-tl*). Severe attacks of renal pain accompanied by scanty, blood-stained urine. Occurs in some cases of movable kidney probably due to kinking of the ureter.

differential blood count (*di-fer-en'-shal*). The determination of the proportion of each type of white cell in the blood, carried out by microscopical examination. Useful in diagnosis.

differential diagnosis. Discrimination between diseases with similar symptoms.

diffusion (*di-fū'-zhon*). The process by which gases and liquids of different densities mix when brought into contact with one another.

digestion (*dī-jest'-chon*). Process of converting food into simple substances capable of absorption into the blood.

digit (*di-jit*). A finger or toe.

digitalis (*dij-i-tā'-lis*). The foxglove; contains the active constituent from which digoxin and related substances are made. It slows, strengthens, regulates the heart beat and increases the cardiac output. It is indirectly a diuretic. It has a cumulative action. Vomiting, slow pulse, or 'coupling' of pulse in patient having this medication should be reported immediately.

dilatation (*dil-a-ta'-shon*). Increase in size, enlargement. The operation of stretching.

dilator (*dī-lā'-tor*). An instrument for dilating any narrow passage, as the rectum, uterus, urethra.

dill. Dried ripe fruit of Anethum graveolens. Its distilled water sometimes given to infants for flatulence.

dilution (*dī-lū-shon*). A solution whose concentration has been lowered by the addition of solvent.

diodone (*dī-ō-dōn*). Intravenous contrast agent; similar to iodoxyl but less irritant.

dioptre (*dī-op'-ter*). The unit of refractive power of lens. A lens of one dioptre has a focal length of 1 metre.

dioxide (*dī-ok'-sīd*). A compound containing two atoms of oxygen, *e.g.* carbon dioxide (CO_2).

diphtheria (*dif-thē'-ri-a*). A serious infectious disease, caused by corynebacterium diphtheriae. Any mucous membrane may be attacked but usually that of the throat or nose. A false, grey membrane develops in the pharynx. There is severe general malaise. An antitoxin is given and the patient kept at rest to avoid heart complications. *D. immunization*, a toxoid is injected prophylactically and all children from a year old should thus be protected against the disease.

diplegia (*dī-plē-ji-ah*). Paralysis of both sides of the body.

diplococci (*dip-lō-ko-kī*). Micrococci which are arranged in pairs. *See* BACTERIA.

diploe (*dip'-lō-ē*). A cellular osseous tissue separating the outer and inner surfaces of the skull.

diplopia (*dī-plō'-pi-a*). Double vision.

dipsomania (*dip-so-mā'-ni-a*). Pathological craving for alcohol.

director (*dī-rek'-tur*). A grooved surgical instrument used to guide another instrument.

Disablement Resettlement Officer. DRO. Officer appointed by Department of Employment and Productivity to provide disabled persons with suitable jobs.

disaccharide (*dī-sak'-ar-īd*). Any carbohydrate formed by the condensation of two monosaccharides, *e.g.* cane sugar.

disarticulation (*dis-ar-tik-ū-lā'-shon*). Amputation at a joint.

disc (*di'-sk*). A circular plate or surface. (1) That part of the optic nerve which is seen with the ophthalmoscope as it enters the eyeball. (2) *Intervertebral d.*, the fibrocartilaginous layer between the vertebrae.

discharge (*dis-charj*). Emission of material, *e.g.* fluid, pus, light, etc.

discission (*dis-sish'-on*). Also called needling. Surgical rupture of the lens capsule of the eye.

discrete (*dis-krēt'*). Separate, distinct; opposed to confluent.

disease (*di-sēz*). A process which disturbs the structure or functions of the body.

disinfectants (*dis-in-fek'-tants*). Agents which destroy micro-organisms; such as sunlight, heat, carbolic acid, sulphur dioxide, chlorine.

disinfection (*dis-in-fek'-shon*). The thorough cleansing with disinfectants in an attempt to destroy micro-organisms.

disinfestation (*di-sin-fes-tā-shon*). Riddance of animal parasites, *e.g.* lice.

dislocation (*dis-lō-kā'-shon*). Displacement of the articular surface of a bone. Treatment, reduction under anaesthesia and immobilization. *Congenital dislocation of the hip joint.* The acetabulum is shallow and does not accommodate the head of the femur. The child has a waddling gait. Treatment must be early and is generally the Lorenz method by which after manipulation the hip is immobilized in plaster for many months. The thigh is abducted at a right angle to the trunk.

disorientation (*dis-or-ien-tā'-shon*). Loss of the ability to locate one's position in the environment, or the mental confusion seen in psychic disorders.

dispensing (*dis-pen'-sing*). The mixing and preparing of medicines.

disproportion (*dis-pro-por'-shon*). General term to indicate that the ratio between the size of the fetal head and the size of the maternal pelvis is abnormally large.

dissection (*dīs-sek'-shon*). A separation by cutting of parts of the body.

disseminated (*dis-em'-in-ā-ted*). Scattered throughout an organ or throughout the body. *D. sclerosis*, a chronic, degenerative disease of the nervous system. Also known as multiple sclerosis and insular sclerosis.

dissociation (*di-sōs-si-ā'-shon*). Abnormal mental state in which the patient fails to recognize certain, frequently unpalatable, facts relating to himself.

dissolution (*dis-so-lū'-shon*). Decomposition.

distal (*dis'-tal*). Situated away from the centre or point of attachment.

distichiasis (*dis-ti-kī'-a-sis*). A double row of eyelashes, causing irritation and inflammation.

distillation (*dis-til-ā'-shon*). The process of vaporizing a substance and condensing the vapour. *Fractional d.* Successive distillations are carried out.

diuresis (*dī-ū-rē'-sis*). An increased secretion of urine.

diuretics (*dī-ū-ret'-iks*). Drugs which increase the volume of urine secreted, *e.g.* caffeine.

diurnal (*dī-er-nal*). Daily.

divaricator (*di-va-ri-kā-tor*). Hinged splint used to treat congenital dislocation of hip.

diverticulitis (*dī-ver-tik-ū-lī'-tis*). Inflammation of a diverticulum. Specially applied to inflammation of diverticula, often very many in number, of the pelvic colon.

diverticulosis (*dī-ver-tik-ū-lō'-sis*). Presence of numerous diverticula of the large intestine.

diverticulum (*dī-ver-tik'-ū-lum*). A pouch-like process from a hollow organ, *e.g.* oesophagus, intestine, urinary bladder.

DNA. *See* DEOXYRIBONUCLEIC ACID.

Döderlein's bacillus (*der-der-līns*). Non-pathogenic bacillus present in secretions of the vagina.

dolor (*dol'-or*). Pain.

domette (*do'-met*). A soft cotton and woollen fabric used for bandages.

dominance (*do'-mi-nanz*). A factor present in the left

cerebral hemisphere of humans, which makes people right- or left-handed. This lateral dominance is established early in childhood.

dominant gene (*do'-mi-nant jēn*). A factor of inheritance that will manifest itself in the next generation.

donor (*dō-nor*). Individual from whom tissue is removed for transfer to another, *e.g.* blood transfusion, grafting.

dorsal (*daw'-sal*). Relating to the back or the posterior part of an organ.

dorsiflexion (*dor-si-flek-shon*). Bending backwards or in a dorsal direction.

dorsum (*daw'-sum*). The back.

dosis (*dō-sis*). A dose.

douche (*doosh*). A shower of water usually used to irrigate a cavity of the body. Hot douche 112° F (44° C); cold douche 60° F (16° C).

Douglas's pouch (*dug'-las*). The peritoneal pouch between the back of the uterus and the front of the rectum.

Down's syndrome. *See* MONGOLISM.

Doyen's gag (*dwah'-yan*). A mouth gag much used by anaesthetists.

Doyen's speculum. A self-retaining speculum for keeping the incision widely open during abdominal operations.

dracontiasis (*dra-kon-tī-a-sis*). Infestation by the guinea-worm, common parasite in tropical countries.

drainage tubes (*drān'-āj*). Tubes made of various materials which are inserted into operation wounds to allow material such as blood to drain from the wound.

drastic (*dras'-tik*). Strong, severe.

draught (*drah-ft*). A quantity of fluid to be taken at one time.

drawsheet (*draw'-shēt*). A sheet so arranged that it can be removed easily from under a patient lying upon it.

Drinker's apparatus (*drin'-kerz*). One of the original mechanical respirators, used to carry out artificial respiration when the respiratory muscles are paralysed, popularly known as the iron lung. The patient lies in a receptacle with his head only outside. A negative pressure is created in the receptacle by means of a suction pump; this draws air through the respiratory passages into the lungs. Now almost obsolete since the use of positive pressure ventilators.

drip, intravenous (*intra-vēn-us*). The administration into a vein of saline, plasma or blood.

drive (*drīv*). In psychology, an urge to satisfy a basic need, such as hunger.

droplet infection. Droplets sprayed from a person's mouth, especially when talking, which infect other people

dropsy (*drop'-si*). Generalized oedema of tissues and fluid in the body cavities, as seen in cardiac failure.

drug. Substance used as a medicine. *D. addiction.* A dependence on drugs which is beyond the subject's control. *D. eruption.* Rash due to sensitivity to a drug. *D. reaction.* General reaction to a drug. This may include fever, malaise, joint pains, rashes, jaundice, etc. *D. resistance.* Strains of micro-organisms resistant to the action of antibiotics.

Duchenne's disease (*dū-shen'*). Progressive muscular atrophy, a disease of muscular tissue.

Ducrey's bacillus (*doo-krā'*). The cause of soft sore or chancroid; a venereal disease. Small oval streptobacillus.

duct. A tube or channel conveying the secretion of a gland, generally lined by simple columnar or cuboidal epithelium.

ductless glands. *See* ENDOCRINE.

ductus (*duk'-tus*). A duct; a little canal of the body. *D. arteriosus*, connects the pulmonary artery and the aorta in fetal life. Occasionally this remains patent.

dum-dum fever. Same as Kala-azar.

dumping syndrome. Palpitations and gastric discomfort sometimes felt by the patient after gastrectomy.

duodenal (*dū-ō-dē-nal*). Belonging to the duodenum.

duodenostomy (*dū-ō-dē-nos'-to-mi*). Surgical establishment of a communication between the duodenum and another structure.

duodenum (*dū-ō-dē'-num*). The first 4cm of the small intestine, beginning at the pyloric orifice of the stomach.

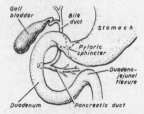

18 The duodenum

Dupuytren's contracture (*dū-pwē'-trenz*). A contracture of the palmar fascia affecting especially the ring and little fingers, which pulls them down into the palm so that they cannot be extended.

dura mater (*dūra mā'-ter*). The outer membrane lining the interior of the cranium and spinal column.

dwarf (*dworf*). Individual of stunted growth.

dys (*dis*). A prefix meaning difficult, painful, abnormal.

dysaesthesia (*dis-es-thē-zi-a*). Partial loss of feeling.

dysarthria (*dis-ar'-thri-a*). Impairment of speech.

dyschezia (*dis-che-si-a*). Painful defaecation.

dyschondroplasia (*dis-kon-drō-plā-si-a*). Multiple enchondromas. Cartilage is deposited in the shaft of some bone(s). Those affected, which are often in the hands and feet, are short and deformed.

dyscoria (*dis-ko-ri-a*). Abnormality in the shape of the pupil.

dyschromatopsia (*dis-krō-mat-op'-si-a*). Loss of vision for colour.

dysdiadokinesis (*dis-dī-a-dō-ki-nē'-sis*). Inability to carry out rapid alternating movements, such as rotating the hands. A sign of cerebellar disease.

dysentery (*dis'-en-ter-i*). Inflammation of the large intestine. There are two kinds of dysentery, bacillary and amoebic; the former due to a bacillus, the latter to the *entamoeba histolytica*.

dysfunction (*dis'-funk-shon*). Abnormal or impaired function.

dyskinesia (*dis-kīn-ē'-zi-a*). Impairment of voluntary movement.

dyslalia (*dis-lā'-li-a*). Mechanical speech defect, *cf.* dysphasia.

dyslexia (*dis-lek-si-a*). Difficulty in reading.

dysmenorrhoea (*dis-men-o-re'-a*). Painful or difficult menstruation.

dysorexia (*dis-o-rek-si-a*). A depraved or unnatural appetite.

dyspareunia (*dis-par-ū'-ni-a*). Painful coitus.

dyspepsia (*dis-pep'-si-a*). Indigestion.

dysphagia (*dis-fā'-ji-a*). Difficulty in swallowing.

dysphasia (*dis-fā-si-a*). Difficulty in speaking.

dysplasia, polyosteotic fibrous (*displā-si-a po-li-os-tē-o-tik fī-brus*). Metabolic defect in the calcification of bone.

dyspnoea (*disp-ne'-a*). Difficult breathing.

dystaxia (*dis-tak-si-a*). Difficulty in controlling voluntary movements. Mild ataxia. *See also* ATAXIA.

dystocia (*dis-tō'-ki-a* or *dis-tō'-*

se-a). A difficult labour (obstetric).

dystrophia adiposo-genitalis (*dis-trō-fia a-di-pō-sō-je-ni-tā-lis*). *See* FRÖHLICH'S SYNDROME.

dystrophy (*dis'-tro-fē*). Defective structure due to shortage of essential factors.

dysuria (*dis-ū'-ri-a*). Painful micturition.

E

E3. Lachesine chloride. Atropine substitute for eye drops in case of atropine irritation.

ear (*ē-r*). The organ of hearing. It consists of external, middle and internal ear.

The *external ear* comprises the auricle and external auditory canal, and is separated from the middle ear by the tympanic membrane.

The *middle ear* is an irregular cavity in the temporal bone. In front it communicates with the Eustachian tube which forms an open channel between the middle ear and the cavity of the nasopharynx. Behind, the middle ear opens into the mastoid antrum, and this in turn communicates with the mastoid cells. There are two openings into the inner ear, the foramen ovale and the

foramen rotunda, both of which are covered with membrane. A string of tiny bones articulating with each other extend from the tympanum to the *foramen ovale* of the internal ear. These bones are, from the tympanum—(1) malleus, (2) incus, (3) stapes.

The *internal ear* comprises (1) the organ of hearing or cochlea in which are the endings of the cochlear branch of the auditory nerve and (2) the organ of equilibrium or balance consisting of the three semicircular canals, arranged at right angles to each other, and supplied by the vestibular branch of the auditory nerve.

ear drum. The tympanum.

ear wax. *See* CERUMEN.

eau (*ō*) water; *eau-de-vie* is brandy.

Eberth's bacillus (*eb-erts bas-il-us*). The typhoid bacillus.

ecbolic (*ek-bol'-ik*). An agent used to stimulate the uterus and thus accelerate the expulsion of the fetus, *e.g.* pituitary extract; it may be used to hasten abortion.

ecchondroma (*ek-on-drō'-ma*). A tumour composed of cartilage.

ecchymosis (*ek-i-mō'-sis*). A bruise; an effusion of blood under the skin.

ECG. *See* ELECTROCARDIOGRAM.

Echinococcus (*e-kī-nō-kok'-us*). One of the species of tape worm. In its adult stage it infests dogs. In its larval stage it produces hydatid cysts in man.

ECHO virus (*e-kō vī-rus*). Enteropathic cytopathic human orphan virus. *See* ADENOVIRUS. May cause benign lymphocytic meningitis and Bornholm disease.

echolalia (*ek-ko-lal'-i-a*). Repetition of everything said.

eclampsia (*ek-lamp'-si-a*). Convulsions arising from severe toxaemia of pregnancy.

ecmnesia (*ek-nē'-zi-a*). A lapse in memory, the memory before and after the lapse being normal.

ECMO virus (*ek-mō vī-rus*). Enteropathic cytopathic monkey orphan virus. *See* ADENOVIRUS.

ecraseur (*ek-rah-ser*). Instrument with wire loop used to remove a polypus.

ECT. *See* ELECTROCONVULSIVE THERAPY.

ectasis (*ek-ta-sis*). Distension, as in bronchiectasis when the bronchial tubes are dilated.

ecthyma (*ek-thī'-ma*). A pustular skin disease, a form of impetigo.

ectoderm (*ek'-tō-derm*). The outer layer of the primitive embryo. From it are developed the skin and its appendages, and the nervous system.

ectogenous (*ek-toj'-en-us*). Originating outside the body.

ectomy (*ek'-tom-i*). A suffix denoting removal.

ectoparasite (*ek-tō-pa-ra-sīt*). Parasite living on the surface of its host.

ectopia (*ek-tō'-pi-a*). Not in the usual place.

ectopic gestation (*ek-top'-ik jes-tā-shon*). Pregnancy in which the fertilized ovum is not situated in the uterus. The ovum may lie in one of the Fallopian tubes or in the

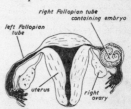

19 Ectopic gestation: fertilized ovum in right Fallopian tube

abdominal cavity. In course of time the gestation sac is apt to rupture, causing profuse haemorrhage into the abdominal cavity and necessitating immediate operation.

ectrodactylia (*ek-trō-dak-til'-i-a*). Absence from birth of one or more toes or fingers.

ectropion (*ek-tro'-pi-on*). Eversion of the eyelid.

eczema (*ek'-ze-ma*). Inflammation of the skin, acute or chronic. There is redness and vesicles may appear which weep and form crusts.

EEG. See ELECTROENCEPHALO-GRAPHY.

effector (*ef-fek-tor*). Nerve endings found in muscles, glands, etc., and which effect a response to a stimulus.

efferent (*ef'-fer-ent*). Conveying from the centre, *e.g.* the motor nerves which convey impulses from the brain and spinal cord to muscles and glands, *cf.* afferent.

effervescent (*ef-fer-ves'-ent*). Bubbling. Giving off small bubbles of gas.

effleurage (*ef-fler'-arj*). Movement performed in physiotherapy. The tips of the fingers or the whole surface of the hand are moved along the course of the blood vessels and lymphatics stimulating the circulation and lymphatic drainage.

effluent (*ef-loo-ent*). Liquid which flows from a source generally referred to sewage.

effort syndrome (*ef-fort sin'-drōm*). Also called da Costa's syndrome, disordered action of the heart, soldier's heart. A form of anxiety neurosis characterized by symptoms referable to the heart.

effusion (*ef-fū'-zhon*). An escape of fluid from one part to another.

egocentric (*ē-gō-sen'-trik*). Self-centred.

Ehrlich's theory. A theory explaining the process of immunity against disease.

ejaculation (*ē-jak-ū-lā'-shon*). Forcible, sudden expulsion, especially of semen.

elastin (*e-las-tin*). Fibrous protein laid down by fibroblasts in connective tissue ground substance. It is structurally similar to collagen and is found particularly in structures which require to withstand mechanical stresses, *e.g.* walls of large arteries.

Elastoplast bandage (*e-las-tō'-plast*). An adhesive bandage containing zinc oxide.

elation (*e-lā-shon*). A happy and exalted state of mind.

elbow (*el'-bō*). The joint between the arm and forearm formed by the humerus above, and the radius and ulna below.

Electra complex (*e-lek-tra kom-pleks*). Excessive love for a father by a daughter who hates her mother. Named after Electra in Greek mythology.

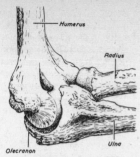

20 The elbow joint

electrocardiogram (*e-lek-trō-kar-di-ō-gram*). ECG. Recording of electrical events occurring in the heart muscle throughout the cardiac cycle. The recording is made by attaching electrodes to the skin and amplifying the electrical signal. The oscillations may be recorded by a pen writer.

electrocardiphonography (*e-lek-trō-kar-di-ō-fō-no'-gra-fi*). Recording of heart sounds electrically by a phonocardiograph.

electroconvulsive therapy (*e-lek-trō-kon-vul-siv the-ra-pi*). ECT. Therapy used especially in depressive mental illness, consisting of passing a low amperage electric current between electrodes placed on the side of the head. The reaction is modified by general anaesthesia and muscle relaxant drugs given before the shock treatment.

electrode (*e-lek'-trōd*). A conductor through which an electric current enters or leaves the battery or the body of the patient.

electro-encephalography (*en-ke-fa-log'-ra-fi*). Recording of electric currents resulting from cerebral activity.

electrolysis (*e-lek-trol'-i-sis*). 1. Separation of ions by placing them in an electric field. 2. Destruction of hair follicles by the passage of an electric current.

electrolytes (*el-ek-trō-līts*). Substances, such as sodium chloride or potassium carbonate, which, dissolved in water, dissociate into ions. The water becomes a conductor of electricity. *E. balance.* Balance of relative amounts of electrolytes, *e.g.* sodium, potassium, chloride, in body fluids, usually blood.

electro-magnetic spectrum (*e-lek-trō-mag-ne-tik spek'-trum*). Wide range of radiations which are transmitted by photons distributed in a frequency pattern known as electro-magnetic waves, including radio waves, light, x-rays and gamma rays.

electromotive force (EMF) (*mō'-tiv*). The measure of the force by which an electric current flows from one point to another. The unit of EMF is the volt.

electromyography (*e-lek-trō-mī-o-gra-fi*). EMG. The recording of electrical events occurring in muscle.

electron (*e-lek-tron*). A negatively charged atomic particle. *E. microscopy*. The use of electrons instead of light to visualize microscopic objects. The apparatus is complex but allows very much greater resolution to be obtained and therefore more details to be seen.

electroplexy (*el-ek-trō-ple'-ksi*). *See* ELECTROCONVULSIVE THERAPY.

electroretinogram (*e-lek-trō-re-ti-no'-gram*). Recording of electrical variations in the retina on exposure to light.

element (*el'-e-ment*). A primary part. A substance which cannot be decomposed further by ordinary chemical means. Two or more elements form a compound.

elephantiasis (*el-e-fan-tī'-a-sis*) or **filariasis**. A parasitic disease of the lymphatic vessels, causing great enlargement of the limb or limbs affected, (usually the leg). It is chronic, and the skin thickens until it somewhat resembles an elephant's hide. The parasite is the *Filaria*.

elevator (*el'-e-vā-ter*). (1) A muscle which raises a limb. (2) An instrument used for raising depressed bone, etc.

elimination (*el-im-in-ā'-shon*). The expulsion of poisons or waste products from the body.

elixir (*e-lik'-ser*). A term sometimes applied to certain preparations of drugs having a sweet taste.

emaciation (*e-mā-sē-ā'-shon*). The act of wasting or becoming thin.

emanation (*em-an-ā'-shon*). The act of flowing out. Applied especially to the rays given out by radioactive substances.

emasculation (*e-mas-kū-lā'-shon*). Castration of the male.

embolectomy (*em-bol-ek'-to-mi*). Removal of an embolus.

embolism (*em'-bo-lizm*). Obstruction of blood vessel, usually an artery by a body, *e.g.* portion of thrombus, fat cells, air, transported in the bloodstream. If the embolus is large enough to block completely any of the valvular orifices of the right side of the heart, sudden death is the result: if small enough to pass through the right side of the heart, the embolus may be arrested somewhere in the pulmonary artery or in one of its subdivisions, giving rise to an infarct of the lung, with symptoms of intense sudden pain in the chest, coughing of blood, and great distress. In certain cases of valvular disease of the heart, pieces of clot formed upon the affected valve break off and are carried away in the bloodstream. When such an embolus reaches an artery too small for it, an embolism results, with symptoms according to the organ affected. Embolism of an artery of the brain may result in immediate death or in paralysis.

embolus (*em'-bō-lus*). A blood clot or other foreign body in the bloodstream.

embrocation (*em-bro-kā'-shon*). A lotion for rubbing on the skin.

embryo (*em'-bri-ō*). Animal in process of development from the fertilized ovum.

embryology (*em-brē-o'-lo-ji*). Science of the development of the embryo.

embryoma (*em-brē-ō'-ma*). Teratoma. An ovarian tumour, often a dermoid cyst.

embryotome (*em'-bri-o-tōm*). An instrument for destroying any part of the child during birth for the purpose of facilitating delivery.

embryotomy (*em'-brē-ot'-o-mi*). Destruction of the fetus.

emesis (*em'-e-sis*). Vomiting.

emetic (*e-met'-ik*). Any means used to produce vomiting. Tickling the throat with a feather; large draughts of tepid water, salt water, mustard and water; ipecacuanha. Apomorphine, given hypodermically.

emission (*ē-mish'-on*). Discharge, especially of semen.

emmetropia (*em-e-trō'-pi-a*). Normal sight.

emollients (*e-mol'-li-ents*). Softening and soothing applications or liniments.

emotion (*e-mō-shon*). A response of mind and body to stimuli; such as anger or fear.

empathy (*em-pa-thi*). The power of projecting one's personality into another person and so fully comprehending that person's situation.

emphysema (*em-fi-sē'-ma*). *Pulmonary e.* The overdistension of the lungs by air resulting in destruction of alveoli. Three types occur: obstructive, compensatory and chronic vesicular emphysema. *Surgical e.* Air bubbles in the subcutaneous tissues following trauma, giving a characteristic 'crackly' feeling when touched.

empirical (*em-pi'-ri-kal*). Term applied to treatment founded on experience only not on reasoning.

emplastrum (*em-plas'-trum*). A plaster.

empyema (*em-pī-ē'-ma*). A collection of pus in a cavity, most commonly referring to the pleural cavity. The term is also used for collections of pus in the maxillary antrum, frontal sinus, and other cavities.

emulsion (*e-mul'-shon*). Fine suspension in a fluid of particles of an immiscible fluid, *e.g.* milk is an emulsion of fat in an aqueous solution.

enamel (*en-am'-el*). The hard outer coating of the tooth. *See* TEETH.

enarthrosis (*en-ar-thrō'-sis*). A ball-and-socket joint.

encephalitis (*en-kef-al-ī'-tis*). Inflammation of the brain. *See* MENINGITIS. *E. lethargica.* Encephalitis associated with profound disturbance of sleep rhythm.

encephalocele (*en-kef'-a-lō-sēl*). Protrusion of the brain through the skull.

encephalography (*en-ke-fal-o'-gra-fī*). Also called ventriculography. The x-ray examination of the brain after air, which is radiolucent, has been introduced into the cerebral ventricles.

encephaloid (*en-kef'-a-loyd*). Brainlike.

encephaloma (*en-ke-fa-lō'-ma*). A brain tumour.

encephalomalacia (*en-kef'-al-ō-mal-ās'-e-ah*). Softening of the brain.

encephalomyelitis (*en-kef'-al-ō-mī-el-ī'-tis*). Inflammation of the brain and spinal cord.

encephalon (*en-kef'-a-lon*). The brain.

encephalopathy (*en-ke-fa-lo'-pa-thi*). Disease of the brain.

encephalotomy (*en-ke-fa-lo-to-mi*). Dissection of the brain.

enchondroma (*en-kon-drō'-ma*). A tumour of cartilage.

encysted (*en-sis'-ted*). Enclosed in a sac or cyst.

endarteritis (*en-dar-te-rī'-tis*). Inflammation of the lining membrane of the arteries.

endemic (*en-dem'-ik*). Occurring frequently in a particular locality.

endocarditis (*en-dō-kar-dī'-tis*). Inflammation of the lining membrane of the heart. The valves are affected in consequence. Often a complication of acute rheumatism, chorea or other fevers. In bacterial or malignant endocarditis, fungating growths develop on the valves.

endocardium (*en-dō-kar'-di-um*). The lining membrane of the heart.

endocervicitis (*en-dō-ser-vi-si'-tis*). Inflammation of the mucous membrane lining the canal of the cervix uteri.

endocolpitis (*en-dō-kol-pī'-tis*). Inflammation of inner coat of the vagina.

endocrine (*en'-dō-krēn*). The term used in describing the ductless glands giving rise to an internal secretion. The endocrines are—suprarenals, thymus, thyroid, parathyroids, pituitary, pancreas, ovaries, and testicles. The pancreas acts as both an endocrine organ and for the secretion of digestive juices. It therefore also has ducts.

endocrinology (*en-dō-krin-ol-o-ji*). Science of the endocrine glands.

endoderm (*en-dō-derm*). Germ layer of embryo composed, as is mesoderm, of cells which have migrated from the surface to the interior of the embryo during gastrulation, and from which the alimentary tract is largely derived.

endogenous (*en-do-jen-us*). Produced within the body, *e.g.* endogenous infection.

endolymph (*en-dō-limf*). Fluid of the membranous labyrinth of the ear.

endometrioma (*en-dō-mē-tri-ō'-ma*). Tumour, from tissue like that of the endometrium, but found outside it in myometrium, ovary, uterine ligaments, rectovaginal septum, peritoneum, caecum, pelvic colon, umbilicus and laparotomy scars.

endometriosis (*en-dō-mē-tri-ō'-sis*). The presence of endometriomata (plural of endometrioma).

endometritis (*en-dō-mē-trī'-tis*). Inflammation of the endometrium.

endometrium. The lining membrane of the uterus.

endoneurium (*en-dō-nū-ri-um*). Fine connective tissue found round each nerve fibre.

end-organ (*end-aw-gan*). Collection of cells connected to the peripheral nervous system which act as a transducer, transforming a stimulus into a nerve discharge (receptor), or a nerve discharge into a stimulus, *i.e.* end-plate.

endoscope (*en'-dos-kōp*). An instrument for the inspection of the interior of a hollow organ.

endosteoma (*en-dos-tē-ō'-ma*). Tumour within a bone cavity.

endosteum (*en-dos'-te-um*). The medullary membrane of bone. *See* BONE.

endothelioma (*en-dō-thē-li-ō-ma*). A malignant growth originating in endothelium.

endothelium (*en-dō-thē'-lē-um*). The lining membrane of serous cavities, blood vessels and lymphatics.

endotoxin (*en-do-toks'-in*). An intracellular toxin, *i.e.* retained within the bacteria. When the bacteria are disintegrated the toxin is liberated.

endotracheal (*en-dō-tra-kē'-al*). Within the trachea.

end-plate (*end plāt*). Accumulation of muscle cytoplasm and nuclei in association with the terminal branches of a motor nerve discharge stimulates contraction of muscle.

enema (*en'-em-a*). An injection into the bowel. It can be given with a rectal tube and funnel but rectal suppositories and disposable enemas are replacing those given by tube and funnel.

enervating (*en-er-vā-ting*). Weakening.

engagement of head (*en-gāj-ment*). Descent of fetal head into the cavity of the pelvis. Normally occurs two to four weeks before term in the primigravida but in multigravida may not occur until labour.

engorgement (*en-gawj'-ment*). Vascular congestion.

enophthalmos (*en-of-thal-mos*). Recession of the eyeball into the orbit.

enostosis (*en-os-tō'-sis*). A tumour in a bone.

ensiform cartilage (*kar'-til-āj*). The sword-shaped process at the lower end of the sternum.

Entamoeba histolytica (*ent-am-ē'-ba his-to-lit-ika*). The parasite which causes amoebic dysentery.

enteral (*en'-ter-al*). Intestinal.

enterectomy (*en-ter-ek'-to-mi*). Excision of part of the intestine.

enteric fevers (*en-te'-rik*). A term now used to include three separate but closely allied diseases: typhoid, paratyphoid A, paratyphoid B fevers.

enteritis (*en-te-rī'-tis*). Inflammation of the small intestine.

Enterobius vermicularis (*en-te-rō-bi-us ver-mi-kū-lā-ris*). Threadworm.

enterocele (*en'-ter-ō-sēl*). Hernia containing a piece of bowel.

enterococcus (*en'-ter-ō-kok-us*). Streptococcus found in intestinal tract.

enterocolitis (*en-te-rō-ko-lī'-tis*). Acute inflammation of the ileum, caecum and ascending colon giving rise to symptoms similar to appendicitis.

enterokinase (*en-ter-ō-kin'-ās*). An activating enzyme of the succus entericus which converts trypsinogen into trypsin.

enterolith (*en'-te-rō-lith*). Stone in the intestines.

enteron (*en-ter-on*). The intestine.

enteropexy (*en-ter-ō-peks'-i*). Suturing of the intestines to the abdominal wall.

enteroptosis (*en-ter-op-tō'-sis*). Prolapse of the intestines due to stretching of the mesenteric attachment, or weakness of the abdominal wall.

enterorrhaphy (*en-te-ro'-raf-i*). The suturing of a rent in the intestine.

enterospasm (*en'-ter-ō-spasm*). Spasm of the intestine. Colic.

enterostenosis (*en-te-rō-ste-nō'-sis*). Stricture of the intestines.

enterostomy (*en-te-ros'-to-mi*). Surgically established opening between the small intestine and another surface, *e.g.* gastro-enterostomy, a connection between the stomach and the small intestine.

enterotomy (*en-ter-ot'-o-mi*). Incision into the small intestine.

enteroviruses (*en-te-rō-vī-ru-sez*). Viruses belonging to the pico RNA virus group. *Es.* enter the body by the alimentary tract and comprise the three polio viruses, the Coxsackie virus causing Bornholm disease and the ECHO viruses causing aseptic meningitis.

entropion (*en-tro'-pi-on*). Inversion of the margin of the eyelid.

enucleation (*e-nū-klē-ā-shon*). (1) Removal of the nucleus. (2) Removal of a central structure, *e.g.* tumour without its surrounding structures. (3) Removal of eye.

enuresis (*en-ū-rē'-sis*). Incontinence of urine. *Nocturnal e.* Bedwetting at night.

environment. The surroundings of a living organism now known to have a profound influence on that organism.

enzyme (*en'-zim*). Protein which acts as a catalyst. There are many different kinds of enzyme which increase the reactivity of certain substances.

eosin (*ē'-o-sin*). An acid dye used extensively for staining histological sections.

eosinophilia (*ē-ō-si-nō-fi-li-a*). (1) Property of being stained by acid dyes such as eosin which combine with basic groups in the tissue. (2) Term used to denote an increase above the normal 2 to 5 per cent in the numbers of polymorphonuclear leucocytes in the blood which stain deeply with eosin.

ependyma (*e-pen'-di-ma*). The lining membrane of the cerebral cavities and spinal canal.

ependymoma (*e-pen-dē-mō'-ma*). A tumour arising from ependymal cells.

ephelis (*e-fe-lis*). A freckle.

epiblepharon (*e-pi-ble-fa-ron*). *See* EPICANTHUS.

epicanthus (*ep-i-kan-thus*). Projection of the nasal fold to the eyelid.

epicardium (*ep-i-kar'-di-um*). Visceral layer of the pericardium.

epicondyle (*ep-i-kon'-dīl*). Bony eminence as upon the femoral condyles.

epicranium (*ep-i-krā'-nē-um*). The integuments which lie over the cranium.

epidemic (*ep-i-dem'-ik*). An infectious or contagious disease attacking a number of people in the same neighbourhood at one time.

epidemiology (*e-pi-dē-mē-ol'-oji*). The study of epidemics.

epidermis (*ep-i-der'-mis*). The outer layer of the skin.

epidermophytosis (*ep-i-der-mō-fī-tō'-sis*). An infection of the skin by fungi, the hands and feet being principally affected. Often termed 'Athlete's Foot' as it is frequently contracted in public gymnasia or swimming baths.

epididymis (*ep-i-di'-di-mis*). A long convoluted tube through which sperm pass between the testis and the vas deferens. It forms a mass at the upper pole of the testis.

epididymitis (*ep'-i-did-i-mī'-tis*). Inflammation of the epididymis.

epididymo-orchitis (*e-pi-did-ē-mō-or-kī'-tis*). Inflammation of the epididymis and testes.

epidural analgesia. *See* CAUDAL ANALGESIA.

epigastrium (*ep-i-gas'-tri-um*). Region of abdomen situated over the stomach.

epiglottis (*ep-i-glot'-tis*). The flap of cartilage which guards the entrance to the glottis or windpipe.

epilation (*e-pi-lā-shon*). Removal of hair with destruction of the hair follicle.

epilepsy (*ep'-il-ep-si*). A disorder of the brain marked by the occurrence of convulsive fits. *Generalised e.*, typical epilepsy, usually idiopathic. In many cases the fit is preceded by a warning or aura. This is usually a sensory disturbance. The two main types are (1) petit mal, momentary loss of consciousness with no convulsion, (2) grand mal, loss of consciousness, tonic and clonic convulsions. *Jacksonian e.* Local spasm, *e.g.* of one limb or one side of the body, due to irritation of the cerebral cortex. Important to observe in which group of muscles the movements start in order that the cerebral lesion may be located.

epileptiform (*ep-i-lep'-ti-form*). Like the convulsions of epilepsy.

epiloia (*e-pi-loy'-a*). Tuberous sclerosis. Inherited defect characterized by sebaceous adenoma of the face, multiple gliomas in the brain and tumours of the heart, kidneys and retina. Fits are the earliest signs of the disease and mental deficiency usually follows.

epimenorrhoea (*e-pē-me-nor-rē'-a*). Menstrual periods of frequent recurrence.

epinephrectomy (*e-pē-nef-rek'-to-mi*). Excision of suprarenal gland.

epineurium (*ep-in-ūr'-i-um*). The sheath of a nerve.

epiphora (*e-pif'-o-ra*). An excessive flow of tears.

epiphysis (*e-pif'-i-sis*). The separately ossified end of growing bone separated from the shaft, diaphysis, by a cartilaginous plate (epiphyseal plate). When growth is completed the epiphysis and diaphysis fuse.

epiphysitis (*ep-if-is-ī'-tis*). Inflammation of an epiphysis.

epiplocele (*ep-ip'-lo-sēl*). A hernia containing omentum.

epiploon (*e-pi-plo-on*). The omentum.

episcleritis (*ep-is-kler-ī'-tis*). Inflammation of the outer layers of the sclera. *See* EYE.

episiotomy (*ep-i-si-ot'-om-i*). Incision of the perineum just at the end of the second stage of labour, sometimes performed to avoid extensive laceration of the perineum.

epispadias (*ep-is-pa'-di-as*). A congenital malformation in which the urethra opens on the dorsum of the penis.

epistaxis (*ep-is-taks'-is*). Bleeding from the nose.

epithelial casts (*ep-ith-ēl'-ial kar-sts*). Filaments of renal epitheulim found in the urine in certain diseases, when examined under the microscope. They are chiefly cylindrical, are finely granular, and the cells have large nuclei. If in considerable quantity, they signify nephritis, or some other disease of the kidneys.

epithelioma (*ep-ith-ēl-i'-ō-ma*). Tumour of epithelium.

epithelium (*e-pi-thē-li-um*). Sheet of coherent cells forming the lining of tubes, cavities and surfaces, except if derived embryologically from mesoderm when it is termed endothelium or mesothelium. Epithelia are classified according to thickness of the sheet and the shape or function of the cells composing them. Epithelium may be mucous, keratinizing, simple (one cell thick), stratified (many cells thick), squamous (flat cells), cubical and columnar (tall cells).

epitrochlea (*ep-i-trok'-lea*). The inner round projection at the lower end of the humerus.

eponym (*e-po-nim*). Name of disease or organ which is called after a person or place, *e.g.* Bornholm disease.

epulis (*e-pū'-lis*). Tumour on the gums.

erasion (*e-rā'-zhon*). Scraping.

Erb's paralysis. The muscles of the upper arm are paralysed due to a lesion of the fifth and sixth cervical nerve roots. May result from excessive traction on the arm during labour. It hangs limply, rotated internally from the shoulder, elbow extended, forearm pronated and palm of hand turned outwards.

erectile tissue (*e-rek'til tis-sū*). Specialized vascular tissue which becomes rigid when filled with blood, *e.g.* penis.

erector (*e-rek-tor*). A muscle which raises a part.

erepsin (*er-ep'-sin*). A ferment of the succus entericus (secretion of the small intestines). It completes the digestion of the proteins.

ergograph (*er'-gō-grarf*). An instrument for recording the amount of work done by muscular action.

ergosterol (*er-go-ster'-ōl*). A sterol found in fats and present in the skin which is converted into vitamin D by irradiation with ultraviolet light.

erosion (*e-rō'-zhon*). Ulceration. *Cervical e.* Vaginal epithelium is replaced by columnar epithelium growing down from the cervical canal. As the secretion of the vagina is acid, this epithelium tends to ulcerate and bleed.

erotic (*e-ro-tik*). Pertaining to sexual love.

eructation (*e-ruk-tā'-shon*). Flatulency, with passage of gas from stomach through mouth.

eruption (*e-rup'-shon*). A breaking out on the skin.

erysipelas (*er-i-sip'-e-las*). Acute streptococcal infection of the skin.

erythema (*e-ri-thē-ma*). Red skin, due to vasodilatation in the dermis. *E. multiforme.* Lesions consisting of raised red lesions of varying size and shape which may blister. The cause is unknown but it may represent an abnormal immune response. *E. nodosum.* Red tender skin nodules on the legs which may occur in certain conditions such as tuberculosis and sarcoidosis.

erythrasmia (*er-ith-raz'-mi-a*). An infection of the skin due to a fungus.

erythroblast (*e-ri-thrō-blast*). Nucleated red blood cell normally found in the bone marrow and which gives rise to a red blood cell.

erythroblastosis fetalis (*erith-rō-blas-tō-sis fē-tā'-lis*). See HAEMOLYTIC DISEASE OF THE NEWBORN.

erythrocytes (*er'-ith-rō-sīts*). Red blood cells.

erythrocythaemia (*e-rith-rō-si-tē'-mi-a*). Increased number of red blood cells.

erythrocytopaenia (*e-rith-rō-sī-tō-pē-ni-a*). Diminished number of red blood cells.

erythrocytosis (*e-rith-rō'-sī-tō'-sis*). See POLYCYTHAEMIA.

erythropoiesis (*e-ri-thrō-pō-ē-sis*). The manufacture of red blood cells.

Esbach's albuminometer (*es'-baks al-bū-min-om'-et-er*). A graduated tube used to estimate the quantity of albumin in urine.

eschar (*es'-kar*). A dry healing scab on a wound; generally the result of the use of caustic. Also the mortified part in dry gangrene.

Esmarch's bandage (*es'-marches*). An india-rubber bandage which is tightly applied to the limb, beginning at the extremity, and when it has reached above the point of operation a stout tube is wound round the limb and fastened. This provides a bloodless surgical field.

esotropia (*ē-so-trō-pi-a*). Converging squint.

ESR. Erythrocyte sedimentation rate. The rate at which red blood cells stick together and sediment to the bottom of a graduated tube. An increased rate is found in infection.

ethics (*e-thiks*). Moral principles governing life.

ethmoid (*eth'-moyd*). A bone of the nose through which the olfactory nerves pass.

ethnology (*eth-nol-o-ji*). The science of the races of mankind.

eugenics (*ū-jen'-iks*). The study of the genetic constitution of the individual by suitable mating, with the aim of improving the genetic constitution of the human race.

eunuch (*ū-nuk*). A castrated human male.

euphoria (*ū-for'-i-a*). Exaggerated sense of well-being.

Eustachian tube (*ū-stā'-shi-an*). The canal from the throat to the ear. See EAR.

euthanasia (*ū-tha-nā'-si-a*). A planned and painless death procured by the use of drugs.

eutocia (*ū-tō'-sē-a*). Easy labour (obstetric).

evacuation (*ē-vak-ū-ā'-shon*). Emptying of contents of an organ *e.g.* stomach, bowel, uterus.

Eve's method. A method of artificial respiration. By placing the patient in a special rocking apparatus, the diaphragm is forced up and down.

eventration (*ē-ven-trā-shon*). Protrusion of the intestines.

eversion (*e-ver'-shon*). Folding outwards.

evisceration (*e'-vis-ser-ā'-shon*). Removal of the abdominal contents.

evolution (*ē-vol-ū'-shon*). Spontaneous evolution means the delivery without obstetric assistance of a fetus in the transverse lie; it is as a rule only possible in the case of a premature or dead fetus.

evulsion (*ē-vul'-shon*). A tearing apart.

Ewing's tumour (*ū-wings tū-mer*). Malignant tumour of bone occurring in young adults.

exacerbation (*eg-zas-er-bā'-shon*). An increase in the severity of symptoms; a paroxysm of disease.

exanthemata (*ek-san-thē-ma'-ta*). Diseases accompanied by specific rashes.

exchange transfusion (*eks-chanj tran-sfu-zhon*). Transfusion of the newborn when the whole circulatory volume of the infant's blood is removed and replaced by donor blood. This is necessary in severe haemolysis of the baby's blood in Rhesus group incompatibility. *See* BLOOD GROUPING.

exarteritis (*eks-ar-te-ri'-tis*). Inflammation of the external coat of an artery.

excipient (*ek-sip'-i-ent*). The substance used as a medium for giving a medicament.

excision (*ek-siz'-zhon*). A cutting out.

excitability (*ek-sī-ta-bi-li-ti*). (1) Reaction to a stimulus. (2) A state of being unduly excited.

excitement (*ek-sit'-ment*). Increased activity of an organ or organism.

excoriation (*eks-ko-rē-ā'-shon*). Abrasions of the skin.

excrement (*eks-kre-ment*). Faecal matter.

excrescence (*eks-kres'-sens*). Abnormal bony outgrowth.

excreta (*ek-skrē'-ta*). The natural discharges from the body, urine, faeces, sweat.

exenteration (*eks-en-ter-ā'-shon*). Removal of all contents. *E. of orbit.* Removal of all contents of the bony orbit. *E. of pelvis.* Removal of pelvic contents and transplantations of ureters into the sigmoid colon.

exfoliation (*eks-fō-lē-ā-shon*). Excessive loss of superficial layers of skin in thin flakes.

exhibitionism (*eks-hi-bi'-shon-izm*). Behaving in a way to attract attention and term used in psychiatry for sex perversion such as indecent exposure.

exhumation (*ek-sū-mā'-shon*). Disinterment of the body.

exogenous (*eks-o'-jen-us*). Due to an external cause.

exomphalos (*eks-om'-fal-os*). Umbilical hernia of congenital origin causing protrusion of intestines through gap in abdominal wall.

exophthalmos, exophthalmia (*eks-of-thal'-mos*). Protrusion of the eyeball. *See also* GOITRE.

exostosis (*eks-os-tō'-sis*). A bony tumour growing from bone.

exotoxin (*ek-sō-tok'-sin*). Toxin released from exterior of an organism, *cf*. endotoxin.

expectorant (*ek-spek'-to-rant*). A drug which increases expectoration.

expectoration (*eks-pek-to-rā'-shon*). The coughing up of sputum.

exploration (*eks-plo-rā'-shon*). Operative surgical investigation.

expression (*eks-pre-shon*). (1) The act of expulsion. (2) Facial appearance.

exsanguinate (*ek-san'-gwin-āt*). To make bloodless.

extension (*ek-sten'-shon*). (1) A certain pull or weight applied to a fractured, dislocated, or contracted limb to keep it straight. There are two methods, (a) Skin traction applied as follows: A long piece of strapping, about 2 in wide, with a stirrup, consisting of a square piece of wood the same width as that of the foot at the ankle, and with a hole in the middle, is required; also some short narrower pieces of strapping. To apply it, the stirrup should be about 4 in below the foot, and the strapping attached to it should be carried up the inside and outside of the leg

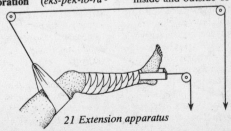

21 Extension apparatus

well above the knee: the short pieces of strapping are put round the leg from the ankle to below the knee. A knotted piece of cord is passed through the hole in the wood over a pulley at the foot of the bed. Weights are attached to the cord, the number varying according to the age of the patient and condition for which it is applied. For a fractured femur ⅟ of the body weight is usually satisfactory. The foot of the bed should be slightly raised. **(b)** Skeletal traction, a Steinmann's pin or Kirschner wire is passed through the lower fragment of the bone or an ice-tong caliper may be inserted. (2) The straightening of a flexed limb or part.

extensor (*eks-ten'-sor*). A muscle which extends a part.

external conjugate (*kon-jū-gāt*). *See* CONJUGATE.

external os. *See* OS EXTERNAL.

external version (*ver-shon*). A method of changing the lie or presentation of the fetus by manipulation of the uterus through the abdominal wall.

extirpate (*ek-ster-pāt*). To remove completely.

extra. Latin for outside.

extracapsular (*eks-tra-kap'-sū-la*). Outside a capsule.

extracellular fluid (*eks-tra-sel-ū-la*). That part of the

body fluid not contained in cells nor the blood.

extract (*ek'-strakt*). Concentrated preparation of a drug: it may be in a liquid or solid form, *e.g.* extract of cascara.

extrapyramidal (*eks-tra-pi-ra'-mi-dal*). Motor nerve tracts and associated centres which do not directly communicate with the main motor pathway (pyramidal tract). It is a very complex system with many functions, one of which is to regulate muscle tone.

extrasystoles (*ek-stra-sis-to-lēs*). Systolic contraction of the heart the impulse for which originates in a focus other than the sinuatrial node, and is therefore outside the normal chain of events in the cardiac cycle.

extra-uterine gestation (*ek-stra-ū'-te-rīn jes-tā'-shon*). Pregnancy outside the uterus. *See* ECTOPIC GESTATION.

extravasation (*eks-trav-a-sā'-shon*). Escape of fluid from its proper channel into surrounding tissue.

extravert (*eks-tra-vert*). *See* EXTROVERT.

extremity (*eks-tre-mi-ti*). The end part of any organ. A limb.

extrinsic (*ek-strin'-sik*). Exter-

nal. From without. *E. factor.*
See PERNICIOUS ANAEMIA.

extrovert (*ek-strō-vert*). Thinking of things other than oneself. The opposite kind of
temperament to introvert.

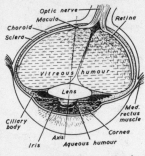

Optic nerve
Macula
Retina
Choroid
Sclera
Vitreous humour
Lens
Med. rectus muscle
Ciliary body
Axis
Cornea
Iris
Aqueous humour

*22 Horizontal section of right
eye*

exudation (*eks-ū-dā'-shon*).
Oozing; slow escape of
liquid.

eye (*ī*). The organ of vision. *See*
illustration.

eye-strain (*ī-strān*). Headache
due to effort required to
focus on near objects when
the refractive properties of
the lens are defective.

eye-teeth (*ī'-tēth*). The canines.

F

F. Abbreviation for
Fahrenheit.

face presentation (*fās pres-en-
tā-shon*). The advance of the
fetus face first into the pelvis
during labour. It is usually
due to some degree of pelvic
contraction. The majority of
such cases are delivered
naturally.

facet (*fas'-et*). One side of a
many-sided body, applied to
a small, smooth, articulating
surface of a bone.

facial (*fā-shi-al*). Relating to
the face. *F. nerve.* Seventh
cranial nerve supplying the
salivary glands and superficial muscles of the face. *F.
paralysis.* Paralysis of the
muscles of the face caused by
injury or disease involving
the facial nerves.

facies (*fa'-si-ēs*). Facial expression particularly applied to
expressions which are diagnostic of certain conditions
e.g. abdominal facies,
adenoid facies.

facultative (*fa-kul-ta-tiv*). Able
to live under varying conditions.

faecal (*fē-kal*). Relating to the
faeces.

faeces (*fē'-sēs*). The discharge
from the bowels. Common
abnormalities to be noted are
Colour—Black may indicate
the presence of altered blood
or the patient may be taking
iron. Green stools occur in
enteritis. Clay-coloured
stools in jaundice. *Consis-
tency*—Loose watery stools

occur in diarrhoea, hard dry stools in constipation. Foreign bodies such as worms may be present. Unaltered blood may be due to haemorrhoids. Mucus and blood may be due to colitis or intussusception.

faecolith (*fē-ko-lith*). Stone-like body composed of compacted faeces.

Fahrenheit (*fa'-ren-hīt*). Temperature scale, *see* p. 13.

faint (*fā-nt*). A state of temporary unconsciousness. Syncope.

falciform (*fal-si-form*). Sickle-shaped. Applied to certain ligaments and other structures.

fallout (*fawl-owt*). Particulate matter containing radioactive material which falls from clouds containing the debris of atomic explosion.

Fallopian tubes (*fal-lo'-pi-an tubes*). Two trumpet-like canals, about 7.5cm long, passing from the ovaries to the uterus. *See* UTERUS and SALPINGITIS.

Fallot's tetralogy (*fa'-loz*). A group of congenital heart defects consisting of dextra-position of the aorta, right ventricle hypertrophy, intra-ventricular septal defect and stenosis of the pulmonary artery.

falx cerebri (*falks se-re-brē*). The fold of dura between the two cerebral hemispheres.

familial (*fam-il'-ial*). Affecting several members of one family.

fanaticism (*fa-na-ti-sizm*). Zeal for some belief or cause carried to excess.

fantasy (*fan'-ta-si*). A world or imagination controlled by the whim of the individual.

Fantus test. Test for the presence of chloride in the urine.

farad (*fa'-rad*). A unit of electrical capacity.

faradism (*far'-a-dizm*). An induced low frequency asymmetrical alternating current used to stimulate muscle where the nerve supply is intact.

farinaceous (*far-i-nā'-shi-us*). Containing flour or grain. Farinaceous diet consists of milk puddings, gruel, bread, and other starchy foods.

fascia (*fa-shi-a*). A fibrous structure separating one compartment of the body from another, or one muscle from another.

fascicle (*fas'-i-kl*). A little bundle of fibres.

fastigium (*fa-sti-ji-um*). The summit or height, *e.g.* of a fever.

fat. An organic compound which is a desirable constituent of human diet. Mother's milk contains about

4 per cent of fat in finely divided globules. Cow's milk contains about 3·6 per cent of fat. Cream contains up to 20 per cent.

fatigue (*fa-tēg*). Tiredness.

fatty degeneration (*dē-jen-e-ră-shon*). Term applied to the appearance of certain cells which as a result of damage take on an appearance of having droplets of fat in their cytoplasm.

fauces (*faw'-sēs*). The cavity at the back of the mouth and leading to the pharynx.

favus (*fā-vus*). A type of ringworm infection.

Fe. Chemical symbol for iron.

febrile (*fe'-bril*). Relating to fever.

fecundation (*fe-kun-dā'-shon*). Impregnation. Fertilization.

fecundity (*fe-kun'-di-ti*). Power of producing young.

feeble-minded. Subnormal mentality. No longer an official classification.

Fehling's solution. Sulphate of copper and potassium hydrate are the chief ingredients; the solution was used as a test for sugar in the urine.

fel. Bile.

felon (*fe-lon*). A whitlow. An inflammation of the finger near the nail.

Felty's syndrome (*fel-tis sin'-drōm*). A kind of rheumatoid arthritis and associated with

leucopenia and splenomegaly.

female (*fē-māl*). Applied to the sex that bears young.

femoral artery (*fem'-o-ral ar'-te-ri*). The artery of the thigh, from the groin to the knee.

femoral canal (*ka-nal'*). The small canal internal to the femoral vein. The site of a femoral hernia.

femoral vein, thrombosis of. See PHLEGMASIA ALBA DOLENS.

femur (*fē'-mer*). The thigh bone.

fenestra (*fen-es'-tra*). A window, applied to certain apertures, *e.g.* fenestra ovalis.

fenestration (*fe-nes-trā'-shon*). Making a window artificially such as that made in the inner ear to help to relieve deafness in otosclerosis.

ferment (*fer'-ment*). See ENZYME.

fermentation (*fer-men-tā'-shon*). Decomposition of organic material by enzymes present in certain organisms, *e.g.* yeasts and bacteria.

ferric (*fe-rik*). Applied to compounds of iron with a valency of more than two.

ferrous. Applied to compounds containing bivalent iron.

ferrum (*fe'-rum*). Iron.

fertility (*fer-ti-li-ti*). Ability to produce young.

fertilization (*fer-ti-lī-zā-shon*). Union of male and female

germ cells whereby repro-
duction takes place.

fester (*fes'-ter*). Inflammation,
with collection of pus.

festination (*fe-sti-nā-shon*).
Propulsive gait as in Parkinsonism.

fetishism. The worship of an
inanimate object which sym-
bolizes a loved person.

fetus (*fē-tus*). The unborn
child. Formerly frequently
spelt foetus.

fetus papyraceus (*pap-ī-rā'-sē-
us*). A fetus which has been
retained within the uterus for
months after its death, and
has undergone a kind of
natural mummification.

fever (*fē-ver*). A rise in body
temperature above normal.
There is generally a quick
pulse, lassitude, often
delirium, and inhibition of
the secretory glands. The
nursing treatment is rest,
freedom from chills, and light
nourishing diet with abun-
dant fluids.

fibre (*fī'-ber*). Threadlike
structure.

fibrillation (*fī-bri-lā-shon*).
Unco-ordinated contraction
of heart muscle. May affect
the atria only (atrial fibrillation) or the ventricles (ventricular fibrillation).

fibrin (*fī-brin*). Protein which
forms a fibrous gel matrix as a
basis for a blood clot. It is

formed from the soluble
plasma protein fibrinogen by
the action of thrombin.

fibrinogen (*fī-bri-nō-jen*).
Blood protein which is converted into fibrin.

fibrinolysin (*fī-bri-nō-lī-sin*).
Enzyme which dissolves
fibrin.

fibro-adenoma (*fī-brō-ad-en-
ō-ma*). A tumour composed
of mixed fibrous and glandular elements.

fibroblast (*fī-brō-blast*). A cell
that forms a new fibrous tis-
sue.

fibrocartilage (*fī-brō-kar-ti-
lāj*). Cartilage with fibrous
tissue.

fibrochondritis (*fī-brō-kon-
drī'-tis*). Inflamed fibrocartilage.

fibrocystic disease (*fī-bro-sis-
tik di-sēz*). See MUCO-
VISCIDOSIS.

fibroelastosis (*fī-brō-ē-las-tō'-
sis*). Rare disorder affecting
the heart. Excess collagen
and elastin form under the
endocardium.

fibroid (*fī'-broyd*). A tumour
composed of fibrous and
muscular tissue. See also
FIBROMYOMA.

fibroma (*fī'-brō-ma*). Benign
tumour of fibrous tissue.

fibromyoma (*fī-brō-mī-ō'-ma*).
A tumour composed of
mixed muscular and fibrous
tissue. Especially common in

the uterus, and commonly spoken of as 'fibroids'.

fibrosis (*fī-brō'-sis*). Decomposition of fibrous connective tissue and usually occurring in regions which have been damaged by some trauma.

fibrositis (*fī-brō-sī'-tis*). Inflammation of fibrous tissue. *See* LUMBAGO.

fibula (*fib'-ū-la*). The small bone on the outer side of the leg.

field of vision (*vi'-zhon*). The area which can be seen without movement of the eye.

filament (*fil'-a-ment*). Threadlike structure.

Filaria (*fil-ar-ia*). Parasitic thread-like worm which may cause lymphatic obstruction. *See* ELEPHANTIASIS.

filiform. Threadlike. *F. bougie.* A slender bougie.

filipuncture (*fil-i-punkt'-ūr*). A method of treating aneurysm by inserting a fine wire thread. This acts as a foreign body, and the blood inside the sac clots.

filter (*fil'-ter*). Device used for removing a certain substance whilst allowing others to pass through. Optical filters made from different types of glass allow only light in certain parts of the spectrum to pass through. Fluid filters, according to their pore-size, are used to remove viruses, bacteria or other suspended impurities.

filterable, filtrable (*fil-trabl*). Able to pass through a filter.

filtration (*fil-trā'-shon*). Passage through a filter.

filum (*fē-lum*). A structure resembling a thread. *F. terminale.* The tapering end of the enlargement of the lumbar spinal cord.

fimbria (*fim-bria*). A fringe, especially the fringe-like end of the Fallopian tube.

finger (*fing'-ger*). One of the digits of the hand.

first intention (*ferst in-ten'-shon*). A surgical term for aseptic healing of a wound by bringing the edges directly together.

first stage (*ferst stāj'*) (of labour). The act of parturition from the first pains to full dilatation of the cervix.

fission (*fi-shon*). Division into two or more parts. *Binary f.* a mode of reproduction for bacteria and protozoa. *Nuclear f.* The splitting of an atomic nucleus, thus releasing energy.

fissure (*fi-sher*). A split or cleft.

fissure in ano (*fi-sher in ā'-nō*). Anal fissure. Small ulcerated cleft in the mucous membrane of the anus.

fistula (*fis'-tū-la*). Any unnatural passage communicating with two epithelialized surfaces. *Fistula in ano*, anal fistula: any sinus connected with the anus and therefore discharging faeces. See ISCHIO-RECTAL ABSCESS. *Faecal fistula*. A communication between the bowel and the surface; this may be a complication of an abdominal operation. General peritonitis seldom occurs, as track of the discharge from bowel to surface becomes walled off by adhesions. They tend to close spontaneously, but take some weeks. *Internal fistula* is an artificial opening between two viscera—*e.g.* (1) biliary fistula, between the gall bladder and intestine. (2) *A vesico-vaginal F.*, a communication between the bladder and the vagina; this may be a complication of an extensive operation on the female generative organs.

fit. Convulsion, usually with loss of consciousness.

fixation (*fĭk-sā-shon*). (1) Focussing the eyes on an object so that the image falls on the retina. (2) Learning something so that it is fixed in the memory or becomes a motor habit, as after learning to ride a bicycle. (3) In psychology abnormal attachment to a thing or person such as a parent so that new interests and attachments do not develop.

flaccid (*flak'-sĭd*). Soft, lacking rigidity.

flagellum (*fla-je-lum*). (Plu. flagella). Fine, thread-like structure projecting from surface of certain cells, *e.g.* spermatozoa, which by a lashing movement propels the cell, *cf.* cilia.

flap. A piece of skin cut to fold over the stump in operation for amputation.

flatfoot. Flattening or total loss of arches of the foot. It then rests completely on the ground, giving characteristic appearance and walk.

flat or **flattened pelvis.** See CONTRACTED PELVIS.

flatulence (*flat'-ū-lens*). Gas in the alimentary canal, usually refers to the stomach. It may be produced by simply swallowing air or by the fermentation of food. Carminatives give relief.

flatus (*flā-tus*). Gas in the alimentary canal, usually refers to the bowel. It may be relieved by passing a flatus tube.

flea (*flē*). The human flea is *Pulex irritans*. It is without wings and sucks blood, giving rise to irritation and sepsis.

flexion (*flek'-shon*). Being bent; the opposite of extension.

Flexner bacillus (*fleks'-ner*). One of the Shigella group of bacteria causing bacillary dysentery.

flexor (*fleks'-or*). A muscle which causes flexion.

flexure (*flek'-sur*). A bend. A curvature of an organ, *e.g. Hepatic f.* Bend of the colon beneath the liver.

floating ribs (*flō'-ting ribz*). The two lower pairs' of ribs not articulating with sternum.

flooding (*flud'-ing*). Excessive bleeding from the uterus.

fluctuation (*fluk-tū-ā-shon*). A wavelike motion felt on palpation of an abscess or a cyst containing fluid.

fluke (*flook*). Any of the trematode class of worm.

fluorescein (*flor-e-sēn*). A coal-tar derivative which stains cornea a vivid green if there is any loss of surface epithelium—*e.g.* in an abrasion or ulcer.

fluorescence (*flo-re sens*). Emission of light at a wavelength which is different from that of the incident light. The emitted light has a lower energy, *i.e.* is of longer wave-length, from the incident irradiation which is absorbed.

fluorescent screen (*flo-res'-ent skrēn'*). A screen coated with materials which fluoresce when exposed to x-rays.

fluoridation (*floor-ī-dā'-shon*). The addition of fluoride, such as when added to drinking water.

fluorine (*floo-o-rēn*). A halogen element. If added in minute quantities to drinking water it may cause a lessened incidence of dental decay.

fluoroscopy (*flo-ro-sko-pi*). Use of fluorescent screen to intensify x-ray images.

flying squad (*flī-ing skwod*). Emergency obstetric unit which can travel rapidly to domiciliary cases of complicated labour.

focus (*fō-kus*). Point of maximum intensity.

foetor (*fē-tur*). Strong unpleasant smell.

foetus (*fē'-tus*). *See* FETUS.

folic acid (*fō-lik a-sid*). Pteroyl-glutamic acid, part of the vitamin B complex found in liver, yeast, spinach, etc. Essential for blood formation.

folie à deux (*fo-lē ah-der*). Delusion shared by two persons.

follicle (*fol'-li-kl*). A minute bag containing some secretion.

follicle stimulating hormone (*fo-li-kl stī-mū-lā-ting hormōn*). FSH. Hormone secreted by the anterior lobe of the pituitary gland. In the female it stimulates the growth of ovarian follicles and the production of oestrogens. In the male it promotes the development of spermatozoa in the testis.

follicular tonsillitis (*fol-lik'-ū-lar*). Pus in the follicles of the tonsils. The tonsils are red and swollen and covered with small yellow spots.

fomentations (*fō-men-tā'-shons*). Lint or flannel wrung out in some boiling fluid and applied for the alleviation of pain. It must be wrung out thoroughly and shaken to allow escape of steam and applied as hot as can be borne; cover lint with a slightly larger piece of jaconet and then a still larger piece of wool, and bandage whole securely.

fomites (*fō'-mīts*). Articles of clothing or bedding which have been in contact with a patient ill with a contagious disease.

fontanelle (*fon-ta-nel'*). A soft space in the skull of an infant before the skull has completely ossified. The anterior fontanelle, or bregma, is where the coronal, frontal and sagittal sutures meet. The posterior fontanelle is where the lambdoid and sagittal sutures meet. The anterior fontanelle is normally closed by 2 years of

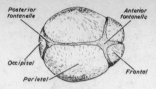

23 The fontanelles

age and delay in closure is a sign of rickets.

food poisoning. Diarrhoea and/or vomiting from eating infected food. Symptoms may be caused by the pre-formed toxins of *Staphylococcus aureus* or *Clostridium welchii* or from infection by organisms of the *Salmonella* group or rarely by *botulinus toxin*. Infected foods are usually meat products or confectionery containing eggs, which have been allowed to remain in warm rooms. Another source of infection may be the unwashed hands of those handling food.

foot. That part of the leg below the ankle.

foot and mouth disease. Virus disease well-known in cattle. It occasionally affects man, causing blistering of the buccal mucosa and similar lesions on the hands and feet, especially round the nails.

foot drop. Inability to keep a foot bent at right angles with the leg. The toes and foot drop and walking becomes difficult. Caused by pressure of bedclothes, or inadequate support to under side of foot when leg is in a splint for a long time, or from paralysis of the muscles which produce dorsiflexion of the ankle.

foramen (*fo-rā'-men*). An opening. *F. magnum*. Opening in the back of the skull through which the spinal cord passes. *F. ovale*. Opening between the right and left atria in the fetus which allows oxygenated venous blood from the placenta to pass into the left side of the heart thus by-passing the pulmonary circulation. It normally closes at birth. *Optic f.*, where the optic nerve enters the skull.

forceps (*for'-seps*). Surgical pincers used for lifting and moving instead of using the fingers.

forebrain. Cerebrum.

forensic medicine (*fo-ren'-sik*). Medicine in so far as it has to do with the law.

foreskin (*for'-skin*). The prepuce, or skin covering the end of the male penis.

formaldehyde (*for-mal'-dē-hīd*). A powerful antiseptic. Its gas is used to disinfect unoccupied rooms.

formication (*for-mi-kā'-shon*). A sensation as of ants creeping over the body. Used almost entirely to denote tingling sensation in a nerve recovering from pressure or injury, and therefore after nerve injury is a sign of regeneration.

formula (*for'-mū-la*). A prescription. Statement of constituents which form a compound.

formulary (*for-mū-la-ri*). A collection of formulae (pl. of formula), for medical preparations such as those found in the British Pharmacopoeia.

fornix (*for'-niks*). An arch. Applied to various anatomical structures, but especially to the roof of the vagina. Pl. **fornices.**

fossa (*fo'-sa*). Little depressions of the body, such as *fossa lacrimalis*, the hollow of the frontal bone, which holds the lacrimal gland. *Iliac fossae*. Concavities of the iliac bones of the pelvis.

Fothergill's operation (*fo'-ther-gilz*). Repair of the anterior and posterior vaginal walls and amputation of the cervix.

fourchette (*foor-shet*). A thin fold of skin behind the vulva.

fovea (*fō'-vea*). A small fossa or cup. In the eye, shallow depression in the retina. It is the site of maximum visual stimulation and the region on which the image is focussed when the eyes are fixed.

fractional distillation (*frak'-shon-al dis-til-ā-shon*). See DISTILLATION.

fractional test meal (*frak-shon-al test' mēl*). Performed to examine the gastric contents and to estimate the rate of emptying of the stomach. A substance is given to stimulate the gastric glands and the resultant secretion of hydrochloric acid is estimated.

fracture (*frak-tūr*). A break in a bone. The symptoms are— pain, swelling, deformity, loss of function, unnatural mobility, shortening, crepitus. A fracture may be: (1) *Simple or closed*, not connected with an external wound. (2) *Compound or open*, communicating with the surface. (3) *Greenstick*, when the bone is fractured half through on the convex side of the bend as in a green twig. Only seen in children. (4) *Comminuted*, where bone is broken into more than two pieces. (5) *Impacted*, where one fragment is driven into the other. (6) *Complicated*, where fracture is combined with injury to another important structure, *e.g.* artery, nerve, or organ. The

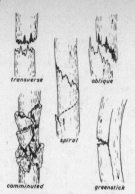

24 Types of fracture

type of break may be: (1) *Transverse*, due to direct violence applied at point of fracture. (2) *Oblique*, due to indirect violence, when a force applied at a distance causes the bone to break at its weakest part. (3) *Spiral*, when a limb is violently rotated. (4) *Depressed fracture*, only of skull, when bone is driven inwards: it may be *guttershaped* with sharp depressed edge, or *pondshaped* with sloping edge; the latter is only in infants and ‾due to birth injury. See COLLES' FRACTURE, POTT'S FRACTURE, SPLINTS, SPONTANEOUS FRACTURE.

fraenum (*frā'-num*). A small membranous fold attached to certain organs, and acting as

a check. *F. linguae.* That
under the tongue.

fragilitas ossium (*fra-jil'-i-tas
os-ium*). Osteogenesis imperfecta. Abnormal brittleness
of the bones. Associated with
abnormal blueness of sclera
of eyes.

framboesia (*fram-bē'-zia*). A
contagious tropical disease
called yaws. Fungus-like
masses are formed on the
face, hands and feet.

free association. In psycho-
analysis, when the patient
gives the first word which a
stimulus brings to his mind,
or a train of ideas.

fremitus (*fre'-mit-us*). A vibration perceived by palpation,
always applied to a vibration
in the chest.

Freud (*froyd*). A famous
Austrian psycho-analyst
(1856–1939).

Freudian (*froy-di-an*). According to Freud's teaching. He
taught that psychological
disorders often resulted from
unconscious sexual im-
pressions during childhood.
These he brought to con-
sciousness through psycho-
analysis. Dreams he said
were the wish-fulfilment of
repressed desires.

Friar's balsam (*fri'-arz*). Compound tincture of benzoin,
often used in steam inhalations.

friction (*frik'-shon*). (1) A circular movement in massage
performed with the tips of the
fingers or thumb as deeply as
possible over joints; the
object being to break down
adhesions. (2) The sound
heard in auscultation when
two dry, roughened surfaces
rub together as in pleurisy.

Friedman's test (*frēd-manz*).
Pregnancy test now obsolete.
The urine of pregnant
women contains an excess of
secretion from the trophoblast, chorionic gonadot-
rophin, or APL principle.
The urine is injected into an
infantile rabbit. The rabbit is
killed in 48 hours. If the
woman is pregnant, characteristic changes will be seen
in the ovaries of the rabbit.

Friedreich's ataxia (*frēd-rīks
a-tak-si-a*). Inherited
degenerative disease of the
nervous system. The onset is
in childhood and is progressive. There is clumsiness,
unsteady gait, weakness,
dysarthria and other
neurological disturbances.

frigidity (*fri-ji-di-ti*). Lack of
sexual desire.

Fröhlich's syndrome (*frer-liks
sin'-drōm*). A disorder with
obesity, sexual infantilism,
disturbances of sleep and
temperature regulation and
diabetes insipidus due to

damage of the pituitary and hypothalamus.

frontal (*frun'-tal*). Relating to the forehead.

frontal bone (*frun'-tal bōn*). One of the bones of the skull. *F. Sinus. See* SINUS.

frostbite (*frost-bīt*). Injury of the skin or a part from extreme cold. There is redness, swelling and pain and necrosis may result.

fructose (*frŭk-toz*). Fruit sugar.

frustration (*fru-strā'-shon*). Disappointment experienced by a person who is thwarted and prevented by circumstances from achieving some desired object.

FSH. *See* FOLLICLE STIMULATING HORMONE.

fugue (*fūg*). A fleeing from reality as in hysteria. The patient has no recollection of his actions during this time.

full time or term. The fetus is said to be at term when it is 20 to 21in long, has both testicles descended (if a boy), and has finger-nails and toe-nails reaching to the ends of the digits. Such a child should weigh anything from 7 lb upwards, and have been developing in the uterus for not less than forty weeks.

Fuller's earth (*ful-erz erth'*). Chiefly consists of silica, alumina, and oxide of iron. Very absorbent.

fulminant, fulminating (*ful'-mi-nā-ting*). Sudden, severe, rapid in course, as fulminant glaucoma.

fumigation (*fū-mi-gā'-shon*). Sterilization of rooms by disinfectant vapour.

function (*funk'-shon*). The normal special work of an organ.

functional disorder (*funk'-shon-al*). The malfunctioning of an organ or organs when no organic disease is present.

fundus (*fun'-dus*). The enlarged part of a hollow organ farthest removed from the orifice; thus the fundus oculi is the interior of the eye behind the lens and pupil, visible with an ophthalmoscope; the fundus uteri is the top of the uterus.

fungi (*fun-gī*) (Sing. fungus). A subdivision of Thallophyta including moulds, mushrooms, rusts, yeasts, etc. Fungi are used as a source of protein and vitamins, certain enzymes, used in baking and brewing and antibiotics, notably penicillin. A few fungi cause disease in man.

fungicide. Any substance used for the destruction of fungi.

funiculitis (*fū-nik-ū-lī'-tis*). Inflammation of the spermatic cord.

funnel chest. Also called pectus excavatum. A developmental deformity in which the sternum is depressed and the ribs and costal cartilages curve inwards.

furuncle (*fū'-rung-kl*). A boil.

furunculosis (*fū-run-kū-lō'-sis*). The appearance of one or more boils.

fusiform (*fū'-zi-form*). Spindle-shaped. Can describe a bacillus. See ANEURYSM.

fusion (*fū-zhon*). Joining together.

G

gag. An instrument for keeping the mouth open. See DOYEN'S GAG.

gait (*gāt*). Manner of walking.

gaiactagogue (*gal-ak'-tag-og*). An agent that causes an increased flow of milk.

galactocele (*ga-lak'-tō-sēl*). A cyst of the breast containing milk.

galactorrhoea (*ga-lak-to-re'-a*). Excessive flow of milk.

galactosaemia (*gal-ak-tō-zē-mea*). A metabolic disorder characterized by presence of galactose in the blood stream.

galactose (*ga-lak'-tōz*). A hexose sugar which, in combination with glucose, forms the disaccharide lactose which is present in breast milk.

gall (*gawl*), or **bile.** A secretion

of the liver; it accumulates in the gall bladder.

gall bladder (*gawl' bla'-der*). The membranous sac which holds the bile. See BILIARY DUCTS.

gallipot (*ga-li-pot*). Small pot for containing medical preparations.

gallon (*ga'-lon*). Liquid measure which equals 8 pints.

gallstone (*gawl'-stōn*). Calculus in the gall bladder. If the stone passes into the cystic or common bile duct there is great pain, and if in the common bile duct, jaundice. See COLIC.

galvanism (*gal'-van-izm*). Therapeutic use of direct electric current, either continuous, or interrupted. Interrupted galvanism is used to stimulate denervated muscle.

galvanometer (*gal-van-om'-e-ter*). An instrument for measuring the flow of an electric current.

gamete (*gam'-ēt*). A sexual reproductive cell, *e.g.* sperm, ovum.

gamgee tissue (*gam'-jē tis-yū*). Absorbent wool between two layers of gauze.

gamma rays (*gam'-a rāz*). Electromagnetic waves of extremely short wave length emitted by radio-active substances; similar to x-rays, but shorter. Employed for dry, cold sterilization of any articles which would be destroyed by moisture or heat.

gammaglobulin (*ga-ma-glo-bū-lin*). Protein fraction of plasma, rich in antibodies against infection.

ganglion (*gang-glē-on*). (1) A collection of nerve cells forming a nerve centre. They are found in the sympathetic nervous system and in other parts of the nervous system. (2) Surgically, a chronic synovial cyst generally connected with a tendon sheath; most common site, back of hand, near the wrist.

ganglionectomy (*gan-glē-ō-nek-to-mi*). Excision of a ganglion.

gangrene (*gang'grēn*). Massive necrosis of tissue as the result of reduced blood supply. *Dry g.* The arterial supply is increasingly diminished, the veins remaining patent. The part becomes dry and mummified. The commonest cause is senility. *Wet g.* is caused by a sudden interference with the arterial supply and the venous return, as may occur if a tourniquet is left on too long or in traumatic conditions. The part readily becomes infected.

Gas g., due to infection by a group of anaerobic gas-forming organisms of which the bacillus Welchii is the best known. Wounds which have been in contact with soil are likely to be infected. The signs are a rise in the pulse rate after recovery from the initial shock, discolouration, oedema, discharge, and gas felt in the tissues. Anti-gas gangrene serum is given as a prophylactic and curative measure. Antibiotics are also prescribed.

gargarisma (*gar'-gar-iz-ma*). A gargle.

gargle (*gar'-gl*). A liquid medicine for washing out the throat.

gargoylism (*gar-goy-lism*). Hurler's syndrome. A defect of skeletal development in which the skull is grossly deformed and the digital bones are bulbous, the hands assuming a claw-like appearance. There is often associated congenital heart disease, enlarged liver and spleen, and intellectual impairment.

gas gangrene (*gas gan'-grēn*). *See* GANGRENE.

Gasserian ganglion (*gas-ē'-rian gan'-gli-on*). A ganglion of the sensory root of the fifth cranial nerve deeply situated in the skull. It is sometimes operated on for the relief of intractable trigeminal neuralgia.

gastrectomy (*gas-trek'-tom-i*). Removal of the stomach.

gastric (*gas-trik*). Relating to the stomach. *G. aspiration*. Also called *g. suction*. Performed postoperatively after operations on the alimentary tract to prevent dilatation of the stomach. A Ryle's tube is passed and the contents aspirated at frequent intervals or continuously. *G. juice*. The digestive fluid of the stomach. *G. lavage*. Washing out the stomach: a procedure used in the treatment of poisoning.

gastric ulcer (*ul-ser*). Ulceration of the mucosa lining the stomach. Acute ulceration may be caused by ingested substances, *e.g.* aspirin. Chronic ulceration may be due to reduced capacity of the epithelium to withstand the acid gastric secretion or to a tumour of the epithelium.

gastrin (*gas-trin*). A hormone released by cells in the wall of the pyloric antrum, when it is distended. This stimulates the secretion of gastric juice by the secretory cells in the rest of the stomach.

gastritis (*gas-trī'-tis*). Inflammation of the epithelium lining the stomach.

gastrocele (*gas'-trō-sēl*). Hernia of the stomach.

gastrocnemius (*gas-trō-knē'-me-us*). A large muscle of the calf of the leg.

gastrocolic reflex (*gas-trō-ko-lik rē-fleks*). Reflex peristaltic contractions in the colon occurring as the result of filling the stomach.

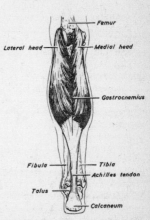

Femur

Lateral head — Medial head

Gastrocnemius

Fibula — Tibia

Achilles tendon

Talus

Calcaneum

25 *The gastrocnemius muscle*

gastroduodenostomy (*gas'-trō-dū-ō-den-ost'-omi*), **gastroenterostomy** (*en-te-ros'-to-mi*), **gastrojejunostomy** (*je-jūn-os'-to-mi*). The operation of making an artificial passage direct from the stomach to the duodenum or the jejunum.

gastroenteritis (*gas'-trō-en-ter-i'-tis*). Inflammation of the stomach and intestines.

gastrogastrostomy (*gas-trō-gas-tros'-to-mi*), **gastrolysis** (*gas-trol'-i-sis*), **gastroplasty** (*gas'-trō-plas-ti*). Operations for the cure of hour-glass contractions of the stomach.

gastrointestinal tract (*gas-trō-in-tes-tī-nal trakt*). The gut including the mouth, oesophagus, stomach, small and large intestine, rectum and anus and the associated structures.

gastropexy (*gas-trō-peks-i*). Fixing a displaced stomach to the abdominal wall by surgery.

gastroptosis (*gas-trop-tō-sis*). Downward displacement of the stomach.

gastroscope (*gas'-tros-kōp*). An instrument for inspecting the cavity of the stomach. It has a light at the end and is passed per oesophagus.

gastrostomy (*gas-tros'-to-mi*). Making an artificial opening into the stomach through which patient is fed by pouring nourishment through a tube directly into the stomach. Performed for stricture, usually malignant, of the oesophagus.

gastrulation (*gas-trū-lā-shon*). Embryological term used to describe the complex movements of cells of the embryo in which the cells which give rise to the internal organs migrate inside the embryo.

Gaucher's disease (*gow-cherz*). A very rare familial disease resulting in enlargement of the spleen with anaemia.

gauze (*gawz*). Open mesh material used in surgical dressings.

gavage (*gav'-ahj*). Forced feeding.

Geiger-Muller counter (*gī-ger moo-ler kown-ter*). Machine which detects and registers radio-activity.

gelatin (*je'-lat-in*). A jelly-like protein obtained by boiling bones, cartilage, and muscle of animals.

gemmellus (*je-mel'-lus*). Twin, the name of two muscles in the buttock.

gene (*jēn*). Chromosomal factor transmitting hereditary characteristics.

general paralysis of the insane. Also called GPI. Dementia due to involvement of the brain in syphilis.

generation (*jen-er-ā'-shon*). (1) Reproduction. The begetting of children. (2) Specific group of individuals resulting from a mating.

genetic (*jen-et'-ik*). Pertaining to genes. Term generally applied to hereditary factors in an individual.

genetics (*je-ne-tiks*). Study of heredity and its variations.

genitalia (*jen-it-ā'-li-a*). The generative organs.

genotype (*je-nō-'-tīp*). The genetic make-up of an individual, *i.e.*, the set of alleles inherited by the individual.

genu (*jen-ū*). The knee.

genu-pectoral position (*jen-ū-pek'-tor-al po-si-shon*). The knee-chest position—the patient resting upon the knees and chest.

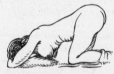

26 The genu-pectoral position

genu valgum (*jen-ū val'-gum*). Knock-knee, knees are bent inwards. *G. varum.* bow-legged.

geriatrics (*je-rē-a-triks*). The study of disease among the elderly.

germ (*jerm*). Term generally applied to pathogenic micro-organisms.

German measles (*jer'-man mēz-lz*). See RUBELLA.

germicide (*jer'-mi-sid*). An agent that destroys micro-organisms, *e.g.* lysol.

gerontology (*je-ron-to-lo-ji*). The study of ageing.

Gesell's development charts (*je-sels*). Charts showing the expected motor activity, manipulation, adaptive behaviour, language, social and play reactions in children at certain ages.

gestation (*jes-tā'-shon*). Pregnancy.

gestation sac. The fetus with its enveloping membranes, decidua, etc. The contents of a pregnant uterus.

Ghon's focus (*gōns fō-kus*). Small focus of infection found in primary infection with tubercle bacillus.

giardiasis (*gi-a-dī-a-sis*). See LAMBLIASIS.

gigantism (*ji-gan'-tizm*). Abnormal overgrowth of the body or of a limb, due to overactivity of the anterior lobe of the pituitary in young people. *See* ACROMEGALY.

Gigli's saw (*jēl-yēs*). An instrument for sawing through bone.

gill (*jil*). Liquid measure, ¼ pint.

gingival (*jin-jī'-val*). Relating to the gums.

gingivitis (*jin-ji-vī'-tis*). Inflammation of the gums.

ginglymus (*jin'-gli-mus*). A hinge joint such as elbow or knee.

girdle (*ger-dl*). Band encircling the body.

glabella (*glá-bel'-la*). Triangular space between the eyebrows.

glairy (*glā-i*). Slimy, albuminous.

gland. A secreting organ. Some have ducts to carry away their secretion, *e.g.* the salivary glands. Others are ductless, *e.g.* the thyroid (*see* ENDOCRINE). Lymphatic glands manufacture leucocytes, filter the lymph and prevent the spread of infection.

glanders (*glan'-ders*). A febrile disease with inflammation of the nasal cavities, communicable to man from the horse, ass and mule. Often fatal.

glandular fever. See INFECTIOUS MONONUCLEOSIS.

glans. Bulbous extremity of the penis and clitoris.

glaucoma (*glaw'-kō-ma*). A disease of the eye with hardening of the globe, due to an increase in the intraocular pressure; acute forms of this disease may lead to complete loss of sight in a few days. *Treatment.* Eserine drops and trephine. *See* TREPHINE.

Glenard's disease (*glā'-narz*). A general slackening of the supporting ligaments in the abdomen, leading to slipping down of the viscera: *e.g.* stomach, kidney, and intestines.

glenoid (*gle'-noyd*). A cavity, a term applied to the socket of the shoulder joint.

glioma (*glī-ō-ma*). A tumour composed of neuroglia, nerve connective tissue. It may develop in the brain or spinal cord.

gliomyoma (*glī-ō-mī-ō'-ma*). A tumour composed of nerve and muscle tissue.

Glisson's capsule (*glis-onz kap'-sūl*). The connective tissue capsule of the liver, enveloping the portal vein, hepatic artery, hepatic ducts.

globulin (*glob'-ū-lin*). Group of proteins widely distributed in the body with numerous specialized functions. One group, the gamma-globulins, are antibodies.

globus hystericus (*glō'-bus histe'-ri-kus*). Hysterical choking feeling as if of a ball in the throat.

glomerulonephritis (*glo-me-roo-lō-nef-rī-tis*). Acute inflammation of the kidney affecting all the glomeruli.

glomerulus (*glo-me-roo-lus*). The filtration unit of a nephron. It consists of a coil of fine capillaries lying in the invaginated blind end of the renal tubule.

glossal (*glos'-sal*). Relating to the tongue.

glossectomy (*glo-sek-to-mi*). Surgical removal of the tongue.

glossitis (*glos-sī'-ṭis*). Inflammation of the tongue.

glossodynia (*glos-sō-di-ni-a*). Pain in the tongue sometimes associated with trigeminal neuralgia but often of unknown origin.

glossopharyngeal (*glo-sō-fa-rin-je-al*). Relating to tongue and pharynx. *G. nerve* is the ninth cranial nerve.

glossoplegia (*glos-sō-plē'-ji-a*). Paralysis of the tongue.

glottis (*glot'-tis*). The aperture between the vocal cords in the larynx.

glucose (*glū'-kōz*). Dextrose. A hexose sugar. *i.e.* a monosaccharide. *c.f.* disaccharide, *e.g.* sucrose; polysaccharide, *e.g.* starch.

gluteal (*glū'-tē-al*). Pertaining to the buttock.

gluteal bandage (*glū'-tē-al ban-dāj*). Triangular bandage of the hip.

gluten (*glū'-ten*). A protein constituent of certain cereals which acts as an antigen in coeliac disease.

gluteus (*glū-te'-us*). *G. maximus, G. medius, G. minimus*—the three large muscles of the buttock.

glycerin (*glis'-er-in*). A sweet, colourless liquid, obtained from oils and fats and byproduct in the manufacture of soap. Used as an emollient in skin preparations.

glycine (*glī-sin*). An amino-acid.

glycogen (*glī'-kō-jen*). A special form of starch which is stored in the liver and muscles and which can be converted to glucose as needed.

glycoside (*glī-kō-sīd*). A compound found in plants containing a carbohydrate molecule. Often the active constituent of a drug, *e.g.* digoxin in digitalis.

glycosuria (*glī-kō-sū-ri-a*). Glucose in the urine, a symptom in diabetes mellitus. Sometimes a transitory state only.

gnathic (*nath'-ik*). Relating to the jaw or cheek.

GNC. Abbreviation for General Nursing Council.

goblet cells (*go'-blet selz*). Pear-shaped cells in mucous membrane which secrete mucin.

goitre (*goy'-ter*). Enlargement of the thyroid gland. *Exophthalmic g.* Activity of the gland is increased, there is protrusion of the eyes, basal metabolic rate is high, increased pulse rate, tremor, sweating, nervousness, diarrhoea. *Parenchymatous g.*, uniform enlargement of the thyroid, very common in young people. *Cystic g.*, may be (1) enlargement of a single vesicle, or (2) liquefaction of an adenoma. *Adenomatous* *g.*, encephaloid masses in gland substance which may be solid or cystic. *Malignant g.*, a malignant growth of the thyroid.

Golgi's cells (*gol-jēs selz*). Nerve cells with short processes found in the brain and spinal cord.

gomphiasis (*gom-fī-a-sis*). Looseness of teeth.

gomphosis (*gom-fō-sis*). Joint when bony eminence fits into a socket.

gonadotrophic (*gon-ad-ō-tro'-fik*). Promoting the activity of the gonads.

gonadotrophins (*gō-na-dō-trō-fins*). Hormones which stimulate the gonads, *e.g.* FSH, LH.

gonads (*gō-nads*). Reproductive glands: ovary of the female, testis of the male.

gonococcus (*gon-o-kok'-us*). The bacterium causing gonorrhoea. It is a Gram negative intra-cellular diplococcus. *See* BACTERIA.

gonorrhoea (*gon-or-rē-'a*). A venereal disease. An acute inflammation, starting nearly always in the cervix or urethra, and due to the gonococcus. This disease is highly contagious. It may cause ophthalmia neonatorum. It may also cause ophthalmia in adults. By an ascending infection, in the female it may pass to the Fallopian tubes and then cause peritonitis. The chief secondary complication of gonorrhoea is gonococcal arthritis, affecting mainly the large joints. The chief symptoms of gonorrhoea are profuse discharge and pain on passing water. Penicillin is administered.

Goodpasture's syndrome (*good-pas-tūrs sin'-drōm*). Haemorrhagic lung disorder and glomerulonephritis.

Gordh needle (*gawd*). Needle through which repeated intravenous injections may be given.

GOT. Glutamic oxalo-acetic transaminase. Increase of transaminase occurs in liver damage and heart muscle damage.

gouge (*gowj*). A grooved instrument of steel used to scoop out dead bone.

gout (*gowt*). Inherited defect of purine metabolism in which uric acid is in excess in the tissues. During acute attacks it is characterized by painful swelling of a joint, classically the big toe.

GPI. *See* GENERAL PARALYSIS.

GPT. Glutamic pyruvic transaminase. The transaminases are increased in acute liver disease.

Graafian follicles (*grah'-fian*).

Small bodies lying on the surface of the ovary, containing fluid and the egg cell. When the egg cell matures the follicle ruptures, setting it free to make its way to the fimbriated end of the Fallopian tube along which it travels.

Graefe's knife (*grāfs*). Small knife used in operations for cataract.

graft (*grahft*). Transplanted living tissue, *e.g.* skin, bone. *Skin g.* may be: (1) *Thiersch*. Large pieces of epidermis with some dermis used chiefly for large areas. (2) *Wolfe*. The whole thickness of the skin is taken, used chiefly for small wounds. (3) *Pedicle*, used to reconstruct after burns or other severe injuries. The skin and underlying tissue is transplanted in stages. The graft retains its blood supply throughout. *Bone g.*, piece of bone removed, usually from the tibia, and secured to replace bone lost elsewhere.

gram (*gram'*). Metric unit of weight; 30 grams are approximately equivalent to 1oz avoirdupois.

Gram's stain. Bacteria which resist decolourization by alcohol after staining with methyl violet and Gram's solution are termed Gram positive, *e.g.* staphylococci, pneumococci. Those which are decolourized by alcohol are term Gram negative, *e.g.* B. coli, gonococci.

grand mal (*gro-mal*). *See* EPILEPSY.

granular (*gra'-nū-la*). Composed of grains or granulations.

granular layer (*gra-nū-la lār*). Region in keratinizing epithelia where the cytoplasm of the cells appears granular.

granulation (*gran-ū-lā'-shon*). The process by which tiny granules of flesh, composed of capillaries and fibroblasts, form on the face of a wound during its healing. Called healing by second intention.

granule (*gran'-ūl*). Small particle or grain.

granuloma (*gran-ū-lō'-ma*). A tumour composed of granulation tissue.

grape sugar. Glucose.

graph (*grahf*). A diagrammatic record of given information, generally numerical.

gravel (*gra'-vel*). A popular term for small concretions formed in the kidney or bladder.

Graves' disease. Exophthalmic goitre. *See* GOITRE.

gravid (*grav'-id*). Pregnant.

gravitational ulcer. Ulcer of lower leg, often a complication of varicose veins.

gravity. Weight. *See* SPECIFIC GRAVITY.

Grawitz tumour (*grah-wits*). A malignant epithelial tumour of the kidney.

gray. The SI unit to replace the rad and the rem. Symbol Gy.

greenstick fracture. *See* FRACTURE.

grey matter. Tissue of the CNS in which are situated numerous cell bodies of nerves, dendritic processes, glial cells, etc.

grid radiotherapy. Irradiation through a sieve-like screen, *e.g.* lead, to improve tissue tolerance in palliative radiotherapy.

grip, grippe. Influenza.

grocer's itch. Eczema of the hands, caused by frequent contact with flour and sugar.

groin (*groyn*). Juncture of the thigh and abdomen.

guaiacum (*gwī-ak-um*). Used to detect presence of blood in the urine.

guillotine (*gil'-lō-tēn*). An instrument for excising the tonsils.

guinea worm (*gi-nee werm*). Nematode worm which may infest man. The female migrates into the subcutaneous tissues.

gullet (*gul'-let*). The oesophagus.

gumma (*gum'-ma*). A soft tumour occurring in the tertiary stage of syphilis. This may ulcerate. The characteristics of a gummatous ulcer are: it has a vertical, punched out edge, the surrounding tissues are healthy, the base is formed by a 'wash-leather' slough; it is painless and very slow to heal. *See* SYPHILIS.

gum resins. Used as antiseptics.

gustatory (*gus'-tā-tor-i*). Pertaining to taste.

gut. The intestine.

gutta. A drop.

guttatim. Drop by drop. Abbreviation, *gtt.*

gutter splints. For limbs, made of wood, tin or some malleable metal, and grooved to fit the limb, and often lined with felt.

gynaecology (*gī-nē-kol'-o-ji*). The study and practice of the management and treatment of disorders affecting female organs, *e.g.* ovaries, uterus, vagina.

gypsum (*jip-sum*). Calcium sulphate (plaster of Paris).

gyrus (*ji'-rus*). A convolution, such as the convolutions of the brain.

H

H. Symbol for hydrogen.

habit. Constant and often involuntary action established by frequent repetition.

habitat. The natural abode of an animal or plant.

haem, haema, haemo, haemato. Prefixes pertaining to blood.

haemangioma (*hē-man-jē-ō'-ma*). Abnormal growth of blood vessels.

haemarthrosis (*hē-mar-thrō'-sis*). Effusion of blood into a joint cavity.

haematemesis (*hē-ma-tem'-ē-sis*). Vomiting blood from the stomach. The blood is dark. non-frothy, generally acid, and is mixed with traces of food. Common causes are ulcers or growths of the stomach.

haematin (*hē'-ma-tin*). The iron containing pigment of haemoglobin.

haematinic (*hē-ma-tin'-ik*). A substance which increases the amount of haemoglobin in the blood, *e.g.* iron.

haematocele (*hē-ma-tō-sēl*). A tumour containing extravasated blood. *Pelvic h.*, a collection of blood in the pouch of Douglas, walled off by adhesions, usually caused by the leaking from a Fallopian tube, the seat of an ectopic gestation.

haematocolpos (*hē-ma-tō-kol'-pos*). Collection of menses in the vagina due to the presence of a septum.

haematocrit (*hē-ma-tō-krit*). Packed cell volume (PCV). A measurement of the proportion of the circulating blood occupied by red blood cells.

haematology (*hē-mat-ol'-o-ji*). The science of the blood.

haematoma (*hē-ma-tō'-ma*). A swelling composed of blood. A bruise.

haematometra (*hē-ma-to-mē'-tra*). Accumulation of blood in the uterus.

haematomyelia (*hē-ma-tō-mī-ē'-le-ah*). Haemorrhage into the spinal cord.

haematoporphyrin (*hē-mat-o-por'-fir-in*). A pigment sometimes present in urine, derived from haemoglobin.

haematorrachis (*hē-ma-tō-ra-kis*). Haemorrhage into the extramedullary region of the spinal cord.

haematosalpinx. Distension of the Fallopian tube with blood.

haematoxylin (*hē-ma-tok-si-lin*). Basic dye prepared from logwood. It stains acid groups in tissue, particularly nucleic acids, and is much used in histology.

haematozoa (*hē-ma-to-zō'-a*). Protozoan parasites in the blood stream.

haematuria (*hē-ma-tū'-ri-a*). Blood in the urine, which may be due to lesions of the kidney, or urinary tract. During menstruation some blood may escape into the urine and thus cause suspicion of true haematuria. In appearance the urine may be bright or dark red if much blood be present, smoky if rather less. Protein will be present.

haemochromatosis (*hē-mō'-krō-ma-tō-sis*). Called also pigmentary cirrhosis or bronzed diabetes. The skin is pigmented due to the deposition of iron which is also present in the liver, heart and pancreas.

haemoconcentration. Concentration of the blood.

haemocytometer (*hē-mō-sīt'-om-et-er*). An instrument to measure average diameter of red blood cells.

haemodialysis (*hē-mō-dī-a'-li-sis*). The removal of waste products such as urea or salt from the blood by circulating it through a dialyser for patients with renal failure.

haemoglobin (*hē-mo-glō'-bin*). The colouring matter of red blood cells, and the agent whereby oxygen is taken up from the air in the lungs and carried to the tissues. The amount of haemoglobin present in the blood can be estimated by a colour test, normal amount (14·6 grams per 100ml) called 100 per cent haemoglobin.

haemoglobinometer (*hē-mo-glō-bin-om'-e-ter*). An instrument for estimating the haemoglobin in the blood.

haemolysin (*hē-mol'-i-sin*). Agent causing the breakdown of the red cell membrane.

haemolytic (*hē-mo-lit'-ik*). Having the power to destroy red blood cells. *H. anaemia*, resulting from destruction of red cells as in forms of poisoning, or by the action of antibodies. *H. disease of the newborn*, jaundice in a Rhesus positive infant caused by red cell destruction by anti-Rhesus antibodies generated in the Rhesus-negative mother's circulation during pregnancy. *See* BLOOD GROUPING.

haemopericardium (*hē-mō-peri-kar'-di-um*). An effusion of blood into the pericardial sac, which may be due to injury or disease.

haemophilia (*hē-mo-fi'-li-a*). A congenital tendency to haemorrhage, the clotting power of the blood being deficient. It occurs only in males, but is transmitted through the females of the family.

haemophiliac. A person suffering from haemophilia.

Haemophilus (*hē-mo-fi-lus*). Bacillus causing respiratory disorders such as the *H. influenzae*. H. pertussis is the cause of whooping cough.

haemophthalmia (*hē-mof-thal-mi-a*). Haemorrhage into the eye.

haemopoiesis (*hē-mō-poy-ē-sis*). The process of formation of the blood cells, particularly the red blood cells. In the fetus, haemopoiesis occurs in the spleen and liver; in the adult, in the bone marrow.

haemopoietin (*hē-mo-poy-ē'-tin*). A hormone produced by the action of the intrinsic factor in the gastric juice on the extrinsic factor, present in food. It is stored in the liver and activates the red bone marrow to manufacture red blood cells.

haemoptysis (*hē-mop'-ti-sis*). Coughing up of blood.

haemorrhage (*hem'or-āj*). A flow of blood. It may be (1) *arterial*, occurring in spurts, and bright red in colour; (2) *venous*, occurring in a steady stream and dark in colour; (3) *capillary*, oozing from a large wound surface. Haemorrhage may be (1) *primary*, at time of injury; (2) *reactionary*, within twenty-four hours of injury due to a rise in the blood pressure; (3) *secondary*, usually within seven to ten days of injury,

due to sepsis. Haemorrhage may be (1) *visible* or (2) *concealed*, into one of the cavities of the body and not appearing at the surface. The symptoms of concealed haemorrhage are pallor of skin and mucous membranes, quick, sighing respiration, rapid, small, weak pulse. Restlessness, subnormal temperature, coldness, sweating and collapse. *See illustration* for pressure points for the arrest of haemorrhage, p. 160.

haemorrhagic disease of new-born (*he-mo-ra-jik*). Congenital abnormality of vitamin K metabolism which results in deficiency of prothrombin in the blood. As a result haemorrhages occur in the body following even slight trauma.

haemorrhoidectomy (*he-mo-roy-dek'-top-mi*). Surgical removal of haemorrhoids.

haemorrhoids (*hem-o-roydz*). Varicose rectal veins (piles).

haemostasis (*hē-mos'-tā-sis*). The prevention of haemorrhage or the measures taken for its arrest.

haemostatic (*hē-mō-sta'-tik*). An agent to arrest a flow of blood.

haemothorax (*hē-mō-tho'-raks*). Escape of blood into the cavity of the chest.

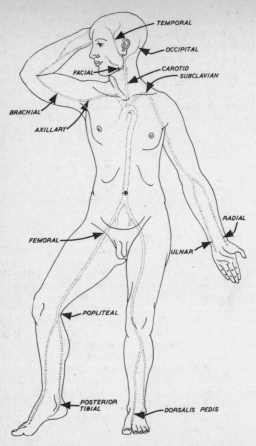

TEMPORAL

OCCIPITAL

FACIAL

CAROTID
SUBCLAVIAN

BRACHIAL

AXILLARY

RADIAL

FEMORAL

ULNAR

POPLITEAL

POSTERIOR
TIBIAL

DORSALIS PEDIS

*27 Arterial system. The arrows indicate points at which
pressure may be applied to check haemorrhage*

hair follicle (*hār fol'-le-kl*). Little pit in the skin in which the root of the hair is fixed.

half-life. The time in which the total radiation emitted by a radio-active substance is reduced by decay to half its original value. It is a constant for each isotope and is independent of the quantity.

halibut liver oil. Oil from the liver of halibut; rich in vitamins A and D.

halitosis (*ha-li-tō'-sis*). Foul breath.

hallucinations (*hal-lū-si-nā'-shons*). The patient perceives something for which there is no sensory stimulus, *i.e.* the sights and sounds are entirely imaginary, *cf.* delusion.

hallucinogens (*ha-lū-si-nō-jens*). Term applied to drugs such as LSD which cause hallucinations.

hallux. The great toe.

hallux valgus. Displacement of the great toe outwards towards the other toes.

halogens (*hal-ō'-jens*). Non-metallic elements of the series fluorine, chlorine, bromine, iodine. They are anionic in solution and combine with metals to form salts.

hamate bone. One of the wrist bones.

hammer toe. A deformity of a toe in which there is permanent dorsal flexion of the first phalanx and plantar flexion of the second and third phalanges.

hamstrings. The tendons traversing the popliteal region.

hand. End of the arm. Its bones are the carpal, metacarpal and phalanges.

handicapped (*hand-di-kapt*). Mentally or physically disabled.

Hanot's disease (*ha-nōz*). A rare type of cirrhosis of the liver of unknown origin.

haploid (*hap-loyd*). Having a set of unpaired chromosomes in the nucleus, characteristic of gametes.

hard chancre (*shan'-ker*). True primary syphilitic sore.

hare lip. A congenital slit in the upper lip, frequently associated with 'cleft palate'.

Harrison's sulcus. A groove extending from the level of the ensiform cartilage towards the axillae. It is produced in rickets.

Hartmann's solution. A saline solution containing sodium lactate. Used in acidosis.

Hashimoto's disease (*ha-shē-mō-to*). A chronic thyroiditis due to autoimmunity to thyroglobulin. It causes myxoedema.

hashish (*hash'-ēsh*). An extract of Indian hemp, a drug

included in the Misuse of
Drugs Act. *See* CANNABIS
INDICA.

haustrations (*haw-strā-shons*).
Sacculations of the colon.

Haversian canals. The minute
canals which permeate bone.

hay fever. Allergic rhinitis
caused by exposure of sensi-
tized respiratory epithelium
to certain dusts and pollens.

head (*hed*). That part of the
body in which is the brain.

headache (*hed-āk*). Pain in the
head.

Heaf test. *See* MANTOUX TEST.

healing (*hē-ling*). Any procedure which cures. The
repair of broken tissue.

health (*helth*). A state of
well-being with mind and
body functioning at their
optimum.

heart. The muscular organ
which pumps the blood
through the system. The
heart is situated behind the
sternum, rather to the left,
the apex of the heart being
under the left breast. If the
ear or a stethoscope be
placed over a healthy heart, a
dull thudding sound is heard,
immediately followed by a
short, sharper, crisper sound;
a short pause follows, and
then the two sounds occur
again. Each pair of sounds
corresponds to one beat of
the heart. *See* DIASTOLE and

SYSTOLE. The heart consists
of four chambers, the right
and left atria and the right
and left ventricles. The
chambers are lined with the
endocardium. Folds of
endocardium form the valves
of the heart. The heart is
enclosed in a membranous
sac, the pericardium. *See* CIR-
CULATION.

heart block. State of partial or
complete prevention of the
passage of the cardiac
impulse through the atrio-
ventricular bundle. It is
characterized by an
extremely slow heart beat
and pulse. *See also* ECG.

heartburn. Burning sensation
at lower end of the
oesophagus, due to acid regurgitation from the stomach.

heart-lung machine. Machine
used in cardiac surgery to
oxygenate the blood.

heat exhaustion (*ek-saws-tyon*).
Condition caused by great
heat when patient has rapid
pulse, dyspnoea and abdominal cramp due to excessive
sweating and loss of sodium
chloride.

heatstroke. Hyperpyrexia due
to failure of temperature-
regulating mechanisms of the
body. Caused by extreme
heat.

hebephrenia (*he-bē-frē-ni-a*).
A form of schizophrenia

sometimes found in young adults.

Heberden's disease (*he-ber-dens*). Generalized form of osteo-arthritis in which there is symmetrical involvement of joints of the hands, knees, jaw and spine. It occurs in postmenopausal women and is characterized by osteo-phytes on the dorsal surface of the terminal phalanges (Heberden's nodes).

Heberden's nodes. Small bony nodules which form at the sides of the finger joints in osteo-arthritis.

hedonism (*hē-do-nism*). Excessive devotion to pleasure.

Hegar's dilators (*hā'-garz*). A series of graduated metal bougies for dilating the cervix and uterus.

Hegar's sign (*hā'-garz*). Spongy feel of the cervix in pregnancy.

helium (*hē'-lē-um*). An inert gas used in certain respiratory tests.

helix (*hē'-liks*). Spiral. Used to describe the configuration of certain molecules, *e.g.* DNA and also the outer rim of the external ear.

Heller's operation. Division of muscle between stomach and oesophagus in cases of dysphagia in cardiospasm.

helminthagogue (*hel-min'-tha-*

gog). Medicine to expel worms.

helminthiasis (*hel-min-thī-a-sis*). Infestation with worms.

helminthology (*hel-min-tho'-lo-ji*). The study of worms.

hemeralopia (*he-me-ra-lō'-pi-a*). Partial blindness; patient can only see in broad daylight.

hemi. Prefix meaning half.

hemianopia (*he-mi-an-ō'-pi-a*). Loss of sight in half of the visual field.

hemiatrophy (*he-mi-at'-ro-fi*). Atrophy of one side of the body only.

hemiballismus (*he-mi-ba-lis-mus*).Violent, flinging sort of involuntary movement due to disease of the basal ganglia.

hemicolectomy (*he-mi-kō-lek-to-mi*). Surgical removal of half the colon, thus right or left hemicolectomy.

hemicrania (*he-mi-krā-ni-a*). Headache on one side of the head. Migraine.

hemiparesis (*he-mi-pa-rē-sis*). Paralysis of one side of the body.

hemiplegia (*hem-i-plē'-ji-a*). Paralysis of one side of the body. The lesion is in the opposite side of the brain.

hemispheres (*hem'-i-sfārs*). Usually cerebral hemispheres, the two sides of the forebrain.

Henoch's purpura (*he-noks per-pū-ra*). A syndrome caused by sensitivity reaction of the vascular endothelium. Blood leaks out of the damaged vessels causing purpuric spots in the skin and other variable symptoms according to which organs are affected. In the *Henoch type* there is abdominal pain; the *Schönlein type* is associated with joint involvement. Often both types co-exist.

hepar. The liver.

heparin (*hep'-ar-in*). An anticoagulant derived from liver tissue. Given by intravenous or subcutaneous injection in doses based on laboratory determinations of patient's blood-clotting time.

hepatectomy (*he-pa-tek-to-mi*). Excision of the whole (in animals) or part of the liver.

hepatic (*he-pat'-ik*). Relating to the liver.

hepatic flexure. The right bend of the colon, under the liver.

hepaticostomy (*he-pa-ti-kos-to-mi*). Operation to make a fistula in the hepatic duct.

hepatitis (*hep-a-tī'-tis*). Inflammation of the liver.

hepatization (*hep-at-īz-ā'-shon*). Conversion into a liver-like substance. A term used to describe the lungs in lobar pneumonia when consolidation occurs.

hepatocele (*hep'-at-ō-sēl*). Hernia containing hepatic tissue.

hepatoma (*hep-at-ō'-ma*). Neoplasm of liver cells.

hepatomegaly (*he-pa-tō-me-ga-li*). An enlarged liver.

hereditary (*he-red'-i-ta-ri*). Transmitted from one's ancestors.

heredity (*he-re-di-ti*). The transmission of genetic characteristics.

hermaphrodite (*her-maf'-rō-dīt*). Abnormality of development in which an individual has tissue capable of producing both male and female gametes. It is associated with ambiguity of secondary sexual characteristics and the individual is generally sterile.

hernia (*her'-nē-a*). Rupture. Protrusion of an organ from its normal position, most common in the case of the bowels. *Inguinal hernia* is through the inguinal canal. *Femoral* through the femoral ring. *Strangulated*, so tightly constricted that gangrene and acute intestinal obstruction results if operation does not relieve. *Scrotal* is hernia descending into the scrotum, and *umbilical* is hernia at the navel. A hernia not amenable to manipulation is termed *irreducible*. If the blood supply to this is interfered with it is termed strangulated. *Hernia cerebri* is protrusion of the brain through a wound in the skull. *Ventral h.*, of the ventral surface of the body such as an umbilical or incisional H., the latter is through an old scar.

hernioplasty (*her-nē-ō-plas-ti*). Operation for hernia when the weak structures are repaired.

herniorrhaphy (*her-ni-or-ra-fi*). Operation to repair a hernia.

herniotomy (*her-ni-ot'-o-mi*). Dividing the constricting band of a strangulated hernia and returning the protruding part.

herpes (*her'-pēz*). Vesicular eruption due to infection by a virus. *H. simplex* virus may reside in epidermal cells without causing any reaction, but under certain circumstances, *e.g.* associated with a cold, an immunological reaction to the virus occurs with blistering and ulceration of the skin known as 'cold sores'. *H. zoster* virus is closely related to, if not identical with, the chickenpox virus and attacks sensory nerves producing pain and vesiculation in the distribution of the nerves (shingles).

Herxheimer reaction (*herks-hī-mer re-ak-shon*). Exacer-

bation of syphilitic lesions for a short period following the commencement of penicillin therapy.

hetero-. Prefix meaning unlike.

heterogeneous (*het-er-ō-jē'-ne-us*). Differing in kind or in nature.

heterogeneous vaccine. Made from some source other than the patient's own organisms; usually from a stock laboratory culture. Opposite to *autogenous*.

heterologous (*he-te-ro'-lo-gus*). Derived from a different species.

heterophoria (*he-te-rō-fo'-ri-a*). Latent squint. A squint which develops only when the patient is tired or in ill health.

heteroplasty (*he-te-rō-plas'-ti*). In plastic surgery when the graft is taken from another person and not from another part of the patient's body.

heterosexual (*he-te-rō-sek-sū-al*). Normal relationship between male and female.

heterotropia (*he-te-rō-trō'-pi-a*). Squint.

hexachlorophane (*hek-sa-klo-rō-fān*). Non-irritant bactericide which can be used in soaps and creams.

Hg. Chemical symbol for mercury.

hiatus (*hī-ā-tus*). An opening or space. *H. hernia*. Hernia of the stomach through the diaphragm at the oesophageal opening.

hibernation (*hī-ber-nā-shon*). To pass the winter in a sleeping state as *e.g.* the tortoise. *Artificial h.* The body temperature is lowered by applying cold externally, to reduce oxygen requirements and to aid as an anaesthetic. *See* HYPOTHERMIA.

Hibitane (*hi-bi-tān*). Proprietary preparation of chlorhexidine diacetate.

hiccup, hiccough (*hi'-kup*). Repeated spasmodic inspiration associated with sudden closure of the glottis which gives rise to the characteristic 'hic' sound. It may be produced by irritation of the diaphragm but in most cases the cause is unknown.

hidradenitis (*hī-drad-en-ī'-tis*). A staphylococcal infection of the skin, occurring usually in the axillae.

hidrosis (*hī-drō'-sis*). Sweating.

Higginson's syringe The ordinary india-rubber syringe, consisting of two tubes, a bulb and valves to maintain flow in one direction only.

hilar (*hī-la*). Relating to the hilum.

hilum (*hī-lum*). Site at which the pedicle of an organ is attached.

hindbrain (*hīnd-brān*). Embry-

ological component which becomes the medulla and cerebellum.

hip. Upper part of thigh where it joins the pelvis.

hip joint. Ball and socket joint between the head of the femur and the acetabulum. *Congenital dislocation of h.j.* Abnormality of development in which the head of the femur does not articulate with the acetabulum. The condition is almost always preventible if recognised within a few days of birth.

Hippocrates (*hip-pok'-ra-tēz*). A Greek physician who lived about 400 B.C. He is the father of modern medicine.

Hirschsprung's disease (*her-sproongz di-zēz*). Developmental abnormality in which there is a defect in the nerve supply to part of the terminal colon which causes an obstruction and results in dilation and hypertrophy of the more proximal segment (congenital megacolon).

hirsute (*her-sūt*). Hairy.

hirsuties (*her-sū-tēs*). Abnormal growth of hair.

hirudo (*hi-roo-dō*). Leech.

His, bundle of. *See* ATRIO-VENTRICULAR BUNDLE.

histamine (*his'-tam-ēn*). An organic base which is released from tissues, esp. mast cells, following injury. It increases the permeability of blood cells and thus initiates the inflammatory reaction.

histidine. *See* AMINO-ACIDS.

histiocyte (*his-ti-ō-sīt*). Connective tissue cell.

histology (*his-tol'-o-ji*). The morphological study of tissues.

histolysis (*his-to-li-sis*). Disintegration of organic tissue.

hives (*hīvs*). Urticaria.

hobnail liver. A liver whose surface is rendered irregular by cirrhosis. A form of CIR-RHOSIS.

Hodge. *See* PESSARY.

Hodgkin's disease. *See* LYM-PHADENOMA.

Hogben's test (*hog-bens test*). A pregnancy test in which the patient's urine is injected into a toad. Now obsolete.

Holger Nielsen method. Method of artificial respiration.

Homan's sign (*hō-mans sīn*). Physical sign of deep vein thrombosis in the leg. Pain is felt in the calf when the toes are dorsiflexed.

homeo, homoeo (*ho-mē-ō*). Prefix meaning similar.

homeostasis (*ho-mē-ō-stā'-sis*). Maintenance of a stable system.

homeothermic (*hō-mē-o-ther-mik*). Term applied to animal when body heat is kept constant regardless of the environment.

homicide (*hom-i'-sīd*). Killing a person.

homoeopathy (*hō-mē-op'-a-thi*). Medicine worked on the system of cures such as those started by Hahnemann. Homoeopathic medicines are mostly given in infinitesimal doses.

homogeneous (*hō-mō-jē'-ne-us*). Of the same kind. Uniform.

homogenized (*hō-mo-je-nizd*). Term applied to substance made into the same consisteney throughout, *e.g.* milk which has its fat evenly distributed.

homolateral (*hō-mō-la'-ter-al*). Relating to the same side.

homologous (*ho-mo'-lō-gus*). Of the same type. Identical in structure.

homosexuality (*ho-mō-sek-sū-a'-li-ti*). A psychological abnormality in which sexual attraction is towards persons of the same sex.

hookworm. *See* ANKYLOSTOMA.

hordeolum (*hor-dē-ō'-lum*). A stye on the eyelid.

hormone (*hor'-mōn*). A substance produced in an endocrine organ which excites functional activity in another organ.

Horner's syndrome (*sin'-drōm*). Unilateral small pupil, ptosis and vasodilation of the cheek with absence of sweating, due to damage to the sympathetic nerves in the neck.

horseshoe kidney. The most important of all serious forms of congenital abnormality of the kidney. The two kidneys are united at their lower poles and form a horseshoe mass generally at a lower level than normal. Possible cause of urinary infection.

Horton's syndrome (*haw-tons sin'-drōm*). Release of histamine in the body causing severe headache.

host (*hōst*). Organism on which a parasite lives.

hourglass contraction. A complication of the third stage of labour, seen especially after prolonged and difficult first and second stages. Postpartum haemorrhage is not uncommonly the result of this condition.

hourglass stomach. A stomach divided by a constriction or spasm into two separate cavities seen after a barium meal x-ray. It may be due to a temporary spasm or the result of fibrosis of a gastric ulcer.

house fly (*hows flī*). The common fly. Latin name, Musca domestica.

housemaid's knee. Inflammation of the bursa patellae, caused by constant kneeling on hard substances. *See* PATELLAR BURSAE.

Houston's folds (*hoos-tonz*). Three oblique folds in the mucous membrane of the rectum.

humanized milk. Cow's milk with reduced fat and increased sugar.

humerus (*hū'-me-rus*). The bone of the upper arm.

humidity (*hū-mid'-it-i*). Moisture. State of being moist.

humour (*hū'-mur*). Any fluid of the body other than blood. *See* VITREOUS HUMOUR.

hunger pain. A symptom of peptic or duodenal ulcer. The pain is relieved on eating.

Huntington's chorea (*ko-rē'-a*). Chronic, progressive chorea. The disease is hereditary.

Hurler's syndrome (*her-lers sin'-drōm*). *See* GARGOYLISM.

Hutchinson's teeth. A condition of the upper central permanent incisors: the cutting edge is smaller than the base, and therefore the teeth are peg-shaped. The edge is deeply notched, a sign of congenital syphilis.

hyaline (*hī'-a-lin*). Transparent like glass. Hyaline cartilage is smooth and pearly. It covers the articular surfaces of bones.

hyaline membrane. Eosinophilic material found in the air passages of the newborn.

It is probably derived from amniotic fluid and may cause collapse of the lungs in the so-called 'pulmonary syndrome of the newborn'. The primary cause, however, is failure of the pulmonary circulation.

hyalitis (*hī-al-ī-tis*). Inflammation of the vitreous humour or the hyaloid membrane of the eye.

hyaloid membrane (*hī'-a-loyd mem'-brān*). The glassy membrane which encloses the vitreous humour of the eye.

hyaluronidase (*hī-al-yūr-on-i-dāz*). An enzyme which, when injected subcutaneously, promotes absorption: in an injection, 500 units aid absorption of 500ml injection solution.

hybrid (*hī-brid*). Offspring resulting from gametes which are genetically unlike.

hydatid (*hī-dat'-id*). Cyst formed by the larvae of certain tapeworms.

hydatidiform mole (*hī-dat-id'-if-orm*). *See* MOLE.

hydragogue (*hī'-dra-gog*). Substance which attracts water, *i.e.* it is osmotically active.

hydramnios (*hī-dram'-nē-os*). Excess of amniotic fluid.

hydrargyrum (*hī-drar'-ji-rum*). Mercury. Symbol Hg.

hydrathrosis (*hī-drar-thrō'-sis*). Accumulation of fluid in a joint, most common in the knee.

hydrate (*hī-drāt*). A chemical compound of a base with water.

hydro (*hī-drō*). Prefix referring to water or hydrogen.

hydroa (*hī-drō-a*). A skin disease causing watery blisters to arise.

hydrocarbon (*hī-drō-kar'-bon*). A compound formed of hydrogen and carbon.

hydrocele (*hī'-drō-sēl*). Swelling containing clear fluid. Most often applied to watery swelling of scrotum.

hydrocephalus (*hī-drō-kef'-a-lus*). A rare congenital disease seen in children. The sutures of the skull do not unite, the cerebrospinal fluid increases, causing the head to swell to an enormous size; often mental symptoms. *Acute h.* Distension of the ventricles, due to a cerebral tumour or meningitis.

hydrochloric acid (*hī-drō-klo'-rik as-id*). Normal constituent of gastric juice: therefore a dilute solution is given when there is a deficiency.

hydrocortisone (*hī-drō-kor'-ti-zōn*). One of the adrenocortical hormones, similar in action to, but more powerful than, cortisone.

hydrogen (*hī'-drō-jen*). A colourless inflammable gas combined with oxygen in the proportions of H_2O forms water.

hydrogen peroxide. H_2O_2. A valuable non-irritating and non-poisonous antiseptic. It effervesces in the presence of pus due to the liberation of oxygen. Usual strength 10 volumes, *i.e.* it contains ten times its volume of available oxygen.

hydrolysis (*hī-drol'-i-sis*). Breakdown of complex substance(s) with the addition of water to give simpler substances.

hydroma (*hī-drō'-ma*). Watery swelling of a limb.

hydrometer (*hī-drom'-e-ter*). An instrument for determining the specific gravities of liquids.

hydrometria (*hī-drō-mē-tri-a*). Abnormal collection of mucus or watery fluid in the uterus.

hydronephrosis (*hī-drō-nef-rō'-sis*). Distension of the pelvis and calyces of the kidney due to obstruction to the ureter. Prolonged back-pressure results in atrophy of the renal substance.

hydropathic (*hī-drō-path'-ik*). Relating to cure by means of water; as by baths.

hydropericardium (*hī-drō-pe-ri-kar'-dē-um*). Fluid in the pericardial sac, *i.e.* pericardial effusion.

hydroperitoneum (*hī-drō-pe-ri-tō-nē'-um*). Peritoneal effusion, *i.e.* ascites.

hydrophobia (*hī-drō-fō'-bi-a*). Rabies. An acute infectious disease contracted from the bite of a rabid dog and accompanied by peculiar mental disturbance. The saliva of a hydrophobia patient is capable of conveying infection.

hydropneumothorax (*hī-drō-nū'-mō-tho-raks*). Fluid and air in the pleural cavity.

hydrops (*hī-drops*). Oedema. *H. fetalis.* Generalized oedema associated with severe haemolytic anaemia in the fetus due to Rhesus incompatibility.

hydrorrhachis (*hī-dror'-a-kis*). Abnormal accumulation of cerebrospinal fluid in the spinal canal.

hydrosalpinx (*hī-drō-sal'-pinx*). Distension of the Fallopian tube by clear fluid.

hydrotherapy. Treatment of disease by the use of water.

hydrothorax (*hī-drō-thaw'-rax*). Fluid in the cavity of the chest.

hydroxyl (*hī-drok-sil*). OH group. The chemical group of one hydrogen atom and one oxygen atom.

hygiene (*hī'-jēn*). The science of the maintenance of health.

hygroma (*hī-grō'-ma*). Cyst in the neck resulting from abnormal development of the lymphatic system.

hygrometer (*hī-grom'-et-er*). An instrument for measuring the moisture in the atmosphere.

hygrosopic (*hī-gro-skop'-ik*). Having the property of absorbing moisture, *e.g.* glycerin.

hymen (*hī'-men*). A fold of membrane at the entrance to the vagina.

hymenotomy (*hī-me-no-to-mi*). Incision of the hymen to increase size of vaginal opening.

hyoid (*hī'-oyd*). Shaped like a V; the name of a bone at the root of the tongue.

hypaemia (*hī-pē'-mi-a*). Lack of blood in a part.

hyper (*hī-per*). A prefix denoting excessive, above, or increased.

hyperacidity (*hī-per-as-id'-it-i*). Undue concentration of acid, as in the gastric juice in some cases of ulcer of the stomach (*hyperchlorhydria*).

hyperactivity (*hī-per-ak-ti-vi-ti*). Over-activity.

hyperaemia (*hī-per-ē'-mi-a*). Excess of blood in a part.

hyperaesthesia (*hī-per-es-thē'-zi-a*). Excess of sensitiveness in a part.

hyperalgesia (*hī-per-al-jē'-si-a*). Excessive sensibility to pain.

hyperasthenia (*hī-pe-ras-thē-ni-a*) Great weakness.

hyperbaric (*hī-per-ba-rik*). Term applied to a gas at greater pressure than normal, *e.g.* H. Oxygen chamber.

hypercalcaemia (*hī-per-kal-sē'-mi-a*). Increase of calcium in the blood.

hypercapnia (*hī-per-kap'-ni-a*). Excess of carbon dioxide in the blood.

hyperchlorhydria (*hī-per-klor-hī'-dri-a*). Excess of hydrochloric acid in the gastric juice.

hyperchromia (*hī-per-krō-mi-a*). Excessively coloured.

hyperemesis (*hī-per-em'-e-sis*). Excessive vomiting. *H. gravidarum*, of pregnancy.

hyperextension (*hī-per-eks-ten-shon*). Over-extension, *e.g.* of a joint.

hyperflexion (*hī-per-flek-shon*). Over-flexion.

hyperglycaemia (*hī-per-glī-sē'mi-a*). Excessive sugar in the blood; occurs in diabetes mellitus.

hyperhidrosis (*hī-per-hī-drō'-sis*). Excess of perspiration.

hyperkeratoses (*hī-per-ke-ra-tō'-sēz*). Callosities and corns of the skin.

hyperkinesis (*hī-per-kī-nē-sis*). Excessive movement.

hypermetropia (*hī-per-me-trō'-pi-a*). Long-sight, a visual affection. The opposite of myopia. Corrected by wearing a biconvex lens.

hypermnesia (*hī-perm-nē'-zi-a*). An exaggeration of memory involving minute details of a past experience. It may occur in mentally unstable individuals after a shock.

hypermotility (*hī-per-mō-ti-li-ti*). Increased motor activity.

hypermyotonia (*hī-per-mī-ō-tō-ni-a*). Increase in muscle tone.

hypernephroma (*hī-per-ne-frō'-ma*). Malignant tumour of kidney also called Grawitz's tumour.

hyperonychia (*hī-per-ō-ni-ki-a*). Thickening of the nails.

hyperostosis (*hī-per-os-tō'-sis*). Hypertrophy of bony tissue.

hyperparathyroidism (*hī-per-par-a-thī'-royd-izm*). Excessive secretion of the parathyroid glands.

hyperphagia (*hī-per-fā-ji-a*). Eating to excess.

hyperphoria (*hī-per-fo-ri-a*). Elevation of one visual axis above the other.

hyperpiesis (*hī-per-pī-ēs'-is*). Abnormally high blood pressure. *See* HYPERTENSION.

hyperpituitarism (*hī-per-pit-ū'-it-ar-izm*). Over-activity of the pituitary gland. Occurring in childhood the patient becomes a giant; in adult life, acromegaly develops.

hyperplasia (*hī-per-plā'-sē-a*). Excessive growth of tissue.

hyperpnoea (*hī-per-pnē'-a*). Respirations increased in rate and depth: a symptom of uraemia.

hyperpyrexia (*hī-per-pī-rek'-si-a*). High fever, arbitrarily above 105° F. or 41° C.

hypersecretion (*hī-per-se-krē'-shon*). Excessive secretion.

hypersensitive (*hī-per-sen-si-tiv*). Abnormally sensitive, *e.g.* to certain foodstuffs.

hypertensin (*hī-per-ten-sin*). Angiotensin.

hypertension (*hī-per-ten-'shon*). Blood pressure above the normal limits, *i.e.* above 140/95 resting BP. Hypertension may be *primary* or *essential*, *i.e.* cause unknown, or *secondary* to artery obstruction, renal disease, endocrine disturbances and other factors.

hyperthermia (*hī-per-ther-mi-a*). Raised body temperature.

hyperthymia (*hī-per-thī-mi-a*). An overactive state of mind with a tendency to perform impulsive actions.

hyperthyroidism (*hī-per-thī'-roy-dism*). Excessive secretion of thyroid hormones.

hypertonia (*hī-per-tō'-ni-a*). Excessive tonicity, as in a muscle or an artery.

hypertonic (*hī-per-to'-nik*). High tone. (1) Increased tone of muscle. (1) Having a higher osmotic pressure than body fluids, *cf.* isotonic, hypotonic saline.

hypertrichosis (*hī-per-trik-ō'-sis*). Excessive growth of hair, or growth of hair in unusual places.

hypertrophy (*hī-per'-tro-fi*). Increase in size in response to demand on the structure, *cf.* hyperplasia.

hyperventilation (*hī-per-ven-ti-lā-shon*). Overbreathing.

hypnosis (*hip-nō'-sis*). Condition resembling sleep in which conscious control of behaviour is reduced. The state is brought about voluntarily in the subject by suggestion.

hypnotic (*hip-not'-ik*). (1) Relating to hypnotism. (2) Drug producing sleep.

hypnotism (*hip-nō'-tism*). Practice of hypnosis.

hypo (*hī-pō*). Prefix denoting below.

hypoaesthesia (*hī-pō-ēs-thē-si-a*). Diminished sense of feeling in a part.

hypocalcaemia (*hī-pō-kal-sē-mi-a*). Diminished amount of blood calcium.

hypochlorhydria (*hī-pō-klor-hī'-dri-a*). Deficiency of hydrochloric acid in the gastric juice.

hypochlorite (*hī-pō-klo'-rit*). A salt of hypochlorous acid. Sodium hypochlorite is used in the treatment of wounds, burns, and the disinfection of food utensils. Sensitive to ultraviolet light, therefore store in brown bottles.

hypochondria (*hī-pō-kon'-dri-a*). An anxiety state about health, the patient suffering from many imaginary ills.

hypochondriac (*hī-pō-kon'-dri-ak*). Person suffering from hypochondria.

hypochondrium (*hī-pō-kon'-drē-um*). Surface anatomy nomenclature relating to the region of the anterior abdominal wall beneath the ribs.

hypochromic (*hī-pō-krō'-mik*). With decreased pigmentation.

hypodermic (*hī-pō-der'-mik*). Below the skin; subcutaneous.

hypogastric (*hī-pō-gas'-trik*). Pertaining to the hypogastrium.

hypogastrium (*hīp-ō-gas'-trium*). Term applied to the region of the abdomen just below the umbilicus. *See* ABDOMEN.

hypoglossal (*hī-pō-glos'-al*). Situated under the tongue. The motor nerve of the tongue, situated under it towards the back.

hypoglycaemia (*hī-pō-glī-sē-mi-a*). Deficiency of sugar in the blood.

hypokalaemia (*hī-pō-ka-lē-mi-a*). Deficiency of potassium in the blood.

hypomania (*hī-pō-mā-ni-a*). Mild form of the affective disorder, mania, in which there is abnormal elation of mood and great energy.

hypomotility (*hī-pō-mō-ti-li-ti*). Decreased movement.

hypoparathyroidism (*hī-pō-pa-ra-thī-roy-dism*). Diminished function of parathyroid glands.

hypophoria (*hī-pō-fo'-ri-a*). Depression of one visual axis below the other.

hypophosphatasia (*hī-pō-fos-fa-tā-si-a*). Inherited deficiency of alkaline phosphatase in the bone cells. As a result there is a failure of the bones to calcify adequately and the serum calcium concentration may rise and there may be anorexia, vomiting and wasting. The amount of alkaline phosphatase in the serum is greatly reduced.

hypophysectomy (*hī-pō-fis-ek-to-mi*). Operation to remove the pituitary gland.

hypophysis cerebri (*hī-po-fi-sis se-re-brē*). Pituitary gland.

hypopiesis (*hī-po-pī-ē'-sis*). *See* HYPOTENSION.

hypopituitarism (*hī-pō-pi-tū'-it-a-rism*). Condition resulting from insufficiency of pituitary secretion.

hypoplasia (*hī-pō-plā'-zi-a*). Tendency to grow to a size smaller than normal.

hypoproteinaemia (*hī-pō-prō-ti-nē-mi-a*). Too little protein in the blood.

hypopyon (*hī-pō'-pi-on*). Pus in the anterior chamber of the eye.

hyposecretion (*hī-pō-se-krē'-shon*). Too little secretion.

hypospadias (*hī-pō-spā'-dē-as*). Malformation of lower wall of the urethra, so that the urethra opens on the under-surface of the penis.

hypostasis (*hī-po-stā-sis*). Deposit: passive congestion.

hypostatic pneumonia (*hī-pō-stat'-ik*). Due to congestion at bases of lungs, often caused by immobility especially in patients confined to bed.

hypotension (*hī-pō-ten-shon*). Low blood pressure.

hypotensive drug (*hī-pō-ten-siv*). Term applied to drug which lowers the blood pressure.

hypothalamus (*hī-pō-thal-a-mus*). A special area of grey matter in the floor of the third ventricle of the brain. Linked with the pituitary gland and also with the thalamus and the autonomic nervous system.

hypothenar eminence. Prominence on the palm below the little finger.

hypothermia (*hī-pō-ther-mi-a*). State of being abnormally cold. *Artificial h.* Technique used in conjunction with major heart surgery, etc., in which the blood is cooled by passing it through a heat exchanger. The body temperature is lowered to about 85° F (29·5° C) at which level the oxygen requirements of tissues, especially the brain cells, are greatly reduced. This enables the circulation to be stopped for a time.

hypothesis (*hī-po'-the-sis*). A suggested explanation of some happening.

hypothrombinaemia (*hī-pō-throm-bi-nē-mi-a*). Deficiency of thrombin in the blood.

hypothyroidism (*hī-pō-thī'-roy-dism*). Insufficiency of thyroid secretion.

hypotonia. Deficient tone.

hypotonic (*hī-pō-to-nik*). (1) Lacking in tone. (2) Of salt solution: having an osmotic pressure less than that of physiological saline (0·9 per cent NaCl). *Cf.* hypertonic.

hypovitaminosis (*hī-pō-vi-ta-mi-nō-sis*). Suffering from lack of vitamins in food intake.

hypoxia (*hī-pok-si-a*). Lacking oxygen.

hystera (*his'-te-ra*). The uterus or womb.

hysterectomy (*his-ter-ek'-to-mi*). Removal of the womb by operation. *Sub-total hysterectomy* is removal of all the womb except the cervix. *Pan h.*, total hysterectomy. *Vaginal h.*, womb removed per vaginam.

hysteria (*his-tā'-ri-a*). A functional neurosis in which there is a reaction, never fully conscious on the part of the patient, to obtain relief from stress by the exhibition and experience of symptoms of illness.

hysterical (*his-te-ri-kal*). Relating to hysteria.

hysterocele (*his'-ter-ō-sēl*). Hernia involving the uterus.

hysteromyoma (*his-te-rō-mī-ō-ma*). Uterine fibroid.

hysteromyomectomy (*his-te-rō-mī-ō-mek-to-mi*). Surgical removal of a uterine fibroid.

hysteropexy (*his-te-ro-pek'-si*). Suturing of the uterus to the abdominal wall to prevent prolapse.

hysteroptosis (*his-ter-op-tō'-sis*). Uterine prolapse.

hysterosalpingography (*his-te-rō-sal-pin-gō-gra-fi*). X-ray examination of the uterus and the Fallopian tubes following the introduction of a contrast medium.

hysterotomy (*his-ter-ot'-o-mi*). Incision into the uterus. The term usually excludes caesarean section.

hysterotrachelorrhaphy (*his-ter-o-trak-el-or'-raf-fi*). Repair of a lacerated cervix uteri.

I

I. Symbol for iodine.

iasis. Suffix used to denote a resulting condition, *e.g.* ankylostomiasis as a result of infection with Ankylostoma duodenale.

ice (*is*). The solid state of water when temperature is lowered to 0° C (32° F). As the water freezes it expands. *I. compress* and *I. poultice* may be used to treat bruises and arrest haemorrhage.

ichthyosis (*ik-thi-ō'-sis*). Inherited defect of keratinization in which the skin is dry and scaly. The so-called acquired ichthyosis is similar in appearance but due to defective nutrition.

icterus (*ik'-ter-us*). Jaundice.

icterus neonatorum (*ik'-ter-us nē-ō-nā-tor'-um*). Jaundice of the new-born child. A slight degree of jaundice is not uncommon a few days after birth, and has no special significance; but serious and fatal cases also arise from umbilical sepsis, haemolytic disease of the newborn, and other causes. *See* JAUNDICE.

id. Unconscious part of personality containing the instinctive impulses.

idea (*i-dēr*). A mental image.

ideation (*ī-dē-ā-shon*). Capacity to form and grasp ideas.

idée fixe (*ē-dā fiks*). One idea dominates all others; a delusion.

identical twins. Twins of the same sex and originating from the same ovum.

identification (*ī-den-ti-fi-kā-shon*). (1) Recognition. (2) Psychiatric emotional attachment to an individual resulting in transposition of behaviour characteristics.

ideo-motor (*i-de-o-mō'-tor*). The association of movement with an idea. Psychologically it is rather like an obsession: an idea that leads to action against the will of the person.

idiocy (*id'-i-o-sē*). Severe mental subnormality. The term has been obsolete since the Mental Health Act of 1959.

177

idiopathic (*id-i-ō-path'-ik*). Without apparent cause.

idiosyncrasy (*id-i-ō-sin'-kra-si*). Individual character or property. Generally used in connection with unusual or unexpected response to drugs.

ileectomy (*ī-lē-ek-tom-i*). Excision of the ileum.

ileitis (*ī-lē-ī-tis*). Inflammation of the ileum. *Regional i.*, Crohn's disease. Characterized by localized regions of non-specific chronic inflammation of the terminal portion of the ileum. Occasionally other parts of the intestine are ,also affected. The cause is not known.

ileocaecal valve (*il'-e-ō-sē'-kal*). Valve at the junction of the large and small intestines.

ileocolitis (*il-ē-ō-ko-lī-tis*). Inflammation of the ileum and colon. A condition not uncommon in children.

ileocolostomy (*il-ē-ō-ko-los'-to-mi*). Surgical anastomosis between the ileum and the colon.

ileoproctostomy (*ī-lē-ō-prok-tos-to-mi*). Operation when the ileum is joined to the rectum.

ileo-rectal (*i'-lē-ō-rek'-tal*). Relating to the ileum and the rectum.

ileosigmoidostomy (*il-ē-ō-sig-moy-dos'-to-mi*). Implantation of the small intestine into the sigmoid flexure.

ileostomy (*i-lē-os-to-mi*). An opening is made into the ileum for the discharge of intestinal contents, thereby bypassing the large bowel.

ileum (*il'-e-um*). The lower portion of the small intestine between the jejunum and caecum. *See* BOWEL.

ileus (*īl'-e-us*). Obstruction of the bowel. Paralytic ileus caused by local inflammation affecting the nerve supply. It may be a complication of abdominal operations, particularly if the bowel has been extensively handled. It may be due to peritonitis.

iliac crest. The highest portion of the ilium. The greatest width from one iliac crest to the other of a normal female adult pelvis should be 27·9 to 29·2cm and should be at least 2·5cm greater than that between the iliac spines.

iliac region. The regions of the abdomen in the neighbourhood of the iliac bones.

iliac spine. The tubercle at the anterior end of the iliac crest.

iliococcygeal (*i-li-ō-kok-si-jē-al*). Relating to the ilium and the coccyx, *e.g.* iliococcygeal ligament: ligament passing between the ilium and coccyx.

iliopsoas (*i-li-ō-sō-as*). The psoas and iliacus muscles.

ilium (*il'-i-um*). The upper part of the innominate bone.

illegitimacy (*i-lej-it-i-ma-si*). Born out of wedlock.

illusion (*il-lū'-zhon*). A deceptive appearance. The misinterpretation of a sensory image.

image. A mental picture of an external object.

imago (*i-mah-gō*). Fantasy woven around someone loved in childhood.

imbalance (*im-ba-lans*). Lack of balance.

imbecility (*im-be-si'-li-ti*). A marked degree of mental incapacity. Obsolete term.

immiscible (*i-mi-ski-bel*). Cannot be mixed together.

immobility (*im-ō-bil'-it-i*). The state of being fixed.

immune (*i-mūn*). Protected against a particular disease as by inoculation.

immunity. State of resistance to infection due to the presence of antibodies capable of combining with antigen(s) carried by the infecting organism and thus damaging the invader or neutralizing enzymes or toxins released by the organism. As well as viruses, bacteria and other parasites the body regards cells from a different individual, *i.e.* different genotype, as infecting organisms. Hence the difficulties of homo-grafting kidneys. In a wider, and less common, usage of the term, immunity applies to all mechanisms, such as impermeability of the skin, antiseptic properties of sebum, disinfection of food by stomach acid, etc., which enable the body to resist infection.

immunization (*im-mū-ni-zā-shon*). Process of increasing the state of immunity, either by contact with the infecting organism or some variant of it which is *Active i.* In *passive i.* there is receipt of an antibody. Active immunization is the principle behind vaccination against smallpox, inoculation against diphtheria, tetanus etc. Passive immunization is temporary. The fetus is passively immunized by antibodies from the maternal blood enabling the new-born baby to resist infection for about six weeks after birth.

immunology (*i-mū-no-lo-ji*). The study of immunity.

immunosuppression (*i-mū-nō-su-pre'-shon*). Deliberate inhibition of normal immune response, especially to permit successful organ grafting.

impaction (*im-pak'-shon*). Wedging or jamming

together, *e.g. impacted fracture* where the bony fragments are jammed together.

impalpable (*im-pal'-pa-bl*). Not capable of being felt.

imperforate (*im-per-'fo-rāt*). Completely closed. *See* ANUS.

impetigo (*im-pe-tī'-gō*). A skin rash of an acute kind, generally a streptococcal and staphylococcal infection. It is contagious.

implantation. The act of setting in; grafting.

implants (*im-plunz*). Pellets of drugs such as testosterone which are inserted under the skin from where they are slowly absorbed.

impotence (*im'-pō-tens*). Absence of power or desire for sexual intercourse.

impregnation (*im-preg-nā'-shon*). The fertilization of an ovum by a spermatozoon. Permeation.

impulse (*im-puls*). A sudden driving force.

inaccessible (*in-ak-se-sibl*). Term applied to a patient with whose mind no contact can be made.

inactivate (*in-ak-ti-vāt*). To destroy activity.

inanition (*in-a-nish'-un*). Exhaustion from want of food.

inarticulate (*in-ar-tik'-ū-lāt*). (1) Without joints. (2) Unable to speak clearly.

incarcerated (*in-kar-se-rā-ted*). Imprisoned. Term applied to a hernia which cannot be reduced, or to a gravid uterus which cannot rise from the pelvis.

incest (*in'-sest*). Sexual intercourse between near relatives.

incidence (*in-si-denz*). Occurrence, such as of a disease.

incipient (*in-si'-pi-ent*). Beginning.

incision (*in-si-zhon*). Act of cutting into with a sharp instrument.

incisors (*in-si'-sers*). Chisel-shaped cutting teeth at the front of the mouth.

inclusion bodies (*in-klus-yon bo-dis*). Intracellular bodies found esp, in affected tissues in virus diseases.

incoherent (*in-kō-hā-rent*). Disconnected. Inconsequent.

incompatible (*in-kom-pa'-tibl*). Not capable of association. Especially applied to drugs which cannot be compounded in the same mixture.

incompetence (*in-kom'-pe-tenz*). Incapable of natural function, *e.g.* aortic incompetence in which the aortic valve of the heart does not close adequately with the result that blood leaks back into the left ventricle.

incontinence (*in-kon'-ti-nens*).

Absence of voluntary control over the passing of urine or faeces.

incoordination (*in-kō-or-din-ā'-shon*). Inability to perform harmonious muscular movements.

incrustration (*in-krus-tā'-shon*). Forming of a scab on a wound.

incubation (*in'-kū-bā'-shon*). Hatching. *I. period.* Time between infection and the appearance of symptoms when it is assumed the infecting organisms multiply.

incubator (*in'-kū-bā-tor*). Apparatus used to provide optimum conditions for incubation.

incus (*in'-kus*). A small anvil-shaped bone of the middle ear. *See* EAR.

index. (1) The forefinger. (2) The ratio of measurement of any quantity in comparison with a fixed standard.

Indian hemp. Cannabis indica. Also called marihuana.

indicanuria (*in-di-ka-nū-ri-a*). Excess of indican in the urine.

indication (*in-di-kā-shon*). Circumstances determining a particular form of treatment.

indicator (*in-di-kā'-tor*). Substance showing a chemical reaction by its change in colour.

indigenous (*in-di'-je-nus*). Native to a particular place.

indigestion (*in-di-jest'-chon*). Failure of the digestive powers; dyspepsia.

indol. A constituent of faeces formed by the putrefaction of protein. In cases of chronic constipation it is absorbed and excreted in urine as indican.

indolent (*in'-do-lent*). A term applied to a painless sore which is slow to heal.

induced current (*in-dūst' kurrent*). A secondary electrical current developed in a conductor by proximity to a primary current.

induction (*in-duk'-shon*). In obstetrics, the artificial production of labour. In electricity, the production of currents in a closed circuit upon the appearance and disappearance of a magnetic or electric field in its neighbourhood.

induration (*in-dū-rā'-shon*). The process of hardening; also, the state of being hardened, as in the early stage of inflammation.

industrial disease. A disease due to a person's occupation, such as silicosis found among silica workers, etc.

inebriety (*in-e-bri-et-i*). Habitual drunkenness.

inertia (*in-er'-sha*). Sluggishness; (1) Resistance to change in motion. (2) In psychiatry, extreme apathy. (3) *Uterine i.* Sluggish contraction of the uterus during labour.

inevitable haemorrhage. Bleeding due to placenta praevia.

in extremis (*in eks-trā-mis*). At the point of death.

infant (*in'-fant*). A newly born child: A term infant should be 50 to 53cm in length. In English law, a person under the age of legal maturity. *I. mortality. See* MORTALITY.

infanticide (*in-fan'-ti-sid*). Murder of an infant.

infantile eczema (*in'-fan-tīl ek-se-ma*). Type of eczema affecting infants and children.

infantile paralysis. Anterior poliomyelitis.

infantilism (*in-fan-ti-lism*). Persistence of childish ways in an adult.

infarct. A wedge-shaped area of dead tissue in an organ. The result of the clogging of an artery by an embolus or thrombus. *See* EMBOLISM.

infection (*in-fek'-shon*). The communication of a disease from one patient to another. *Droplet i.* In the fine spray which is ejected from the mouth on talking, sneezing, coughing.

infectious disease (*in-fek-shus*). A communicable disease.

infectious mononucleosis (*in-fek-shus mo-nō-nū-kle-ō-sis*). Glandular fever. Probably a virus infection and characterized by malaise, pyrexia, muscle pains, sore throat, enlargement of lymph glands and the spleen and an increase in the numbers of mononuclear white blood cells. Occasionally there is enlargement of the liver, jaundice and rash.

inferior (*in-fē-ri-or*). Lower.

inferior vena cava. The chief vein of the lower part of the trunk of the body.

inferiority complex (*in-fē-ri-o-ri-ti kom-pleks*). Aggressive, extrovert behaviour compensating for feeling of inferiority.

infertility (*in-fer-ti-li-ti*). Inability to reproduce. It may affect either the male or the female.

infestation (*in-fes-tā-shon*). The invasion of the body by parasites such as lice.

infiltration (*in-fil-trā'-shon*). (1) An effusion of fluid into the connective tissue. (2) Local spread of a malignant tumour.

inflammation (*in-flam-mā'-shon*). The response of the tissues to an injury. The signs are heat, redness, swelling, pain, loss of function.

inflation (*in-flā'-shon*). Blown out and expanded by air or gas.

influenza (*in-floo-en'-za*). Virus infection affecting the epithelium of the respiratory tract.

infra (*in-fra*). Below.

infra-red (*in-fra-red*). Electro-magnetic waves with longer wave length than visible red light, *i.e.* photons with a lesser frequency than the lower end of the visible spectrum. Because it is easily absorbed infra-red radiation transfers heat to the absorbing material and is used therapeutically for this purpose.

infundibulum (*in-fun-dib'-ū-lum*). (1) A funnel-shaped orifice or passage. (2) Outgrowth of floor of brain forming part of the pituitary gland.

infusion (*in-fū'-zhon*). (1) Fluid allowed to flow into a vein (intravenous infusion) or under the skin (subcutaneous infusion) by the force of gravity. (2) Crude extract of material using boiling water, *e.g.* tea is an infusion of tea leaves.

ingestion (*in-jes-tyon*). The taking in of food or other substances into the body.

ingrowing toe-nail. Lateral extension of the nail bed.

inguinal (*in'-gwi-nal*). Pertaining to the groin. *Inguinal canal*, about 1½in in length, lies in groin, and is occupied in the male by the spermatic cord, and in the female by the round ligament, with their corresponding vessels and nerves. The exit from the abdomen of these structures is at the internal abdominal ring or upper extremity of the inguinal canal. This is a potential source of weakness, and may be the point of exit of a hernia which, pushing its way below the muscles roofing over the canal, appears at the external abdominal ring as a tender swelling.

inhalation (*in-ha-lā'-shon*). Act of breathing in vapour or fumes by the mouth or nose, a form of treatment frequently ordered in disorders of the throat or chest.

inhaler (*in-hā'-ler*). Apparatus for administering steam inhalation. The drug and boiling water are put into the container and the patient inhales through the mouthpiece.

inherent (*in-hār'-ent*). Inborn.

inhibition (*in-hi-bish'-on*). Restraint. The term is used ubiquitously to imply the prevention of some activity;

thus psychological inhibition, enzymatic inhibition, nerve inhibition, etc.

initial (*in-i'-shal*). Beginning.

injected (*in-jek'-ted*). Congested.

injection (*in-jek'-shon*). Introduced material under pressure into tissues.

innate (*i-nāt*). Congenital, inborn.

innervation (*in-ner-vā'-shon*). The supply of nerves or the conveyance of nervous impulses to or from a part. *Reciprocal i.* One set of muscles contracts whilst those opposing it relax.

innocent (*i-nō-sent*). Not malignant.

innocuous (*i-no'-kū-us*). Harmless.

innominate artery (*in-om'-in-āt*). The large artery which arises from the arch of the aorta and divides into the right common carotid and right subclavian arteries.

innominate bone. Bone forming anterior walls and sides of the pelvic cavity.

innoxious (*i-nok-sē-us*). Not harmful.

inoculation (*in-ok-ū-lā'-shon*). Introduction of micro-organisms into tissue or culture media etc.

inorganic (*in-or-ga'-nik*). Mineral as opposed to living material or its products.

inositol (*i-no-si-tol*). Substance in vitamin B complex found in muscle and other animal tissue and also in seeds.

inquest (*in-kwest*). A judicial inquiry into the cause of death.

insanity (*in-san'-i-ti*). Madness. Severe mental disorder (an absolute term).

insecticide (*in-sek-ti-sīd*). A preparation for destroying insects.

insemination (*in-se-mi-nā'-shon*). Introduction of semen into the vagina. *Artificial i.* Injection of semen into vagina or uterus.

insertion (*in-ser'-shon*). The attachment of a muscle to the part it moves.

insidious (*in-sid'-ē-us*). (1) Cunning. (2) Disease in which there are no perceptible signs or symptoms.

insight (*in-sit*). An awareness of one's own mental state and behaviour.

in situ. In position.

insolation (*in-so-lā'-shon*). Exposure to the sun's rays.

insomnia (*in-som'-ni-a*). Sleeplessness; often a troublesome complication during convalescence.

inspiration (*in-spir-rā'-shon*). Drawing air into the lungs.

inspissated (*in-spi-sā'-ted*). Thickened by evaporation.

instep. Arch on the dorsal surface of the foot.

instillation (*in-stil-lā'-shon*). Pouring in drop by drop, *e.g.* into eye.

instinct. An inborn organization of perception, feeling and action, *e.g.* the sight of something which threatens life arouses the emotion of fear and the instinct of flight.

insufflation (*in-sūf-flā'-shon*). Blowing powder into a cavity of the body. The instrument used has a long tube or nozzle with a rubber bulb attached to the distal end.

insula (*in'-sū-la*). Small part of the cerebral cortex lying deeply in the lateral sulcus.

insulation (*in-sū-lā'-shon*). Material preventing loss of or access to internally situated structure of heat, light, electrical current, water, etc.

insulator (*in-sū-lā'-tor*). A substance which does not conduct electricity.

insulin. Secretion of the islets of Langerhans in the pancreas which exerts control over the metabolism of glucose in the body. Used as a subcutaneous injection for reduction of blood sugar in diabetes.

insulinase (*in-sū-li-nās*). Enzyme which inactivates insulin.

insulinoma (*in-sū-li-nō-ma*). An adenoma of the islet cells of the pancreas.

integument (*in-teg'-ū-ment*). The skin.

intellect (*in-te-lekt*). Reasoning power whereby we can think logically.

intelligence (*in-tel-li-jentz*). Certain mental ability involving reasoning and recognition of pattern, etc., as distinct from memorization of information or other mental functions.

intelligence quotient. The ratio of mental age to chronological age.

intelligence tests. Tests not based on a person's knowledge but on his ability to learn. *See* INTELLIGENCE.

intention tremor. Tremor which occurs only during active movement, symptomatic of Parkinsonism.

inter (*in'-ter*). A Latin prefix meaning 'between' and used with many medical terms, such as *intercostal*, between the ribs; *intermittent* fevers, in which there are regular pauses between the attacks.

interarticular (*in-ter-ar-tik'-ū-la*). Between the joints.

intercellular (*in-ter-se-lū-la*). Between cells, *e.g.* intercellular fluid.

intercostal. Between the ribs.

intercourse (*in-ter-kors*). Communication. *Sexual i.* Coitus.

intercurrent (*in-ter-ku'-rent*).

Occurring between. *I. infection*. Another infection occurring in a patient already suffering from some other one.

intermenstrual (*in-ter-men-strū-al*). Between the monthly periods.

intermittent. Occurring at intervals. When applied to the pulse, signifies that some of the beats of the heart fail to reach the wrist. *I. claudication*. Literally intermittent limping due to ischaemia of the muscles of the legs.

internal (*in-ter'-nal*). Inside.

internal os. The junction of the cavity of the cervix uteri with that of the body of the uterus. *See also* UTERUS.

internal version. Version by inserting one hand completely into the uterus, and so changing the presentation or lie of the fetus.

interosseous (*in-ter-os-sē-us*). Between two bones.

intersex (*in-ter-seks*). Imperfect sexual differentiation of an individual into either male or female.

interstitial (*in-ter-sti'-shal*). Between parts, *i.e.* in connective tissue.

interstitial keratitis (*ke-ra-ti'-tis*). Manifestation of syphilis consisting of inflammation of the cornea.

intertrigo (*in-ter-trī'-gō*).

Eczematous condition of deep crevices or folds of skin, due to retention of perspiration.

intertrochanteric (*in-ter-trō-kan-te-rik*). Between the trochanters.

interventricular (*in-ter-ven-tri-kū-la*). Between the ventricles.

intervertebral (*in-ter-ver-te-bral*). Between the vertebrae.

intestinal malabsorption. Malabsorption syndrome. Failure to absorb digested foodstuffs.

intestinal obstruction. Obstruction to the passage of food or faeces through the intestine. Either due to physical blockage or absence of peristalsis.

intestines (*in-tes'-tinz*). The alimentary canal from the duodenum to the anus.

intima (*in'-ti-ma*). Inner coat of arteries consisting of endothelium and its elastic fibre attachment to the connective tissue of the media.

intolerance (*in-tol'-er-ans*). Constitutional incapacity to endure or benefit by a remedial agent.

intoxication (*in-tok-si-kā-shon*). Poisoning; drunkenness.

intra. Within.

intra-abdominal (*in-tra-ab-do-mi-nal*). Within the abdominal cavity.

intra-articular. Within the capsule of a joint.

intracellular (*in-tra-sel-lū-la*). Within a cell.

intracerebral (*in-tra-se-re-bral*). Between the two cerebral hemispheres.

intracranial (*in-tra-krā-ni-al*). Within the skull.

intradermal (*in-tra-der-mal*). Within the skin.

intradural (*in-tra-dū'-ral*). Within the dura mater.

intragastric (*in-tra-gas-trik*). Within the stomach.

intrahepatic (*in-tra-he-pa'-tik*). Within the liver.

intralobular (*in-tra-lo'-bū-la*). Within a lobule.

intramedullary (*in-tra-me-du-la-ri*). Within the bone marrow.

intramuscular (*in-tra-mus'-kū-la*). Within a muscle. Many injections are given intramuscularly but care must be taken with choice of site, because of danger of damaging nerves and blood vessels.

intranasal (*in-tra-nā'-sal*). Within the nasal cavity.

intraocular (*in-tra-o-kū-la*). Within the globe of the eye.

intra-osseous (*in-tra-os-sē-us*). Within a bone.

intraperitoneal (*in-tra-pe-ri-to-nē-al*). Pertaining to the peritoneal cavity.

intrathecal (*in-tra-thē'-kal*). Pertaining to the lumen of a sheath or canal, usually meaning the spinal canal.

intratracheal (*in'-tra-trak-ē'-al*). Inside the trachea. Thus *intratracheal cannula*. Those used for the administration of anaesthetic are known as *endotracheal* tubes.

intra-uterine (*in'-tra-ū'-ter-in*). Within the uterus. *I. contraceptive device* (IUD). A small device of plastic or stainless steel placed in the uterus by the doctor to prevent pregnancy.

intravenous (*in-tra-vē-nus*). Within the lumen of a vein.

intrinsic (*in-trin-sik*). Inherent, peculiar to a part.

intrinsic factor. Castle's antipernicious anaemia substance. Factor present in normal gastric juice which enables the absorption of cyanocobalamin (B_{12}) to take place. It is probable that it is an enzyme.

introitus (*in-trō'-it-us*). An entrance, applied to the inlets of the pelvis and vagina.

introspection (*in-tro-spek-shon*). State of mental self-examination.

introvert (*in-trō-vert'*). An individual whose attention centres on himself rather than on outside things. Opposite to an extrovert.

intubation (*in-tū-bā'-shon*). Insertion of a tube into a passage or organ, esp. tracheal intubation.

intumescence (*in-tū-mes'-sens*). Swelling, increase.

intussusception (*in-tus-sus-sep'-shon*). The reception of one part of the intestine (the intussusceptum) into another (the intussuscipiens); occurs most often between 3 and 9 months, and causing intestinal obstruction, with the passage of blood and mucus rectally and frequent vomiting. The treatment is immediate laparotomy.

in utero (*in ū-te-rō*). Within the uterus.

invagination (*in-vaj-i-nā'-shon*). Turning inwards to form double-layered pouch.

invasion (*in-vā-zhon*). Onset, esp. of a disease.

inverse (*in-vers*). Inverted in position, etc. The direct opposite.

inversion (*in-ver-shon*). Turning upside down or inside out.

invertase (*in-ver-tās*). Enzyme in intestinal juice converting cane sugar into glucose and laevulose.

in vitro (*in vē-trō*). Literally in glass, *i.e.* in the test-tube as opposed to in life, *cf.* IN VIVO.

in vivo (*in vē-vō*). In the living body.

involucrum (*in-vo-lū-krum*). Layer of new bone ensheathing a sequestrum.

involuntary (*in-vo-lun-ta-ri*). Independent of the will. *I. muscles* are innervated by the autonomic nervous system.

involute (*in'-vo-lūt*). Rolled inward from the edges; becoming smaller.

involution (*in-vo-lū'-shon*). (1) A turning in. (2) The shrinking of the uterus and surrounding structures after labour. The uterus, from weighing 1kg at labour, shrinks in six weeks to the weight of 50g. Arrest of this process is called subinvolution.

involutional melancholia (*in-vo-lū-sho-nal me-lan-kō-li-a*). Depression due to hormonal changes at the menopause. A similar syndrome occurs in males.

iodine (*ī'-ō-dēn*). A poisonous element obtained from the ashes of seaweed. A useful antiseptic for the skin.

iodism. Iodine poisoning. Symptoms are those of a cold in the head with a pustular rash.

ion (*i'-on*). Electrically charged atom or group of atoms. Many substances ionise in solution forming cations (+ve) and anions (−ve).

ionizing radiation (*i-o-nī-zing*

rā-di-ā-shon). High energy radiation capable of producing ions in materials exposed to it.

ionization (*ī-on'-ī-zā-shon*). The process of producing ions in a substance.

ipsilateral (*ip-si-la-te-ral*). On the same side.

IQ. Abbreviation for intelligence quotient.

iridectomy (*ir-i-dek'-to-mi*). Cutting off a piece of the edge of the iris to make an artificial pupil to the eye.

iridocele (*ī-ri-dō-sēl*). Protrusion of a portion of iris through a wound in the cornea.

iridocyclitis (*ir'-id-ō-si-klī'-tis*). Inflammation of the iris and uveal tract.

iridodialysis (*i-ri-dō-dī-a-li-sis*). A pathological state in which the ciliary border of the iris is separated from its attachment.

iridoplegia (*ī-ri-dō-plē'-ji-a*). Paralysis of the muscle which constricts or dilates the pupil.

iridotomy (*ī-ri-do-to-mi*). An incision into the iris.

iris (*ī'-ris*). The coloured circle surrounding the pupil of the eye. *See* EYE.

iritis (*ī-rī'-tis*). Inflammation of the iris.

irradiation (*i-rā-di-ā-shon*). Exposure to electro-

magnetic waves or charged particles (α and β rays).

irreducible (*ir-re-dū'-si-bl*). Incapable of being returned to its proper place by manipulation; usually term applied to a hernia.

irrigation (*ir-ri-gā'-shon*). Washing out.

irritant (*ir'-ri-tant*). Agent causing irritation, *i.e.* resulting in a response.

ischaemia (*is-kē'-mi-a*). Diminished supply of blood to a part.

ischaemic contracture (*is-kē-mik con-trak-tūr*). Volkmann's contracture. Permanent shortening of muscle by fibrosis resulting from impairment of blood supply.

ischio-rectal abscess (*is'-kē-ō*). A collection of pus in the fatty cavity on one or other side of the rectum. May burst externally through the skin or internally into rectum when a fistula-in-ano results.

ischium (*is'-kē-um*). The lower and hind part of the innominate bone.

Ishihara test (*i-shi-hah-ra*). Colour charts used to test for colour blindness.

islets of Langerhans. *See* LANGERHANS' ISLETS.

isolation (*ī-sō-lā'-shon*). The act of setting apart; an isolation room or ward is one kept for contagious or infectious diseases, and the nurse has to follow strict rules to prevent the spread of the disease.

isomers (*ī-sō-mers*). Compounds made up of the same elements in the same proportions but having different arrangements of their atoms which gives them differing physical or chemical properties, e.g. butyl alcohol.

isometric (*ī-sō-me-trik*). Of equal measure. Static.

isotonic (*ī-sō-ton'-ik*). Having the same osmotic pressure. Thus a solution which is isotonic with blood serum neither attracts fluid from the vessels nor itself tends to pass through into them.

isotopes (*ī-zō-tōps*). Differing forms of the same element with different atomic weights but the same chemical properties. *Radioactive i.* Isotopes with radioactive properties, emitting beta rays and sometimes gamma rays. Used to diagnose and treat disease.

isthmus (*is'-mus*). The neck or constricted part of an organ.

itching. Sensation, probably due to sub-threshold pain stimuli, which is characterized by the *scratch* reaction.

-itis (*ī'-tis*). Suffix meaning inflamed, *e.g.* dermatitis, inflammation of the skin.

** īUD.** *See* INTRA-UTERINE.

J

Jacksonian epilepsy. *See* EPILEPSY.

Jacquemier's sign (*jak-mē-āz sīn*). Blueness of the vaginal walls seen in early pregnancy.

jaundice (*jawn'-dis*). A syndrome characterized by increased levels of bile pigments in the blood and tissue fluids. These pigments are taken up by the tissues giving rise to a yellow colour of the sclera, skin and mucous membranes. The cause of jaundice may be obstructive, hepato-cellular or haemolytic (excessive destruction of red blood cells). Hepato-cellular jaundice includes conditions such as infective hepatitis, a virus disease affecting the liver; toxic damage to the liver cells, *e.g.* acute yellow atrophy 'and other condition which reduce the efficiency of the liver in excreting bile pigments. Obstruction to any portion of the biliary tree may result in jaundice. The commonest cause of obstruction is gall stones.

jaw bone. *See* MAXILLA.

jejunectomy (*je-jū-nek-to-mi*). Excision of part of the jejunum.

jejunostomy (*je-jū-nos'-to-mi*). Making an artificial opening into the jejunum.

jejunum (*je-jū'-num*). That portion of the small intestine which lies between the duodenum and the ileum. *See* BOWEL.

jerk. A sudden contraction of muscle.

jigger. A tropical sand flea (*Dermatophilus penetrans*) which is parasitic in man, burrowing into the toes. Another name is chigoe.

joint (*joynt*). Point of contact of two or more bones. An articulation.

jugular (*jug'-ū-lar*). Relating to the neck.

jugular veins. Two large veins in the neck which convey most of the blood from the head.

Jung's method (*yoongs*). Psychoanalysis.

jurisprudence, medical. *See* MEDICAL J.

justo minor pelvis. Form of CONTRACTED PELVIS.

juxtaposition (*juks'-ta-po-si-shon*). Placed alongside or next to.

K

K. Chemical symbol for potassium.

Kahn test (*karn*). A method of investigating the serum of patients suspected of syphilis. It is more convenient, simpler, and quicker than the Wasserman Reaction, but should confirm rather than supplant it, the WR on the whole being more reliable.

kala-azar (*ka-la-ā'-za*). A tropical disease transmitted from man to man by sand-flies and is caused by the protozoon *Leishmania donovani*. There is enlargement of the spleen, fever and anaemia.

kangaroo ligature. Suture material from the tendons of a kangaroo's tail.

kaolin (*kā-ō-lin*). China clay; a hydrated silicate of aluminium. It is an ingredient of cataplasma kaolini. *Heavy k.* is used to prepare k. poultice. *Light k.* is an adsorbent and demulcent and is used in mixtures for diarrhoea.

karyokineses (*ka-re-ō-kīn-ē'-sis*). Indirect cell-division, *i.e.* division preceded by complicated changes in the nucleus of the cell.

katabolism (*kat-ab'-ol-ism*). *See* METABOLISM.

katathermometer. A wet and dry bulb thermometer for measuring the cooling and drying powers of the atmosphere, thus it is a test of the efficiency of the ventilation.

katatonia (*ka-ta-tō-ni-a*). *See* CATATONIA.

kathode (*ka-thōd*). *See* CATHODE.

kation (*ka-ti-on*). *See* CATION.

Kayser Fleischer rings (*kā-ser flī-sher*). Brownish pigmented rings seen in the cornea of patients with Wilson's disease.

Keller's operation. Operation to correct hallux valgus.

keloid (*kē'-loyd*). A connective tissue growth of the skin, arising always in a scar of some previous injury.

keratectasia (*ke-ra-tek-tā'-si-a*). Protrusion of the cornea.

keratectomy (*ke-ra-tek'-to-mi*). Surgical removal of part of the cornea.

keratin (*ke-ra-tin*). Fibrillar protein. It is produced by epithelial cells and is found in horns, hooves, hair and the protective covering of the skin.

keratitis (*ker-a-tī'-tis*). Inflammation of the cornea.

keratolytics (*ke-ra-tō-li-tiks*). Agents such as salicylic acid which break down keratin.

keratoma (*ke-ra-tō'-ma*). A callosity or horny overgrowth.

keratomalacia (*ker-at-ō-ma-lā'-ki-a*) Softening of the cornea which may lead to ulceration and blindness. Occurs in association with vitamin A deficiency.

keratome (*ker'-at-ōm*). Surgical knife used for incisions of the cornea.

keratometer (*ke-ra-to-me-ter*).

Ophthalmometer, for measuring corneal astigmatism.

keratoplasty (*ke-ra-tō-pla-sti*). Corneal graft.

keratosis (*ke-ra-tō-sis*). Skin disease with excess of horny tissue.

kerion (*ke'-ri-on*). A term for crusted ringworm.

kernicterus (*ker-nik'-te-rus*). Many areas of the brain, particularly the basal ganglia, central cerebellar nuclei, the medulla and hippocampus are stained yellow with bilirubin. The brain cells are damaged. A complication of haemolytic jaundice of the new born.

Kernig's sign. A sign of meningitis. It consists of an inability to extend the knee joint when the thigh is flexed to a right angle with the trunk.

ketogenic diet (*kē-tō-je-nik di-et*). Diet with high fat producing ketosis.

ketonaemia (*kē-tō-nē-mi-a*). Ketone bodies in the blood.

ketone (*kē-tōn*). Acetone. *K. bodies.* Oxybutyric acid, aceto-acetic acid and acetone, the last two being products of incomplete fat metabolism in the body as a result of insufficient catabolism of carbohydrates.

ketonuria (*kē-to-nū-ri-a*). Ketone bodies in the urine.

ketosis (*kē-tō'-sis*). Acidosis.

The condition in which ketones are found in excess in the body.

ketosteroids (*kē-tō-ste-royds*). Androgens secreted in the adrenals and testes, whose presence in the urine is an indication of the activity of these glands.

kettle. A bronchitis or croup kettle has a long spout coming out of the lid, so that the steam can be directed well out into the room. A roll of brown paper added to the spout of an ordinary kettle does in an emergency.

kidneys. Two organs in the region of the hollow of the back which secrete the urine. *Artificial k.* Apparatus through which blood is passed and allowed to dialyse, across a membrane, usually a coiled tube, placed in a warm bath of saline. This process allows waste products and other materials to be removed from the blood and simulate the function of the kidneys.

Killian's operation. For suppuration in the frontal sinus. Removal of part of frontal bone to allow of complete drainage.

kilogram (*kil'-lo-̄gram*). A thousand grams, equivalent to 2·2 lb.

Kimmelstiel-Wilson disease

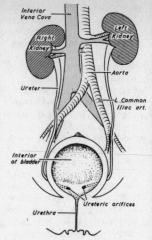

28 Anterior view of urinary tract

(*ki-mel-stēl wil-son di-sēz*). Disease with glycosuria, nephrotic symptoms, proteinuria and oedema.

kinaesthesis (*kin-ēs-thē'-sis*). The sense of muscular movement.

kinase (*kī-nāz*). Substances in the tissues which make proenzymes become enzymes.

kinematics (*kī-ne-ma-tiks*). The study of motion.

kineplasty (*kīn'-e-plas-ti*). A plastic amputation with the object of making the stump useful for locomotion.

kinesis (*kī-nē-sis*). Movement.

kinetics (*kī-ne-tiks*). The study of movement or change.

Kirschner wire (*ker-shner*). Wire used in orthopaedic surgery to apply skeletal traction to a fractured bone.

kiss of life. Mouth-to-mouth artificial respiration.

Klebs-Loeffler bacillus (*lerf'-ler*). The bacillus of diphtheria. Also known as corynebacterium diphtheriae.

Klebsiella (*kleb-si-e-la*). Genus of bacteria which may cause respiratory infections.

kleptomania (*kelp-tō-mā'-ni-a*). Obsessional neurosis manifested by compulsive stealing.

Klinefelter's syndrome (*klīn-fel-ters sin'-drōm*). Chromosome abnormality causing infertility in the male due to congenital malformation of gonads.

Klumpke's paralysis (*kloomp-kers pa-ra-li-sis*). Paralysis of the flexor muscles to the wrist and fingers caused by injury to the eighth cervical and first dorsal nerves.

knee (*nē*). The joint between the femur and the tibia.

knee cap. Patella.

knee-elbow position. *See* GENU-PECTORAL.

knee jerk. A jerk of the leg elicited by tapping on the patel-lar tendon when the knee is flexed. May be absent or exaggerated in diseases of the nervous system.

knock-knee. Genu valgum.

knuckle (*nukl*). Dorsal aspect of a phalangeal joint.

Koch's bacillus (*koks ba-si-lus*). Mycobacterium tuberculosis.

Koch-Weeks bacillus (*kok-wēks ba-si-lus*). Micro-organism causing acute conjunctivitis.

Köhler's disease (*ker-lers dis-ēz*). Osteochondritis affecting the scaphoid bone in the foot which becomes compressed and sclerotic. Occurs in children.

koilonychia (*koy-lō-ni-ki-a*). Spoon-shaped nails found in iron deficiency anaemia.

Koplik's spots. Small white spots to be found on the inner surface of the cheeks in measles, often before the skin rash appears.

Korsakow's syndrome (*kor'-sa-kovs sin'-drōm*). A confusional state especially as to recent events due to brain injury or toxic causes such as chronic alcoholism.

kraurosis vulvae (*kraw-rō'-sis*). Senile degeneration of the skin of the vulva. *See* LEUKO-PLAKIA.

Kretschmer's types (*kret-ch-mers tūps*). Classification of potential psychopathic tendencies in relation to physical characteristics, *e.g.* pyknic type is short and fat with a tendency to manic-depressive psychosis. Aesthetic type is tall and thin with a tendency to schizophrenia.

Krukenberg's tumour (*kroo-ken-bergs tū-mer*). A secondary carcinoma in the ovary, the primary usually occurring in the stomach.

Küntscher nail (*koon-cher*). An intramedullary nail used to fix fragments of fractured long bone in alignment.

Kupffer's cells (*koop-fers sels*). Star-shaped cells in the liver. Part of the reticulo-endothelial system.

kwashiorkor (*kwa-shi-aw-kor*). Disease with wasting, oedema, anaemia and enlargement of the liver due to lack of protein in the diet.

kyphoscoliosis (*kī-fō-skō-li-ō'-sis*). Combined anteroposterior deformity (kyphosis) and lateral curvature (scoliosis) of the spine.

kyphosis (*kī-fō-sis*). Humpback, angular deformity of the spine. May be caused by Pott's disease.

L

labia majora (*lā-bi-a ma-jo-ra*). (*Sing.* labium). Two large folds at the mouth of the

pudendum; called also the *labia pudendi*.

labia minora (*lā-bi-a mi-nor'-a*). Two smaller folds within the majora. *Syn.* nymphae.

labial (*lā-bi-al*). Relating to the lips or to the labia.

labile (*lā-bīl*). Unstable.

laboratory (*lab-or'-a-to-ri*). A place where scientific experiments and investigations are carried on.

labour (*lā'-ber*). The progress of the birth of a child. There are three stages. (1) The dilatation of the cervix. (2) The passage of the fetus through the canal and its birth. (3) From the birth of the child to the expulsion of the placenta.

labyrinth (*lab'-i-rinth*). The internal ear. *See* EAR.

labyrinthitis (*lab'-i-rin-thī'-tis*). Inflammation of the labyrinth of the ear causing vertigo.

laceration (*las'-er-ā-shon*). A lacerated wound with torn or irregular edges; not clean cut.

lacrimal (*lak'-ri-mal*). Relating to tears and the glands which secrete them.

lacrimal apparatus. *See* p. 195.

lacrimation (*lak-ri-mā'-shon*). Flow of tears.

lactagogue (*lak'-ta-gog*). *See* GALACTAGOGUE.

lactalbumin (*lak-tal-bū'-min*). The albumin of milk. A protein.

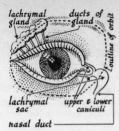

lachrymal ducts of
gland gland
outline of orbit
lachrymal upper & lower
sac caniculi
nasal duct

29 The lacrimal apparatus

lactase (*lak'-tāz*). An enzyme of
the succus entericus which
converts lactose into glucose.

lactate. A salt of lactic acid.

lactation (*lak-tā'-shon*). The
process or period of suckling.

lacteals (*lak'-te-als*). The lymphatic vessels, which convey
the chyle from the small
intestine.

lactic acid. An acid produced by
the fermentation of lactose.
The souring of milk is
accompanied by the forma-
tion of this acid.

lactiferous ducts (*lak-tif'-er-us
dukts*). The canals of the
mammary glands.

lactifuge (*lak-ti-fūj*). Lessening
the secretion of milk.

lactobacillus (*lak-tō-ba-si-lus*).
A non-pathogenic Gram-
positive bacterium.

lactogenic (*lak-tō-jē'-nik*). Promoting the flow of milk. *L.
hormone.* Prolactin. A hormone released from the
anterior pituitary which
causes milk production
following parturition.

lactose (*lak-tōz*). A disaccharide sugar, composed of
glucose and galactose, which
occurs in milk.

lacuna (*la-kū'-na*). A space.

Laennec's cirrhosis (*la-neks
si-rō-sis*). The commonest
type of cirrhosis of liver
commonly attributable to
damage to the liver by high
consumption of alcohol.

laevulose. *See* LEVULOSE.

laked (*lākt*). Describes haemo-
lysed blood.

lalling. Baby talk when the
letter 'l' is used instead of the
letter 'r'.

lambdoid (*lam-'doyd*). Like
Greek letter λ, chiefly
applied to the suture between
the occipital and parietal
bones.

lambliasis (*lam-blī-a-sis*). Also
called giardiasis. Parasitic
infection of small intestine.

lamellae (*la-mel'-lē*). Thin
sheets of tissue, *e.g.* bone.

lamina (*lam'-i-na*). A thin layer.

laminectomy (*lam-in-ek'-to-
mi*). Excision of some of the
vertebral laminae to gain
access to the spinal cord, or to
relieve pressure on nerve
roots as in prolapsed intervertebral disc.

lancet (*lan'-set*). A sharp
pointed two-edged surgical
knife.

Lancefield's groups (*larnts-fēlds groops*). A classification of streptococci into groups of which Group A includes the common pathogenic haemolytic streptococcus.

lancinating (*lan-si-nā-ting*). Cutting or tearing, often applied to pain.

lanette wax. A self-emulsifying wax used in water-miscible ointment bases.

Langerhans' islets. Small areas of special cells in the pancreas. They secrete insulin. *See* INSULIN and DIABETES.

lanolin (*lan'-ō-lin*). Purified wool-fat. Used as the basis for various ointments.

Lansing virus. A strain of poliomyelitis virus.

lanugo (*lan-ū'-gō*). The downy growth which covers an infant from the fourth month of gestation, but has mostly disappeared by term.

laparotomy (*lap-ar-ot'-o-mi*). Opening the abdominal cavity. Usually for investigation.

lardaceous disease (*lar-dā'-she-us*). Degeneration of the tissues till they resemble wax. Amyloid disease.

laryngeal (*la-rin'-je-al*). Relating to the larynx. *L. stridor.* Gasping respiration due to spasm of the glottis.

laryngectomy (*lar-in-jek'-to-mi*). Removal of the larynx.

laryngismus stridulus (*la-rin-jis-mus stri-dū-lus*). Croup. Laryngeal spasm due to tetany in an infant. There is apnoea and then a crowing sound.

laryingitis (*lar-in-jī'-tis*). Inflammation of the larynx, causing loss of voice, and in acute cases, with much oedema, threatening suffocation.

laryngology (*la-rin-go-lo-ji*). Science of anatomy and diseases of the larynx.

laryngopharynx (*la-rin-gō-fa-rinks*). The lower part of the pharynx.

laryngoscope (*la-rin'-go-skōp*). Instrument for examining a larynx.

laryngostenosis (*la-rin'-gō-ste-nō'-sis*). Stricture of the larynx.

laryngotomy (*la-rin-go-to-mi*). *See* TRACHEOSTOMY.

laryngo-tracheo-bronchitis (*la-rin-gō-tra-kē-ō-bron-kī-tis*). Acute viral inflammatory disease affecting the respiratory tract. Often occurs during influenza epidemic and affects principally young children.

larynx (*lar'-rinks*). The upper part of the windpipe containing vocal cords. Voice sounds may be produced during expiration.

laser (*lā-zer*). A very narrow

and intense beam of light that will cut through metals.

Lassar's paste. Ointment containing zinc oxide, starch, salicylic acid, soft paraffin. Used for skin eruptions.

lassitude (*la-si-tūd*). Feeling of weakness, a frequent feature of debilitating diseases such as anaemia.

latent (*lā-tent*). Not visible, lying hidden for a time. *L. heat.* The heat absorbed or released in a change of state without an alteration in temperature, e.g. water into steam and vice versa. *L. period.* Incubation time.

lateral (*lat-er-al*). On the side. For *lateral sinus, see* SINUS.

lavage (*lav-ahj*). Washing out.

laxative (*laks'-a-tiv*). A mild purgative.

lead (*led*). A soft heavy metal whose salts are poisonous. *L. poisoning* may occur in children due to chewing cots and toys covered with paint containing lead. The symptoms and signs include malaise, colic, peripheral neuropathy and sometimes encephalitis. Pallor is often marked and a blue line on the gums is characteristic.

leather-bottle stomach. Loss of elasticity in the stomach wall resulting from infiltration by neoplastic cells.

lecithin (*les'-i-thin*). A phospholipid.

leech (*lētsh*). Aquatic worm which is able to suck blood from the skin.

leg. Anatomically the part of the lower limb from knee to ankle. *White l.* Condition caused by venous thrombosis in the lower limb. Sometimes seen after childbirth. *See* PHLEGMASIA.

legumin (*le-gū-min*). A globulin derived from the seeds of various plants such as peas and beans.

Leishman-Donovan body. Eosinophilic bodies representing rounded forms of leishmania donovani found in the cells parasitized by kala-azar.

Leishmaniasis (*lēsh-ma-nĭ-a-sis*). Infection with organisms of the type which cause kala-azar and oriental sore.

Lembert's suture. Special suture used in stitching up the peritoneal coat of the intestine or other abdominal organs after any incision or injury.

Lennander's incision. An abdominal incision to the right or left of the middle line down to the rectus; the inner edge of this muscle is then retracted and the posterior layer of its sheath incised as well as the peritoneum.

lens (*lenz*). Transparent refractile tissue of the eye (*see* EYE), which focuses the image on the retina.

lenticular. Pertaining to a lens.

lentigo (*len-tī-go*). A freckle.

Leon virus. A strain of poliomyelitis virus.

leontiasis ossea (*lē-on-tī'-a-sis os'-se-a*). A disease in which the bones of the face are deformed and greatly increased in size; sometimes found in leprosy.

leproma (*le-prō-ma*) (plu. lepromata). Swelling in the skin found in certain cases of leprosy.

leprosy (*lep'-ro-si*). An infective disease, cutaneous in its earlier stages, but afterwards involving both soft tissue and bone. The first stage may last days or months; there are pains in the limbs, lassitude, and feverish attacks. The second stage is eruptive, and the blotches on the skin come and go. In the third stage the disease becomes either nodular (*lepra tuberculosa*) or blotched (*lepra maculosa*); if the blotches become white and anaesthesia sets in, it is called white leprosy. Leprosy, also called Hansens's disease, was formerly treated with chaulmugra oil. Modern treatment is sulphone therapy, which can cure leprosy in its early stages.

leptomeningitis (*lep-tō-men-in-jī-tis*). Inflammation of the pia mater and arachnoid coverings of the brain, distinguished from pachymeningitis, in which the dura mater is the seat of inflammation.

leptospira (*lep-tō-spī'-ra*). Type of spirochaete. Notably *L. Icterohaemorrhagicae* which causes Weil's disease.

Leriche syndrome (*le-rēsh sin'-drōm*). Obstruction to the flow of blood at the lower end of the aorta giving rise to intermittent claudication.

lesbianism (*les-bi-a-nism*). A female homosexual relationship.

lesion (*lē-'zhon*). Any injury or morbid change in the function or structure of an organ.

lethal (*lē-thal*). Deadly, fatal.

lethargy (*le'-tha-ji*). Drowsiness.

leucin (*lū'-sin*). An amino-acid.

leucocyte. A white blood cell. *See* BLOOD COUNT.

leucocythaemia (*lū-kō-sī'-thē'-mi-a*). Morbid increase of the white cells of the blood. Same as leukaemia.

leucocytolysis (*lū-kō-sī-tol'-is-is*). Destruction of leucocytes.

leucocytosis (*lū-kō-sī-tō'-sis*). An increase of white cells of the blood; usually occurs in sepsis and is then a defensive mechanism.

leucoderma. A condition in which there are patches of skin which are defectively pigmented, and consequently pale in colour.

leuco-erythroblastic anaemia (*lū-ko-e-ri-thrō-blas-tik a-nē-mi-a*). Descriptive term applied to the appearance of nucleated red cells and primitive white cells in the circulation. It is due to neoplastic infiltration of bone marrow.

leuconychia (*lū-ko-nik'-i-a*). Curved white lines on the finger-nails showing interrupted nutrition.

leucopenia (*lū-kō-pē'-ni-a*). Diminution of the number of white cells in the blood.

leucopoiesis (*lū-kō-poy-ē-sis*). Formation of white blood cells.

leucorrhoea (*lū-kor-re'-a*). A whitish mucoid discharge from the vagina.

leucotomy (*lū-ko-to-mi*). Transection of nerve fibres passing to and from a lobe of the brain. Usually *Prefrontal leucotomy*, an operation undertaken to relieve certain types of mental disorder in which the prefrontal lobes are surgically isolated from the rest of the brain.

leukaemia (*lū-kē'-mi-a*). A dis-

ease of blood-forming organs, characterized by increase of white cells of the blood. *Lymphatic l.* That in which large numbers of primitive lymphocytes appear in the blood. *Myeloid l.* That in which primitive polymorphonuclear leucocytes appear in large numbers. *Monocytic l.*, *Eosinophilic l.*, as for the other forms, but exhibiting monocytes and eosinophils respectively. *See* BLOOD.

leukoplakia (*lū-kō-plā-ki-a*). A smooth glazed white state of the tongue which may precede cancer of that organ. A similar condition of the vulva is also found in women.

levator (*le-vā'-tur*). A muscle which lifts up a part. *Levator ani*: muscle of the pelvis which plays an important part in keeping pelvic viscera in position. *Levator palpebrae superioris*: muscle which raises the upper eyelid.

levulose (*lev'-ū-lōs*). Fruit sugar or fructose. *L. tolerance test.* In the normal individual there is little or no rise in the blood sugar taken 1 hour after 100 grams of levulose. In hepatic insufficiency the blood sugar will show an increase of 30mg per 100ml in the first half-hour and may later rise much higher.

libido (*li-bi-dō*). The drive to obtain satisfaction through the senses. Term sometimes used for sexual desire.

lice (*līs*). Plural of louse.

lichen (*li-'ken*). A term for skin diseases of which the striking feature is chronic inflammatory papules. *Lichen planus*: showing papules, which are angular, lilac in colour, often with a depression in their centre and in some lights shiny. Usually affects flexor aspects of forearms, back of neck, and inner side of thighs.

lie of fetus. The position of the fetus in the uterus is termed its lie, *i.e.* transverse lie, vertical lie.

Lieberkühn's glands (*lē'-berkūn*). Tubular glands of the small intestine, which secrete the intestinal juice.

lien (*lē-en*). The spleen.

lienculus (*lē-en'-kū-lus*). An accessory spleen.

ligament (*lig'-a-ment*). A tough band of fibrous tissue connecting together the bones at the joints.

ligation (*lig-ā'-shon*). The application of a ligature.

ligatures (*lig'-a-tūrs*). Threads of silk, wire, catgut, fascia, nylon, etc., used to tie arteries, stitch tissue, etc.

light adaptation. The adaptation of the pupil of the eye to light incident on the retina. Also termed light reflex.

lightening (*lī-te-ning*). Relief of pressure in upper part of abdomen during last few weeks of pregnancy when fetal head enters the pelvis.

lightning pains (*līt'-ning pānz*). Shooting, cutting pains felt in some cases of tabes dorsalis.

limbus. A border. Junction of cornea and sclera.

lime (*līm*). Calcium oxide. Lime salts increase the coagulability of the blood; they take part in the formation of bone, and are a component part of many tonic medicines.

lime water (*līm' wor'-ter*). A solution of calcium hydroxide in distilled water. Used as a diluent for milk, and generally to counteract acidity.

liminal (*li-mi-nal*). The lowest threshold at which stimuli can be perceived.

linctus (*link'-tus*). A syrup, usually applied to a cough mixture to be taken in small doses.

linea alba (*line-e-a al'-ba*). The white line down the centre front of the abdomen. It is formed by the tendons of the abdominal muscles.

lineae albicantes (*lin'-e-ē al-*

bik-an'-tēz). *See* STRIAE
GRAVIDARUM.

linea nigra (*lin'-e-a nē-gra*). A
pigmented line seen in pregnant women running in mid-
line from above the umbilicus
to the symphysis pubis.

lingual (*ling'-gwal*). Relating to
the tongue.

liniment (*lin'-i-ment*). A liquid
preparation for application
to the skin with friction.

linolenic acid (*li-nō-le-nik*). A
constituent of vegetable fats,
essential for health.

linseed (*lin-sēd*). Seeds of the
flax plant.

lint. Loosely woven cotton
material, having one side
smooth and the other rough.
The smooth side is applied
next to the skin. Used for
surgical fomentations and
kaolin poultices.

lipaemia (*lip-ē'-mi-a*). Presence
of excess of fat in the blood.

lipase (*lī-pāz*). An enzyme in
the pancreatic secretion
which splits fat into glycerin
and a fatty acid. *Syn.* steapsin.

lipo-atrophy (*lī-pō-a-trō-fi*).
Loss of subcutaneous fat. A
complication which may arise
in sites of insulin injections.

lipochondrodystrophy (*lī-pō-
kon-drō-dis-tro-fi*). Term
sometimes used to describe
gargoylism or Hurler's syndrome.

lipodystrophy (*li-po-dis-tro-fi*).
A disorder of fat metabolism
which most commonly affects
women who show little fat
above the waist but are obese
around the buttocks and legs.

lipoidosis (*li-poy-dō-sis*). Disturbance in metabolism of
lipoids.

lipoids (*li-poyds*). Substances
(*e.g.* lecithin) which resemble
fats, in being dissolved by
organic solvents such as
alcohol and ether. They
occur in living cells.

lipoma (*li-pō'-ma*). Tumour of
fat cells.

lipotrophic substances (*lī-pō-
trō-fik*). Factors such as
choline and methionine,
found in the diet and preventing excess of fat being deposited in the liver.

liquefaction (*li-kwe-fak-shon*).
Being converted into a liquid.

liquor amnii (*lī-kwor am-nē-ē*).
The watery fluid by which the
fetus is surrounded.

liquor folliculi (*lī-kwor fo-li-
kū-lē*). Fluid in a Graafian
follicle.

liquores (*lī-kwor-ĕz*). Solutions
of active substances in water.
Liquor calcis saccharatus,
lime-water.

Listerism. The principles of
antiseptic surgery.

Liston's splint (*lis'-tonz splint*).
To immobilize the hip; made
of wood. Little used now.

lithagogues (*lith-'a-gogs*). Drugs which expel or dissolve stones.

lithiasis (*lith-ī-a-sis*). Formation of stone.

litholapaxy (*li-thō-la-paks'-ē*). Operation for crushing a stone in the bladder and removing the fragments at the same time.

lithopaedion (*lith-ō-pēd'-ion*). A calcified fetus in the abdominal cavity.

lithotomy (*li-tho-to-mi*). Operation of cutting into a bladder to remove a stone.

lithotomy position. Patient supine with thighs and knees flexed. The hips must be abducted.

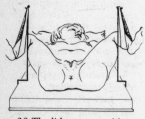

30 The lithotomy position

lithotrite (*lith'-ō-trīt*). An instrument for crushing stones in the bladder. It is passed through the urethra.

lithotrity (*lith-ot'-ri-ti*). Operation of crushing a stone in the bladder.

lithuria (*lith-ū-ri-a*). Passing gravel or crystals of uric acid with the urine.

litmus (*lit'-mus*). A blue pigment turned red by acids. *L. paper.* Paper impregnated with litmus; used for testing urine and gastric secretion. A red litmus paper is turned blue by an alkali.

litre (*lē-ter*). Metric measure of volume. The volume of 1kg water at 4° C; approximately 1·76 pints.

Little's disease. Spastic paraplegia or diplegia of infants due to birth injury or faulty development of the brain.

Littré's hernia (*lē-trā*). A diverticular hernia.

liver (*liv'-er*). Large organ occupying the upper right portion of the abdomen. It has many important functions including the secretion of bile, the manufacture of serum albumin and the storage of glycogen, etc.

livid (*li'-vid*). Blue-grey in colour.

Loa Loa. One of the parasites causing filariasis.

lobar (*lō'-ba*). Pertaining to a lobe.

lobe (*lōb*). Rounded division of an organ.

lobectomy (*lō-bek'-to-mi*). Excision of a lobe.

lobule (*lo-būl*). Small lobe.

localized (*lō-kal-īzd*). Limited

to a certain area; not widespread.

lochia (*lo'-ki-a*). The vaginal
discharge following delivery.
For the first day or two is
almost pure blood, but in
normal cases becomes
rapidly brown and then paler
and ceases in a few weeks.

lock-jaw. *See* TETANUS.

locked twins. The condition of
twins when some part of one
absolutely prevents the birth
of the other by causing complete impaction.

locomotor ataxia (*lō-kō-mō-tor
a-tak'-sia*). Impaired gait in
walking. A chronic disease
due to degeneration of parts
of the spinal cord and nerves.
See TABES DORSALIS.

loculated (*lok'-ū-lā-ted*). Divided into many cavities.

locum tenens (*lō-kum tē'-nens*).
A practitioner who tem-
porarily takes the place of
another.

loin (*loyn*). The lateral portion
of the back between the
thorax and pelvis.

longevity (*lon-gev'-i-ti*). Long
life.

long sight. Hypermetropia.

lordosis (*lor-dō'-sis*). Undue
curvature of the spine with
the convexity forwards; an
exaggeration of the normal
curve of the lumbar part of
the spine.

Loreta's operation (*lo-ret-az*).

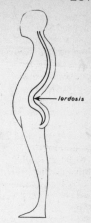

31 Lordosis

Forcible dilatation of the
pylorus for stricture.

lotion. A medicinal solution for
external use.

loupe (*loop*). Magnifying lens
used in ophthalmology.

louse (*lows*). *See* PEDICULUS.

Lovset's manoeuvre (*luv-sets
ma-noo-ver*). An obstetrical
manoeuvre used to deliver
breech presentations with
extended arms.

lower motor neurone disease.
Disease affecting the lower
motor neurone fibres. They
arise from cell bodies in the
anterior horns of the spinal
cord and pass to the motor
end plates of the muscles
which they innervate.

Lesions of the lower motor neurones result in paralysis and wasting of the muscles.

lower uterine segment (*lō-wer ū'-te-rīn seg'-ment*). That portion of the uterus, consisting of the cervix and the lower end of the body, which undergoes dilatation during labour.

LSD. Lysergic acid. One of the hallucinogenic group of drugs.

lubricant (*loo-bri-kant*). Any substance, such as an oil, which makes a surface slippery.

'lubb-dupp'. The heart sounds. The first is heard when the atrio-ventricular valves close, the second on closure of the semilunar valves.

lucid (*loo'-sid*). Clear.

Ludwig's angina (*lood'-vig's an-jī'-na*). An acute inflammatory condition in the sublingual and submaxillary regions.

lumbago (*lum-bā'-gō*). Painful condition of the lumbar muscles, due to inflammation of their fibrous sheaths. May be caused by a displaced intervertebral disc.

lumbar (*lum'-ba*). Pertaining to the region of the loins.

lumbar puncture (*pungk-cher*). This is the operation of tapping the cerebrospinal fluid in the lumbar region.

lumbar sympathectomy (*lumba sim-pa-thek-to-mi*). Operation to remove the sympathetic chain in the lumbar region.

lumen (*lū-men*). The cavity inside a tube.

lungs. The two organs of respiration, situated in the right and left sides of the cavity of the chest.

lunula (*lū'-nū-la*). White crescent at the root of the nail.

lupus erythematosus (*e-rith-em-a-tō-sus*). A disorder classed with the so-called collagen diseases. A localized form may affect the skin of exposed regions. The generalized form is known as systemic lupus erythematosus. The clinical manifestations of the disease are very varied. The criterion of diagnosis is the presence of LE cells in peripheral blood. LE cells are white cells which have ingested nuclear material.

lupus vulgaris (*loo-pus vul-ga-ris*). Tuberculosis affecting the skin.

luteinizing hormone (*lū-ti-nī-zing*). Hormone of the anterior pituitary gland stimulating the formation of corpus luteum in the ovary.

luteotrophin (*lū-tē-ō-trō-fin*). Pituitary hormone responsible for subsequent growth and development of the corpus luteum, after its formation by the follicle-stimulating hormone and the luteinizing hormone.

luteus (*loo'-tē-us*). Latin word for yellow. *See* MACULA LUTEA and CORPUS LUTEUM.

luxation (*luk-sā'-shon*). Dislocation of a joint.

lying-in (*lī-ing in'*). The puerperium.

lymph (*limf*). That part of the blood plasma which has passed through the walls of the capillaries, bathing the tissue cells, giving them nourishment and taking away waste products. It is also found in the lymphatic vessels and serous cavities.

lymphadenitis (*lim-fad-en-ī'-tis*). Inflammation of the lymphatic glands.

lymphadenoid goitre (*lim-fa-de-noyd goy-ter*). *See* HASHIMOTO'S DISEASE.

lymphadenoma (*lim-fa-de-nō'-ma*). Also called Hodgkin's disease. Serious disease characterized by enlargement of the lymphatic glands, and progressive anaemia, usually with enlargement of the spleen. There are often remissions, and it can be checked for a time by chemotherapy, X-rays, and surgical removal of localized groups of glands.

lymphangiectasis (*lim-fan-jē-ek'-ta-sis*). Dilated state of lymphatic vessels.

lymphangioma (*lim-fan-jē-ō'-ma*). Tumour composed of lymphatic vessels.

lymphangioplasty (*lim-fan-jē-ō-pla'-sti*). An operation for the relief of lymphatic obstruction.

lymphangitis (*lim-fan-jī-tis*). Inflammation of lymphatic vessels.

lymphatic leukaemia (*lim-fat-ik lū-kēm-ia*). *See* LEUKAEMIA.

lymphatics (*lim-fat'-iks*). Small vessels pervading the body, and containing lymph.

lymphocytes (*lim'-fō-sīts*). One of the normal varieties of white blood cells. *Lymphocytosis*, excess of these cells in the blood; found in leukaemia, whooping cough, tuberculosis and lymphadenoma. *Lymphopenia*, deficiency of lymphocytes.

lymphocythaemia (*lim-fō-sī-tē'-mea*). Increase of lymphocytes in the bloodstream.

lymphocytosis (*lim-fō-sī-tō'-sis*). Lymphocythaemia.

lymphogram. The method of demonstrating the lymphatic system following the injection of contrast medium opaque to x-rays.

lymphogranuloma inguinale (*lim-fō-gra-nū-lō-ma in-gwi-na-lā*). A venereal disease found esp. in the tropics.

lymphoid (*limf-oyd*). Having the character of lymph. *L. tissue*, adenoid tissue.

lymphoma (*lim-fō'-ma*). Tumour of lymphatic tissue.

lymphosarcoma (*lim-fō-sar-kō'-ma*). A sarcoma originating in lymphatic tissue.

lysergic acid (*lī-ser-jik*). *See* LSD.

lysine (*lī-sēn*). *See* AMINO-ACIDS.

lysins (*lī'-sins*). Antibodies able to dissolve cells. *Haemolysins*, those able to dissolve red blood cells. *Bacteriolysins*, those able to dissolve bacteria.

lysis (*lī-sis*). Dissolution. Decline of a fever.

lysozyme (*lī-sō-zīm*). Bactericide found in tears, nasal mucus and other secretions.

M

m. Abbreviation for metre.

McBurney's point. On line from umbilicus to anterior superior iliac spine, at outer edge of rectus muscle; corresponds to base of the appendix, and pressure here will give rise to pain when appendix is inflamed.

maceration (*mas-e-rā'-shon*). The softening of a solid by soaking it in a liquid; or of a

fetus which has died some time before delivery.

Mackenrodt's ligaments (*ma-ken-rōtz li-ga-mens*). Also called transverse cervical or cardinal ligaments. One of the chief supports of the uterus.

MacNaughton rules. In English law provisions necessary to establish diminished criminal responsibility on the grounds of insanity.

macro (*mak-rō*). Prefix meaning large.

macrocephalous (*mak-rō-kef'-a-lus*). Having a large head.

macrocheilia (*ma-krō-kī-li-a*). Excessively large lips.

macrocytes (*mak'-ro-sīts*). Abnormally large red cells, present in the blood in certain types of anaemia, including pernicious anaemia.

macrodactyly (*mak-rō-dak'-ti-li*). Enlargement of the fingers.

macroglossia (*mak-rō-glos'-ia*). Hypertrophy of the tongue.

macromastia (*mak-rō-mas'-ti-a*). Abnormally developed breasts.

macrophage (*ma-krō-fāj*). Wandering scavenger cells which form part of the reticulo-endothelial system. Their function is to engulf tissue debris and foreign particles. In connective tissue they are termed *histiocytes*

207 MAL

and in the blood they are known as *monocytes*. The engulfment of material is termed phagocytosis.

macroscopic (*mak-rō-skop'-ik*). Visible to the naked eye.

macula (*mak'-ū-la*). A spot discolouring the skin. *M. lutea*, central spot of the posterior surface of the retina, just lateral to the optic disc marked by a small depression, and where vision is most acute.

maculopapular (*ma-kū-lō-pa'-pū-la*). A rash having both macules and papules.

Madura foot (*mad-ū-ra*). *See* MYCETOMA.

Magendie, foramen of (*maj-en-di*). An opening in the roof of the fourth ventricle through which the cerebrospinal fluid passes into the subarachnoid space.

mal. Sickness. Mal de mer, sea sickness. Grand mal, major epilepsy. Petit mal, minor epilepsy.

malabsorption (*ma-lab-sorp-shon*). Reduced ability to absorb substances in the food from causes such as intestinal hurry, loss of absorbing surface as in extensive bowel resections, and diseases affecting the bowel wall including tropical sprue, coeliac disease and idiopathic steatorrhoea.

malacia (*mal-ā'-ki-a*). Pathological softening.

maladjustment (*mal-a-just'-ment*). Not in line, as with a badly set bone. In psychology, poorly adapted to circumstances.

malaise (*mal'-āz*). A general feeling of illness or discomfort.

malar (*mā'-lar*). Relating to the cheekbone.

malaria (*ma-lār-ia*). A disease due to a parasite introduced into the blood by certain mosquitoes. *See* ANOPHELES.

male fern. Filix mas.

malformation (*mal-faw-mā-shon*). Congenital deformity.

malignant (*ma-lig'-nant*). Virulent, fatal. A *malignant tumour* or *growth* is one which if not totally removed will spread locally and also cause similar growths in other parts of the body until the patient dies, *e.g.* carcinoma, sarcoma.

malignant hypertension. Hypertension associated with papilloedema and renal failure.

malignant pustule. Anthrax contracted from cattle, causing gangrenous carbuncle.

malingering (*ma-ling'-ger-ing*). Shamming sickness.

malleolus (*mal-le'-ō-lus*). The projection of the ankle-bone. The inner malleolus is at the lower extremity of the tibia. The outer one at the lower extremity of the fibula.

mallet finger. Deformed finger with flexion of distal phalanx.

malleus (*mal'-le-us*). A hammer-shaped bone of the middle ear. *See* EAR.

malnutrition (*mal-nū-tri'-shon*). A state of undernourishment or imperfect nutrition.

malocclusion (*ma-lo-kloo-zhon*). Bad contact between the masticating surfaces of the upper and lower teeth.

Malpighian corpuscle (*mal-pig-ian kor-pusl*). Mesh of capillaries which act as a filtering coil for blood passing through the kidneys.

malpresentation (*mal-prez-en-tā'-shon*). Any presentation, other than the vertex, of the fetus at the onset of labour.

malt (*mawlt*). Grain of barley which has begun to sprout and has then been dried. It contains a ferment (malt diastase) which converts starch into sugar.

Malta fever. *See* UNDULANT FEVER.

maltase (*mawl-tāz'*). An enzyme of the succus entericus which converts maltose into glucose.

maltose (*mawl-tōz*). A disaccharide composed of two molecules of glucose.

malunion (*mal-ū'-ni-on*). Faulty union of divided tissues, as of the fragments of a broken bone.

mamilla (*ma-mil'-la*). The nipple.

mammae (*mam'-mē*). The breasts, or milk-supplying glands.

mammaplasty (*ma-ma-pla'-sti*). Plastic surgery on the breasts.

mammary (*mam'-ma-ri*). Relating to the breasts.

mammography. To demonstrate tissue changes in the breast—xeroradiography frequently used for this technique.

Manchester repair. A type of gynaecological operation for uterovaginal prolapse.

mandible (*man'-di-bl*). The lower jaw.

Mandl's paint (*man'-dlz pānt*). An antiseptic paint containing tincture of iodine, used in tonsillitis.

mania (*mā'-nia*). Pathological combination of elation and energy. The patient is uncontrollably excited.

manic depressive psychosis (*sī-kō-sis*). A mental illness when intense excitement alternates with depression.

manipulation (*ma-nip-ū-lā'-shon*). Handling and working with the hands to procure some healing result.

mannerism (*ma'-ne-rizm*).

Habitual expression or actions of an individual which are characteristic of him. Under stress they may become exaggerated.

manoeuvre (*ma-noo'-ver*). Special movement by the hand or with an instrument for a particular purpose.

manometer (*man-om'-e-ter*). An instrument for measuring the pressure of gases and liquids.

Mantoux test (*man-too'*). Test of the body's reaction to antigenic material prepared from tubercle bacilli. This material called tuberculin is injected intradermally in serial dilutions (1 in 10,000; 1 in 1,000; 1 in 100). A localized inflammatory reaction within 48 hours signifies a positive response. *Heaf test.* A similar test for the same purpose. Tuberculin is injected by special 'gun'.

manual (*man'-nū-al*) (adjective). Done by hand.

manubrium sterni (*man-ū'-bri-um ster'-nē*). The uppermost part of the sternum.

manus (*ma-nus*). Latin for hand.

marasmus (*ma-ras'-mus*). Progressive emaciation.

marble bone disease. Disease which may be familial, with osteosclerosis of the entire skeleton, the spongy part of

the bone becoming compact. There is also anaemia.

Marfan's syndrome (*mar-fans sin'-drōm*). *See* ARACHNO-DACTYLY.

marihuana (*ma-roo-ah-na*). *See* CANNABIS INDICA.

Marmite (*mar'-mit*). A proprietary preparation of dried yeast rich in vitamin B. Can be used for soups or sandwiches.

marrow (*ma'-rō*). The soft substance which fills the medullary canal of a long bone and the small spaces in cancellous bone. The red cells of the blood are formed in the red bone marrow. Yellow marrow contains fat.

marrow puncture (*ma-rō pung-cher*). Investigative procedure involving the aspiration of marrow cells, usually by puncturing the sternum with a needle.

masochism (*ma'-zo-kism*). A delight in being tortured or humiliated from which a sexual pleasure may be derived.

Mason's gag (*mā'-sonz*). A mouth gag.

massage (*ma'-sahj*). Manipulation and rubbing of body designed to promote blood flow.

masseter (*mas-sē'-ter*). A strong facial muscle which moves the lower jaw.

mastalgia (*mas-tal-ji-a*). Pain in the breast.

mast-cells. Cell containing heparin and histamine, lining the walls of small blood vessels.

mastectomy (*mas-tek-to-mi*). Surgical removal of the breast. *Radical m.* The breast is removed together with the lymph glands of the axilla and the pectoral muscle.

mastication (*mas-tik-ā'-shon*). Chewing.

mastitis (*mas-tī'-tis*). Inflammation of the breast.

mastodynia (*mas-tō-di-ni-a*). Pain in the breasts often in the premenstrual phase.

mastoid (*mas'-toyd*). Literally, breastlike. The *mastoid process* is the projecting portion of the temporal bone behind the ear; it contains numerous air spaces including the *mastoid antrum.*

mastoidectomy (*mas-toy-dek'-to-mi*). Excision of the inflamed mastoid cells.

mastoiditis (*mas-toyd-ī'-tis*). Inflammation of the mastoid antrum and cells.

mastoidotomy (*mas-toy-do-to-mi*). Incision of cells of mastoid process.

masturbation (*mas-ter-bā'-shon*). Excitation of one's own genitals to produce an orgasm.

materia medica (*mat-er-ia med'-ik-a*). Branch of medical study dealing with the nature and use of drugs, *i.e.* pharmacology and therapeutics.

matrix (*mā-triks*). Continuous medium in which structures are embedded.

matter. Any substance. Pus is sometimes referred to as matter. *Grey m.* The nerve cells or non-medullated nerve fibres. *White m.* Medullated nerve fibres which are enveloped by a white sheath.

mattress suture. A continuous stitch through both the skin edges.

maturation (*mat-ū-rā'-shon*). Ripening: the process of becoming fully developed.

maxilla (*mak-si'-la*). The upper jaw bone.

maxillary (*mak-sil'-a-ri*). Pertaining to the maxilla.

mean (*mēn*). The average.

measles, morbilli (*mē-zels*). An infectious disease common in children. Incubation period 10 to 12 days. Early symptoms are those of a cold, sore throat, cough and rise in temperature, Koplik's spots. The rash appears on the fourth day, about the neck and behind the ears, gradually spreading to the rest of the body and extremities. The normal is reached about the seventh or ninth day.

Most infectious period is before the rash appears. *German measles*, Rubella.

meatus (*mē-ā'-tus*). An opening into a passage.

mechanism of labour (*mek'-an-izm*). The series of forces which act upon the fetus while it is being driven through the birth canal, with the resistances to those forces, and the resulting effects of both upon the attitude and movements of the fetus.

Meckel's diverticulum (*me-kels dī-ver-tik'-ū-lum*). A small blind protrusion occasionally found in the lower portion of the ileum. In rare cases it produces acute intestinal obstruction by strangulating an adjacent coil of gut.

meconium (*me-kō'-ne-um*). A black, sticky substance voided from the bowels of an infant during the first day or two after its birth.

medial (*mē-di-al*). The middle.

median (*mē-di-an*). In the middle. *M. line*, an imaginary longitudinal line dividing the body down the centre. *M. nerve*, one of the nerves of the arm.

mediastinum (*mē-di-as-tī'-num*). The space in the chest between the two lungs. It contains the heart, glands and great vessels.

medical jurisprudence (*jūris-prū'-dens*). Medicine as it is connected with the law; for instance, in case of suicide or murder.

medicament (*med-ik'-a-ment*). Any medicinal drug or application.

medicated (*me-di-kā-ted*). Impregnated with a medicament.

medication (*me-di-kā'-shon*). Giving a medicine to a patient. *Pre-operative m.* One given before an operation as a basal anaesthetic.

medicinal (*me-di'-si-nal*). Pertaining to the science of medicine or to a drug.

medicine (*me'-di-sin*). The treatment of disease. A drug used to prevent or treat disease. Term often used for diseases for which surgery is not required.

medico-chirurgical (*me-di-kō-ki-rur-ji-kal*). Relating to both medicine and surgery.

medico-social worker. Specially trained worker in hospital concerned with the patient in the community. Formerly called hospital almoner, now known as a hospital social worker.

Mediterranean fever (*med-it-e-rān-ian*). *Same as* UNDULANT FEVER, MALTA FEVER.

medium (*mē'-di-um*). Material used to nourish cultures of tissues, cells and micro-organisms.

medulla (*med-ul'-a*). Latin for marrow. Term also applied to central part of various organs *e.g.* kidney, adrenal gland.

medulla oblongata. The lowest part of the brain where it passes through the foramen magnum and becomes the spinal cord. It contains the vital centres which govern circulation and respiration.

medullary (*me-dul'-la-ri*). Relating to the marrow.

medullated (*mē'-du-lā-ted*). With an enveloping medulla or marrow.

medullated nerve fibre. Nerve fibre surrounded by a myelin sheath.

medulloblastoma (*me-du-lō-bla-stō'-ma*). Malignant tumour, from embryonic cells of neuro-epithelial origin, occurring in the cerebellum.

megacephaly (*me-ga-ke'-fa-li*). An abnormally large head.

megacolon (*meg-a-kō'-lon*). Hirschsprung's disease.

megakaryocytes (*me-ga-ka-ri-ō-sīts*). Large multi-nucleated bone marrow cells which produce the blood platelets.

megalo (*me-ga-lō*). Prefix meaning large.

megaloblast (*me-ga-lō'-blast*). An abnormally large nucle-ated blood cell. Megaloblasts occur in the blood in pernicious anaemia. Also known as macrocytes.

megalokaryocytes (*me-ga-lō-ka'-ri-ō-sīts*). *See* MEGAKARYOCYTES.

megalomania (*meg-al-ō-mā'-nia*). Mental condition with delusional ideas of personal greatness.

Meibomian glands (*mī-bō'-mian*). Sebaceous glands of the eyelids, *M. cyst,* Chalazion.

Meigs' syndrome (*mīgs sin'-drōm*). Ascites and hydrothorax associated with ovarian fibroma.

meiosis (*mī-ō-sis*). (1) Division of diploid cell to yield haploid gametes. The gametes (spermatozoa, ova) must have their chromosome number reduced by half in order to compensate for the doubling which occurs by fertilization. (2) Contraction of pupil of eye.

mel. Honey.

melaena (*mel-ē'-na*). Black tar-like stools, due to the presence of blood which has undergone changes in the alimentary tract. The blood is often from a gastric or duodenal ulcer.

melancholia (*mel-an-kō'-li-a*). Morbid depression, a form of mental illness. There is often a strong suicidal tendency.

melanin. A name for the dark pigments found in the eye, skin, hair; pigmentation may be markedly increased in Addison's disease.

melanoma (*mel-an-ō'-ma*). A tumour containing black pigment, melanin. May start as innocent pigmented wart, but possesses tendency to malignancy.   (Malignant melanoma or melanotic carcinoma.)

melanosis (*mel-an-ō'-sis*). Black spots in the tissues.

membrane (*mem-brān*). A thin layer of tissue.

menapthonum. Vitamin K.

menarche (*me-nar-kā*). The beginning of menstruation.

Mendel's law (*men'-delz lor*). A theory of heredity which laid the foundation for the theories of genetic inheritance.

Ménière's disease (*mā-nē-ārs*). Giddiness resulting from disease of the internal ear or the equilibrating mechanism of the brain.

meningeal (*men-in-jē'-al*). Pertaining to the meninges.

meninges (*me-nin'-jēz*). The membranes surrounding and covering the brain and spinal cord. They are, from without: the dura mater, the arachnoid, the pia mater.

meningioma (*me-nin-jē-ō'-ma*). Tumour derived from the meninges.

meningism (*men-in-jis'-m*). Syndrome characterized by symptoms and signs of meningitis but occurring in the absence of any causative organism. Probably a non-specific inflammatory reaction of the meninges to circulating toxins or some other trauma.

meningitis (*men-in-ji'-tis*). Inflammation of the meninges due to infection by organisms. Acute bacterial or viral meningitis is characterized by fever, headache, vomiting, backache and development of a stiff neck. Stupor, coma, convulsions may follow. A more insidious onset is sometimes seen in tuberculous meningitis.

meningocele (*men-in'-jō-sēl*). Protrusion of meninges from a bony defect usually in the spine, *e.g.* spina bifida.

meningococcus (*men-in'-jō-kok'-us*). A micro-organism, the cause of cerebrospinal fever.

meniscectomy (*me-nisk-ek-to-mi*). Removal of a semilunar cartilage from the knee joint.

meniscus (*me-nis-kus*). (1) A semilunar cartilage. (2) A lens. (3) The crescent-like surface of a liquid in a narrow tube.

menopause (*men'-ō-pawz*). Cessation of menstruation. Ovulation stops and reproductive life ends. It usually occurs between 40 and 50 years of age and is associated with alterations in hormonal balance which sometimes produce troublesome symptoms such as hot flushes, etc.

menorrhagia (*men-o-rā'-ji-a*). Excessive menstrual bleeding.

menses (*men-sēz*). The menstrual flow.

menstruation (*men-stroo-ā'-shon*). Monthly discharge of uterine mucosa with resultant bleeding which occurs in the absence of pregnancy in sexually mature women.

mental (*men'-tal*). (1) Pertaining to the mind. (2) Pertaining to the chin.

menthol (*men'-thol*). A local anodyne.

mento-anterior (*an-te'-rē-or*). The ordinary kind of face presentation, with the chin to the front; *i.e.* towards the maternal pubes.

mento-posterior (*pos-tār-ior*). Having the chin behind. A term applied to a variety of face presentation. *See* FACE PRESENTATION.

meralgia paraesthetica (*me-ral'-ji-a par-ēs-thet-'i-ka*). An affection of the nerves of the lumbar plexus giving rise to pain and sensory disturbances in the legs.

mercurialism (*mer-kū'-ri-al-ism*). Chronic poisoning by mercury. Occurs in workmen who labour with the metal, or inhale its vapours. *Symptoms:* (1) soreness of gums and loosening of teeth; (2) increased salivation; (3) foetor of breath; (4) griping and diarrhoea.

mesarteritis (*mes-ar-ter-ī'-tis*). Inflammation of the middle coat of an artery.

mesencephalon (*mes-en-kef'-a-lon*). The midbrain.

mesenchyme (*me-sen-kīm*). Embryonic connective tissue which forms bone, cartilage, connective tissue and blood, etc.

mesenteric (*mes-en-ter'-ik*). Pertaining to the mesentery.

mesentery (*mes'-en-ter-i*). A large fold of the peritoneum to which the small intestines are attached.

mesmerism (*mez'-mer-izm*). Hypnosis.

meso-appendix (*mes-ō-ap-en'-diks*). The mesentery of the appendix vermiformis.

mesocolon (*mes-ō-kō'-lon*). The fold of the peritoneum attached to the colon.

mesoderm (*mes'-o-derm*).

Germ layer of cells which have migrated from the surface of the developing embryo during gastrulation and which is situated between the ectoderm and the endoderm. The mesoderm gives rise to muscle, blood and connective tissues, etc.

mesometrium (*mes-ō-mē'-tri-um*). The broad ligaments which attach the uterus to the sides of the pelvis.

mesosalpinx (*mes-ō-sal'-pinks*). The part of the broad ligament which lies immediately below the Fallopian tubes.

mesothelium (*me-sō-thē-li-um*). General term applied to the epithelium lining serous cavities.

mesovarium (*mes-ō-vār'-i-um*). A short peritoneal fold connecting the ovary to the posterior layer of the broad ligament.

metabolic (*met-a-bol'-ik*). Pertaining to metabolism.

metabolism (*met-a'-bol-izm*). The biochemical processes taking place in the tissues of a living organism. Building up processes known as anabolism. Breaking down processes known as katabolism.

metacarpals (*met-a-kar-pals*). The five bones of the hand joining the fingers to the wrist.

metacarpophalangeal (*me-ta-kar-pō-fal-an-jē-al*). Relating to the metacarpus and the phalanges.

metamorphosis (*me-ta-mor-fō'-sis*). Transformation.

metaphysis (*me-ta'-fi-sis*). Part between the shaft, diaphysis, and the end, epiphysis, of the long bones.

metaplasia (*met-a-plā'-zi-a*). Conversion of one tissue into another.

metastasis (*me-tas'-ta-sis*). Transfer or spreading of a disease from one organ to another which is remote. A malignant growth is spread in this way.

metatarsalgia (*met'-a-tar-sal'-ji-a*). Pain in the fore part of the foot.

metatarsals (*met-a-tar'-sals*). The five bones of the foot between the tarsus and the toes.

meteorism (*mē-tē-or-ism*). Distension of the intestines by gas.

methaemoglobin (*met-hē-mō-glō-bin*). Altered haemoglobin producing cyanosis.

methaemoglobinuria (*met-hē-mō-glō-bin-ū'-ri-a*). The presence of methaemoglobin in the urine.

methandienone (*me-than-di-e-nōn*). An anabolic steroid derived from testosterone.

methionine (*me-thē-ō-nīn*). An

essential amino-acid containing sulphur. Used in liver damage and hepatitis.

methyl (*me-thil*). The chemical radical—CH_3.

methylated spirit (*me-thi-lā-ted*). Ordinary ethyl alcohol to which some methyl alcohol has been added in order to give it a nauseous taste and odour.

metra (*me'-tra*). The womb.

metre (*mē'-ter*). A measure of length, containing 100 centimetres, and equal to 39·37in.

metric system (*met'rik sis-tem*). System of weights and measures employing the metre and the gram as standard units which are multiplied or divided by powers of ten.

metritis (*me-trī-tis*). Inflammation of the womb.

metrocolpocele (*met-rō-kol'-pō-sēl*). Protrusion of the uterus into the vagina, the wall of the vagina being pushed in advance.

metropathia haemorrhagica (*me-trō-pa'-thia hē-mō-ra'-ji-ka*). Excessive menstrual bleeding due to excess of oestrin and associated with follicular ovarian cysts.

metroptosis (*met-rop-tō-sis*). Prolapse of the womb.

metrorrhagia (*met-ro-rā'-ji-a*). Bleeding from the uterus, other than at the menstrual period. It should always be investigated, as it is usually due to some pathological condition.

Mg. Chemical symbol for magnesium.

Michel's clips (*mi-chels*). Small metal clips used for suturing skin wounds after surgical operations. A special forceps is necessary for their removal.

micro (*mī-krō*). Prefix meaning small.

microbe (*mī-krōb*). Microorganism. *See* BACTERIA, VIRUS.

microbiology (*mī-krō-bī-o-lo-ji*). The study of microorganisms.

microcephalic (*mī-krō-kef-al'-ik*). Having an abnormally small head.

micrococci (*mī-krō-kok'-kī*). Genus of bacteria.

microcyte (*mī-krō-sīt*). A small red blood cell.

microcythaemia (*mī-krō-sit-hē'-mi-a*). Circulation of abnormally small erythrocytes in the blood.

microcytic anaemia (*mī-krō-si-tik*). Due to iron deficiency. The red cells in the blood are smaller than normal. The treatment is to give large doses of iron.

microgram (*mī-kro-gram*). μg. One millionth part of a gram.

micrometer (*mī-krom'-e-ter*). Instrument for measuring very small distances.

micron (*mī'-kron*). A millionth part of a metre, represented by the Greek letter μ.

micro-organism (*mī-krō-or'-gan-izm*). Any microscopic plant or animal.

microphthalmos (*mī-krof-thal'-mos*). Abnormal smallness of the eyes.

microscope (*mī-kro-skōp*). An instrument which magnifies minute objects invisible to the naked eye.

microsporon (*mī-krō-spo'-ron*). A fungus causing disease of the skin and hair.

microtome (*mī'-krō-tōm*). An instrument "for cutting fine sections for microscopic examination.

micturition (*mik-tū-rish'-on*). The act of passing urine.

midbrain (*mid-brān*). Small part of the brain between the forebrain and hindbrain.

midriff (*mid'-rif*). The diaphragm.

midwife (*mid'-wīf*). A woman who conducts the confinement of another.

midwifery (*mid'-wif-ri*). The art and science of the conduct of pregnancy, labour and the puerperium.

migraine (*mē-grān'*). Paroxysmal attacks of headache, usually with nausea and often preceded by disorders of vision. Migraine is usually unilateral.

miliaria papillosa (*mi-lē-ā-ri-a pa-pi-lō-za*). Prickly heat; an affection due to a disorder of the sweat glands. Their ducts are obstructed.

miliary (*mil-i-a-ri*). Like millet seed. Thus *miliary tuberculosis* is an acute form of infection in which the tissues are studded with small tubercles so as to resemble a mass of millet seeds.

milium (*mil'-i-um*). Small white round tumour, the size of a pin's head, which results from obstruction of the duct of a sebaceous gland. Occurs chiefly on forehead, eyelids, cheeks.

milk. The secretion of the mammary glands. The average composition is:

	Human Milk	Cow's Milk
Protein:	%	%
Lactalbumin	1·4 } 2	·75 } 4
Casein	·6	3·25
Fat . .	4	4
Carbohydrate	6	4
Salt . .	·2	·7
Water .	87·8	87·3

Human milk is neutral or slightly alkaline. Cow's milk is usually slightly acid by the time it reaches the consumer. Specific gravity 1026 to 1036.

milk sugar. *See* LACTOSE.

milk teeth. The first set of teeth. *See* TEETH.

Miller-Abbott tube. A double-bore rubber tube which is passed via the mouth into the duodenum so that intestinal suction can be applied in obstruction of the upper intestinal trace.

milliampere (*mil-i-ahm-pār*). One thousandth part of an ampere.

millicurie (*mi-li-kū-ri*). Unit of radioactivity, one thousandth of a curie.

milligram (*mil'-i-gram*). One thousandth part of a gram.

millilitre (*mil-i-lē-tr*). One thousandth part of a litre. Abr. ml. It is taken as equivalent to a cc.

millimetre (*mi-li-mē-tr*). One thousandth part of a metre.

Millin's prostatectomy (*mil-lins pro-sta-tek-to-mi*). In this operation the bladder is not incised but the prostate gland is enucleated from around the neck of the bladder. Also called retropubic prostatectomy.

Milton (*mil'-ton*). Proprietary antiseptic containing sodium hypochlorite.

miner's nystagmus. Nystagmus due to insufficient light striking the retina.

minim (*min'-im*). The sixtieth part of a fluid drachm; practically one drop.

miosis (*mī-ō-sis*). *Syn.* meiosis.

miotic (*mī-ō-tik*). *Syn.* meiotic. Term applied to a drug which contracts the pupil of the eye.

miscarriage (*mis-ka'-rāj*). *See* ABORTION.

Misuse of Drugs Act 1971. This Act supersedes the Dangerous Drugs Act. It controls possession and supply of certain habit-forming narcotic drugs and others producing profound effects on the central nervous system. All drugs coming under the Act and its Regulations are known as Controlled Drugs.

mitosis (*mī-tō'-sis*). A method of cell division in which the number of chromosomes remains unchanged.

mitral valve (*mī-tral val'v*). The valve of the heart between the left atrium and the left ventricle. Disease of this valve may give rise to *mitral stenosis* when there is narrowing of the orifice of the valve or *mitral regurgitation* or *incompetence* when the valve fails to close properly.

mittelschmerz (*mi-tel-shmā-rz*). Pain occurring at the time of ovulation allegedly due to peritoneal irritation by blood from the ruptured follicle.

ml. Millilitre.

modiolus (*mō-di-ō'-lus*).
Central axis of the cochlea.

molar teeth (*mō'-lar tēth*). The
grinders. *See* TEETH.

mole (*mōl*). (1) Pigmented
raised area of skin, which
may also be hairy. (2) In obstetric practice, a tumour
composed of coagulated
blood, fetal membranes and
the embryo; due to haemorrhage into a gestation sac,
and followed sooner or later
by abortion. *Carneous* or
fleshy m. When mole is
retained in utero for some
time, the fluid part of the
blood clot becomes absor-
bed, leaving solid fleshy
masses, in the midst of
which traces of the embryo
may or may not be found.
Hydatidiform or *vesicular m.*
Degeneration of the chorion
in the early weeks of pregnancy, resulting in the death
of the embryo and the conversion of the chorionic villi
into beadlike cysts or vesicles
which may attain the size of a
grape. Two prominent symptoms are (*a*) undue enlargement of the uterus for the
period of amenorrhoea, (*b*) a
watery pink discharge which
may contain vesicles. No fetal
parts are felt and no fetal
heart heard, and the uterus
feels softer than in a normal
pregnancy. As soon as diag-

nosed the uterus should be
emptied. The villi may
become malignant, and in-
vade the wall of the uterus. It
is then known as *chorion-
epithelioma*.

molecule (*mol'-e-kūl*). The
smallest possible particle of a
substance consisting of one
or more atoms of one or more
elements. Thus one atom of
sodium with one atom of
chlorine forms one molecule
of sodium chloride.

molluscum (*mol-us-kum*). Skin
disease, either *contagiosum*,
common in childhood, or
fibrosum, involving the formation of overgrowths of
fibro-cellular tissue.

Mönckeberg's arteriosclerosis
(*mernk-bergs   ar-tār'-ē-ō-
skle-rō'-sis*). Sclerosis of the
medium and small arteries
with extensive degeneration
of the middle muscle lining,
with atrophy and calcareous
deposits in the muscle
cells.

mongolism (*mon-go-lism*).
Down's syndrome. Due to
abnormality of chromosome
21 occurring during meiosis.
A chromosome pair fails to
separate with the result that
the child has a chromosome
too many, *i.e.* 47 instead of
46. Mongols usually have
slanting eyes, short head,
hypotonia and a low IQ.

Monilia (*mo-ni'-lia*). A yeast, which is liable to infect mucous membranes, giving rise to thrush.

monitoring. A recording, usually by automatic means, of the patient's blood pressure, temperature, pulse and respiration.

mono (*mo-nō*). Prefix meaning one.

mono-amine oxidase inhibitor. Drug which relieves depression by preventing breakdown of serotonin and other amines in brain tissue, *e.g.* phenelzine. During treatment, alcohol and foods rich in tyramine, *e.g.* cheese, should be avoided.

monocular (*mo-nok'-ū-lar*). Relating to one eye only.

monocyte (*mo-nō-sīt*). A type of white cell.

monocytosis (*mo-nō-sī-tō-sis*). Term employed when monocytes comprise more than 8 per cent of the total white cell count.

monograph (*mon'-ō-graf*). Book on one subject only.

monomania (*mon-ō-mā'-ni-a*). A neurosis when the patient has fixed ideas on one particular subject.

mononuclear (*mo-nō-nū-klē-a*). With one nucleus.

monoplegia (*mon-ō-plē'-ji-a*). Paralysis of one limb.

monorchid, monorchis (*mon-or'-kid*). Having only one testicle.

monosaccharide (*mon-ō-sak'-ar-īd*). Simplest sugar, *e.g.* glucose.

Monro's foramen (*mun-rōz*). Interventricular foramen. The communication between the two lateral ventricles and the third ventricle of the brain.

monster (*mon'-ster*). An abnormal individual owing to fetal maldevelopment.

mons veneris (*monz ven'-e-ris*). The eminence over the os pubis in women.

Montgomery's glands (*munt-gum'-er-ēz glanz*). Small prominences about the nipple, which become more evident during pregnancy and lactation. *See also* AREOLA.

Mooren's ulcer (*moo-renz*). Basal cell carcinoma affecting the cornea.

morbid (*mor'-bid*). Diseased, disordered, pathological.

morbilli (*mor-bil-ē*). Measles.

morbus (*mor'-bus*). Latin for disease.

Morgagni, hydatids of (*maw-ga-nyi hī-da-tids*). Small translucent cysts arising from the embryonic pronephros which occur attached by pedicles to the fimbriated end of the Fallopian tubes.

moribund (*mor'-i-bund*). In a dying state.

morning sickness. *See* VOMITING OF PREGNANCY.

moron (*maw'-ron*). Feeble-minded person.

morphine (*mor'-fin*). An alkaloid obtained from opium, used as a sedative or anodyne.

morphinism (*mor'-fin-izm*). Chronic poisoning from indulgence in the drug.

morphoea (*maw-fē-a*). Scleroderma affecting the skin only. Patches of atrophic, depigmented skin overlie connective tissue which has lost its elasticity.

morphology (*mor-fol-o-ji*). The science of form and structure of organisms.

mors (*mawz*). Latin for death.

mortality (*maw-ta'-li-ti*). Death rate. The annual death rate in this country is the no. of registered deaths × 1,000 divided by the mid-year population. The *Infant M. Rate* is the no. of deaths of infants under 1 year × 1,000 divided by the no. of registered live births. The *Maternal M. Rate* is the no. of deaths of women ascribed to pregnancy or childbearing × 1,000 divided by the no. of registered live and stillbirths.

mortuary (*mor'-tū-a-ri*). A place where dead bodies are kept.

morula stage (*mo-rū-la stāj*). Early stage found in developing ovum.

motile (*mō-til*). Able to move independently.

motions (*mō'-shons*). The evacuations of the bowels. *See* FAECES.

motor end plate. An accumulation of nuclei and cytoplasm of muscle fibres at the termination of motor nerves.

motor nerves (*mō'-ter*). Those nerves which, passing *from* a nerve centre, effect a response in the motor organ (a muscle or a gland); the opposite to sensory nerves, which, passing *to* a nerve centre, convey a sensation.

motor neurone disease (*mō-ter nū-rōn di-sēz*). Disease of unknown cause characterized by degeneration of the anterior horn cells of the spinal cord, the motor nuclei of the cranial nerves and the corticospinal tracts; also called progressive muscular atrophy and amyotrophic lateral sclerosis.

mould (*mō'-ld*). Any minute fungus.

moulding (*mōl'-ding*). The alteration in shape of the infant's head produced by the pressure it is subjected to whilst being driven through the birth canal.

mountain sickness (*mown'-tān*).

Vomiting, tachycardia, breathlessness.

movements (fetal) (*moov-mentz*). *See* QUICKENING.

moving beam radiotherapy. Technique employed to increase the dose incident on the target tissue while reducing the skin dose by rotating the beam in an arc with its centre in the target.

mucilage (*mū'-sil-lāj*). Aqueous solutions of gum or starch.

mucin (*mū'-sin*). An albuminoid constituent of mucus.

mucocele (*mū'-kō-sēl*). A cyst distended with mucus, as of the gall bladder or lacrimal sac.

mucoid (*mū'-koyd*). Resembling mucus.

mucolytic (*mū-kō-li-tik*). Drug which helps to soften mucus.

mucopurulent (*mū-kō-pu-roo-lent*). With mucus and pus.

mucosa (*mū-kō'-za*). A mucous membrane.

mucous membrane (*mū'-kuss*). A surface which secretes mucus. The lining of the alimentary canal, air passages, and urinogenital organs: merges into true skin at the various orifices of these canals. *Mucous polypus*, a small outgrowth from the mucous surface of the cervix uteri or of the nose.

mucoviscidosis (*mū-kō-vis-ki-dō-sis*). Fibrocystic disease of the pancreas. A recessively inherited disorder of salt secretion in which there is an inability of secreting glands to reabsorb sodium. As a result the mucous secretions are extremely viscous and obstruction to the ducts of glands results with consequent dilation, stasis, infection and fibrosis. The extent of the involvement by the disease is variable but usually affects the pancreas and lungs.

mucus (*mū'-kus*). A viscid fluid of the body secreted by the mucous membranes. Mucus in the urine shows as a transparent, cloudy sediment, easily dispersed by shaking the vessel.

multigravida (*mul-ti-gra'-vi-da*). Also multipara. A pregnant woman who has previously had one or more pregnancies.

multilocular (*mul-ti-lok'-ū-lar*). Having many locules.

multipara. *See* MULTIGRAVIDA.

multiple myeloma (*mul-ti-pl mĭ-e-lī-ma*). Neoplasm of plasma cells which infiltrate and replace the bone marrow. Characteristic features are anaemia, bone pains, and large quantities of circulating globulins of an abnormal type which may be excreted

in the urine. *See* BENCE JONES
PROTEIN.

multiple pregnancy (*mul-ti-pl*).
Twins, triplets, or any larger
number of fetuses gestated
together by one mother.

mumps (*mu'-mpz*). Infectious
parotitis, inflammation of the
parotid glands. Long incubation period, twelve to
twenty-eight days, and
quarantine must therefore be
most carefully enforced. A
complication not uncommon
is acute swelling of the testes
with great pain; and
occasionally acute ovaritis in
females.

murmur (*mer'-mer*). Abnormal
sound of the heart or the
lungs heard upon auscultation.

Murphy's sign. If continuous
pressure is exerted over an
inflamed gall bladder while
the patient takes a deep
breath it causes him to 'catch'
the breath just before the
zenith of inspiration.

Musca domestica (*mus'-ka
dō'-mes-ti-ka*). The common
fly.

muscae volitantes (*mus'-kē*).
Spots or filaments which float
in the vitreous humour of the
eye and which are visible to
the patient.

muscarine (*mus'-kar-in*). A
poisonous alkaloid which is a
product of putrefaction and is

occasionally found in mushrooms.

muscle (*mus'-sl*). Specialized
tissue composed of highly
contractile cells. There are
three varieties of muscle in
the body: (1) Striated, voluntary muscle. (2) Smooth,
involuntary, and (3) Cardiac
muscle. *M. atrophy peroneal.*
Charcot-Marie-Tooth dis-
ease. An inherited condition
in which there is degeneration of the anterior horn cells
of the peroneal nerves, *M.
dystrophy.* A group of conditions also known as
myopathies in which there is
degeneration of groups of
muscles without apparent
nerve involvement.

musculo-spiral nerve (*mus-kū-
lō-spī-ral nerv*). A nerve of
the arm.

mustard (*mus'-tud*). Plant of
which the crushed seeds are
used.

mutant (*mū-tant*). An individual possessing characteristics due to a genetic change.

mutation (*mū-tā'-shon*). Genetic change, producing change
in the individual of the
species.

mute (*mūt*). Without the power
of speech. Dumb.

myalgia (*mī-al'-ji-a*). Pain in the
muscles. *M. epidemic.* Bornholm disease. Characterized
by sudden onset of fever and

intercostal or diaphragmatic pain. It is thought to be caused by a virus.

myasthenia (*mī-as-thē'-ni-a*). Debility of the muscles.

myasthenia gravis (*mī-as-thē-ni-a grah'-vis*). A progressive loss of power in groups of muscle. Relieved by injections of prostigmine and surgical removal of the thymus gland.

myatonia (*mī-a-tō-ni-a*). Lack of muscle tone.

mycelium (*mī-sē'-li-um*). The filaments of fungus forming an interwoven mass.

mycetoma (*mī-se-tō'-ma*). Also known as Madura foot. A tropical disease due to infection with a vegetable parasite akin to that of actinomycosis. The part affected—most commonly the foot—becomes the seat of chronic inflammatory swelling with formation of ulcers and sinuses.

Mycobacterium (*mī-kō-bak-tā-rē-um*). A Gram positive genus of bacteria. *M. leprae* causes leprosy and *M. tuberculosis*, tuberculosis.

mycosis (*mī-kō'-sis*). Disease caused by fungus.

mydriasis (*mid-ri'-a-sis*). Increase in the size of the pupil of the eye.

mydriatics (*mid-rē-at'-iks*). Drugs which dilate the pupil

of the eye, *e.g.* atropine, homatropine.

myelin (*mī-el-in*). Medullary sheath of a nerve.

myelitis (*mī-e-lī-tis*). Inflammation of the spinal cord.

myelocele (*mī-e-lō-sēl*). A spina bifida in which the sac contains a portion of the spinal cord.

myelocyte (*mī-e-lō-sīt*). Bone marrow cell.

myelogram (*mī-el-ō-gram*). Radiograph of the spinal cord.

myeloid (*mī'-e-loyd*). Of the marrow. *M. tissue.* Tissue giving rise to the cellular elements of the blood, *viz.* red cells, white cells and platelets.

myeloma (*mī'-el-ō'-ma*). Neoplasm of plasma cells.

myelomatosis (*mī-e-lō-ma-tō-sis*). *See* MULTIPLE MYELOMA.

myelosclerosis (*mī-el-ō-skle-rō-sis*). Replacement of bone marrow by fibrous tissue.

myocardial (*mī-ō-kar'-di-al*). Pertaining to the muscle of the heart.

myocarditis (*mī-ō-kar-di'-tis*). Inflammation of the muscular tissue of the heart. Often follows acute rheumatism.

myocardium (*mī-ō-kar'-di-um*). The heart muscle.

myogenic (*mī-ō-je'-nik*). Originating from muscular tissue.

myoglobin (*mī-ō-glō-bin*). A

specialized haemoglobin found in muscle which has slightly different dissociation characteristics from that in the blood so that oxygen is transferred from the blood to the muscle.

myoma (*mī-ō'-ma*). Any tumour composed of muscular tissue.

myomectomy (*mī-ō-mek'-to-mi*). Removal of a myoma; usually referring to a fibroid from the uterus.

myometrium (*mī-ō-mē-tri-um*). The uterine muscle.

myopathy (*mī-op'-ath-i*). Any disease of a muscle.

myope (*mī'-ōp*). A short-sighted person. *Myopic*, pertaining to shortsightedness.

myopia (*mī-ō'-pi-a*). Short-sightedness; corrected by wearing a biconcave lens.

myosarcoma (*mī-ō-sar-kō'-ma*). A malignant tumour of muscle.

myosin (*mī-ō-sin*). Protein found in muscle.

myosis (*mī-ō'-sis*). Contraction of the pupil of the eye.

myositis (*mī-ō-sī'-tis*). Inflammation of a muscle. *M. ossificans*. May follow stretching of an injured muscle. Its fibres and haematoma are replaced by cancellous bone. the condition can be prevented by resting the injured muscle.

myotics (*mī-ot'-iks*). Drugs which cause the pupil to contract, *e.g.* eserine. *Syn.* meiotics, miotics.

myotomy (*mī-ot'-o-mi*). Cutting through a muscle.

myotonia (*mī-o-tō'-ni-a*). (1) Tonic muscular spasm. (2) Muscle stretching.

myringa (*mir-in'-ga*). The tympanic membrane of the ear.

myringitis (*mir-in-jī'-tis*). Inflammation of the tympanic membrane of the ear.

myringotome (*mir-in-go-tōm*). Knife used for myringotomy.

myringotomy (*mir-in-got'-o-mi*). Incision of the tympanic membrane of the ear, performed when the presence of pus is suspected in the middle ear.

myrrh (*mer*). An astringent gum-resin of pleasant odour, used in mouthwashes.

myxoedema (*miks-e-dē'-ma*). Syndrome due to hypothyroidism and characterized by dry atrophic skin, swelling of the limbs and face and retardation both physical and mental. The metabolic rate is diminished and the patient dislikes the cold intensely.

myxoma (*miks-ō'-ma*). Tumour of connective tissue containing mucoid material.

myxosarcoma (*miks-ō-sar-kō'-ma*). A malignant myxoma.

N

N. Chemical symbol for nitrogen.

Na. Chemical symbol for sodium.

Naboth's follicles (*nah'-bōt*). Small cystic bodies resulting from infection of *N. glands*.

Naboth's glands. Small glandular bodies situated in the neck of the uterus.

NaCl. Chemical symbol for sodium chloride, *i.e.* common salt. It is present in all the body fluids.

Naegele's obliquity (*nā'-gēl-e*). Tilting of the fetal head towards one or other shoulder as it enters the brim of the pelvis; by this attitude a slightly smaller transverse diameter of the head is presented to the brim.

naevus (*nē'-vus*). A birthmark due to a mass of dilated veins or arteries, usually very tiny ones.

nail (*nāl*). Horny plate found at the tip of finger or toe.

nape (*nāp*). The back of the neck.

napkin rash. Inflammation of the 'napkin area' in a baby. Caused by alkalis, dampness, friction or infection. The nappies should not be washed in detergents as this is a frequent cause of the rash.

narcissism (*nar-sis'-izm*). An abnormal love for oneself; named after Narcissus, who fell in love with the reflection of himself.

narco-analysis (*nar-kō-a-na'-li-sis*). In psychotherapy, the patient is made to talk freely, bringing repressed matter to consciousness after having had an injection of a sedative drug.

narcolepsy (*nar-ko-lep-si*). A condition characterized by sudden attacks of sleep occurring repeatedly during the day.

narcosis (*nar-kōs'-is*). A state of unconsciousness produced by the use of narcotics.

narcotic (*nar-kot'-ik*). A drug which produces unconsciousness, *e.g.* paraldehyde, the barbiturates.

nares (*na'rēz*). The nostrils.

nasal (*nā-'sal*). Relating to the nose.

nascent (*nās'-sent*). At the moment of birth.

nasogastric (*nā-zō-gas-trik*). Relating to the nose and stomach. *N. tube.* Used in artificial feeding.

nasolacrimal (*nā-zō-la'-krimal*). Relating to the nose and lacrimal apparatus.

nasopharyngeal (*nā'-zō-far-in-je'-al*). Pertaining to the naso-pharynx.

nasopharynx (*nā'-zō-far'-inks*). The space between the posterior nares, the base of the skull, the soft palate, the upper end of the oesophagus, and the epiglottis.

nates (*nā'-tēz*). The buttocks.

natural childbirth. A school of opinion concerning childbirth which advocates the minimum of medical interference with the process of delivery.

nausea (*naw'-sē-a*). A feeling of sickness.

navel (*nā'-vel*). The umbilicus, the point of connection of the umbilical cord.

navicular (*na-vi-kū-la*). The boat-shaped tarsal bone.

nebula (*neb'-ū-la*). A cloud or mist. Term applied to filmy corneal opacities.

nebulae (*ne-bū-lē*). Plural of nebula. Used to describe sprays of very fine particles used, for example, to facilitate absorption of inhaled substances.

nebulizer (*neb'-ū-li-zer*). *See* ATOMIZER.

neck (*nek*). Narrow part near the end of an organ, *Derbyshire n.* Goitre. *Wry n.* Torticollis.

necrobiosis (*ne-krō-bī-ō-sis*). Death of tissue. *Red n.* A type of degeneration occurring in a fibroid of the uterus if pregnancy takes place. After labour, the fibroid can recover its vitality.

necropsy (*ne-crop'-si*). Examination of a body after death.

necrosis (*ne-krō'-sis*). Death of tissue.

necrotic (*ne-krot'-ik*). Relating to necrosis.

needle holder (*nē'-dl hōl-der*). Instrument for holding surgical needles.

needling. Perforation with a needle especially in cataract. *See* DISCISSION.

negativism (*neg'-a-tiv-izm*). A state of mind in which the ideas and behaviour of an individual are in opposition to those of the majority and contrary to suggestion.

Neisseria (*nī-se-ri-a*). Genus of diplococci. *N. gonorrhoeae* causes gonorrhoea; *N. meningitidis* causes epidemic cerebrospinal meningitis.

Nelaton's line (*ne-la-tons*). Line from the anterior superior iliac spine to the tuberosity of the ischium.

nematodes (*ne-ma-tōds*). Worms including round worms, threadworms and eelworms. Some of these are parasitic to man, *e.g.* hookworm.

neonatal (*nē-ō-nā-tal*). Relating to the first four weeks of life.

neonate (*nē-ō-nāt*). Term applied to a child during the first month of life.

neoplasm (*nē'-ō-plasm*). A tumour. An abnormal local

multiplication of some type of cell. A neoplasm may be either *benign* if it shows no tendency to spread, or *malignant* if the growing cells infiltrate surrounding tissues and invade other parts of the body.

nephrectomy (*nef-rek'-tō-mi*). Removal of a kidney.

nephritis (*ne-frī'-tis*). Inflammation of the kidney. The term nephritis is used to describe a large number of widely differing conditions affecting this organ.

nephro- (*nef-rō*). Pertaining to the kidney.

nephroblastoma (*ne-frō-bla-stō'-ma*). Wilms' tumour. A neoplasm of the kidney which occurs in children.

nephrocalcinosis (*ne-frō-kal-si-nō'-sis*). A complication of hyperparathyroidism in which calcium becomes deposited in the renal tubes.

nephrocapsulectomy (*nef-rō-kap-sū-lek'-to-mi*). Operation to remove the kidney capsule.

nephrography (*nef-ro-gra-fi*). X-ray examination of the kidney.

nephrolithiasis (*nef-rō-lith-ī'-as-is*). Stone in the kidney.

nephrolithotomy (*nef'-rō-lith-ot'-o-mi*). Removal of a stone from the interior of the kidney.

nephroma (*nef-rō'-ma*). Tumour of the kidney.

nephron (*nef'-ron*). A unit of the kidney. It consists of a glomerulus, with the secreting part of its tubule. One kidney has about a million nephrons.

nephropexy (*nef'-rō-pek'-si*). Stitching a movable kidney into a firm position.

nephroptosis (*nef-rop-tō'-sis*). Downward displacement of the kidney.

nephrosis (*nef-rō'-sis*). Chronic progressive degenerative disease of the renal tubes.

nephrostomy (*nef-ros-to-mi*). Surgical opening into the kidney to drain it.

nephrotic syndrome (*nef-ro-tik sin'-drōm*). Degenerative disease of renal tubules characterized by heavy proteinuria, with reduction of plasma protein and oedema. Prognosis variable.

nephrotomy (*ne-frot'-o-mi*). Cutting into the kidney.

nephro-ureterectomy (*nef-rō-ū-rē-te-rek'-to-mi*). Operation to remove both kidney and ureter.

nerve (*nerv*). A bundle of fibres, conveying the impulses of movement and sensation to and from the organs. *See* MOTOR NERVES, SENSORY NERVES, VASOMOTOR.

nerve root. Each spinal nerve

arises from the spinal cord by two roots; the dorsal root carries the sensory fibres and the ventral root the motor fibres.

nervous (*ner'-vus*). Pertaining to the nerves. May also mean anxious and excited.

nettle-rash. Urticaria.

neural (*nū-ral*). Relating to nerves.

neuralgia (*nū-ral'-ji-a*). Pain in the distribution of a nerve. *e.g. trigeminal n.* Severe pain in the distribution of the trigeminal nerve. *Sciatica* is neuralgia of the sciatic nerve distribution. The cause may be irritation of the nerve by some bony structure or a tumour, but frequently the cause cannot be ascertained. For intractable pain interruption of the sensory fibres of the nerve is often helpful.

neurapraxia (*nū-rā-prak'-si-a*). There is a temporary block to nerve conduction as after giving a local anaesthetic.

neurasthenia (*nū-ras-thē'-ni-a*). Nervous exhaustion.

neurectomy (*nū-rek'-to-mi*). Excision of part of a nerve.

neurilemma (*nū-ri-lem'-a*). The sheath of a nerve fibre.

neurinoma (*nū-ri-nō-ma*). Tumour of a neurilemma.

neuritis (*nū-rī-'tis*). Inflammation of a nerve.

neuroblast (*nū-rō-blast*). Embryonic nerve cell.

neuroblastoma (*nū-rō-blas-tō'-ma*). Malignant growth of sympathetic nerve ganglia, *esp.* adrenal medulla. Strictly a tumour of neuroblasts.

neurodermatitis (*nū-rō-der-ma-ti-tis*). Characteristic hyperkeratosis associated with habitual scratching.

neuroepithelium (*nū-rō-ep-i-thē'-li-um*). Specialized nerve epithelium, *e.g.* the retina, which consists of nerve endings, rod and cone-shaped cells of the optic nerve.

neurofibroma (*nū-rō-fī-brō'-ma*). Tumour arising from connective tissue surrounding peripheral nerves.

neurofibromatosis (*nū-rō-fī-brō-ma-tō-sis*). Von Recklinghausen's disease. Generalized distribution within the body of neurofibromata.

neuroglia (*nū-rō-glī-a*). Connective tissue cells of the central nervous system are collectively known as *glia*. Neuroglia are cells with long fibrous processes which are derived from embryonic nervous tissue and are closely related to Schwann cells; their exact supportive function is not known. *Microglia* are similar to macrophages.

neurolemma (*nū-rō-lem-ma*). *See* NEURILEMMA.

neuroleptic (*nū-rō-lep-tik*). Drug affecting the nervous system.

neurologist (*nū-ro'-lo-jist*). Physician who specializes in neurology.

neurology (*nū-ro'-lo-ji*). Medical science of diseases of the nervous system.

neuroma (*nū-rō'-ma*). A tumour composed of nerve tissue.

neuron (*nū'-ron*). A nerve cell and its processes.

neuronotmesis (*nū-ron-ot-mē-sis*). Severance of a nerve.

neuropathic (*nū-'ro-path'-ik*). Relating to nervous disorder.

neuropathy (*nū-ro-pa-thi*). Disease of the nervous system.

neuroplasty (*nū-rō-plas-ti*). Operation to repair a nerve.

neurosis (*nū-rō'-sis*). A disorder of mental function whereby patients are abnormally emotionally vulnerable but retain external reality; *cf.* psychosis. Neuroses include behaviour disorders such as hysterical and obsessive compulsive reactions and disturbances of 'affect', as for example, in anxiety states.

neurosurgery (*nū-rō-ser'-je-ri*). Surgery of peripheral and central nervous system.

neurosyphilis (*nū-rō-si'-fi-lis*). Involvement of the central nervous system by syphilis.

neurotic (*nū-ro-tik*). Relating to a neurosis.

neurotmesis (*nū-rot-mē'-sis*). The nerve trunk is severed or crushed and there can be no useful recovery without surgery.

neurotomy (*nū-ro-to-mi*). Division of a nerve.

neurotripsy (*nū-rō-trip-si*). The crushing of a nerve.

neurotropism (*nū-rō-tro-pism*). Predilection of an infecting organism for nervous tissue.

neutral (*nū'-tral*). Neither acid nor alkaline.

neutropaenia (*nū-trō-pē'-ni-a*). Insufficiency of neutrophil polymorphonuclear leucocytes in the blood.

neutrophil (*nū-trō-fil*). Predilection for neutral dyes, *i.e.* not acidophil or basophil. Term used to describe the majority of polymorphonuclear leucocytes which do not demonstrate any characteristically staining granules in their cytoplasm, *cf.* basophil, eosinophil.

nicotine poisoning. Result of over-indulgence in smoking due to an alkaloid in tobacco leaves. Cardinal features are the paralysis of autonomic ganglia and constriction of coronary arteries.

nicotinic acid (*ni-kō-tin'-ik*). Pellagra-preventing factor of

vitamin B complex. *See* VITA-
MINS.

nictitation (*nik-ti-tā'-shon*). Involuntary blinking of the
eyelids.

nidation (*ni-dā-shon*). Implantation.

Niemann-Pick's disease. A
lipoid storage disease in
which lecithin is deposited.
An inherited defect of phospholipid metabolism which
leads to widespread deposition of lecithin in the tissues.
It is associated with mental
retardation.

night-blindness (*nīt-blīnd'-
ness*). *See* NYCTALOPIA.

nigrescent (*ni-gres'-sent*).
Growing black.

nigrites (*ni-grish'-i-ēz*). Black-
ness. *N. linguae*, a condition
in which the filiform papillae
of the tongue are hyper-
trophied and darkly pig-
mented.

nihilism (*ni-hi-lism*). Psychiatric term denoting feeling of
hopelessness in the patient.

nipple (*nip'-pl*). Small eminence in the centre of each
breast.

nipple shields. Covering of glass
or india-rubber put on the
nipples to protect them when
they are sore.

Nissl's granules (*nis-lz gran-
ūlz*). Granular substances
found in the cell body of a
neuron.

nit. The egg of the louse.

nitrate (*nī'-trāt*). A salt of nitric
acid.

nitric acid (*nī'-trik as'-id*). A
corrosive fluid used in testing
for protein, etc.

nitrite (*nī'-trīt*). A salt of nitrous
acid.

nitrogen (*nī-trō-jen*). A colourless inert gas, forming about
78 per cent of the atmos-
phere and acting as a diluent.
Nitrogenous foods. *See* PRO-
TEIN.

nitrous oxide (*nī-trus ok'-sīd*).
Laughing gas; an anaesthetic.

Nobecutane (*nō-bek'-ū-tān*).
Resinous spray used to form
a covering over wounds.

nocturia (*nok-tū-ri-a*). Passing
urine at night. May be a
symptom of cardiac failure.

nocturnal (*nok-ter-nal*). At
night. *N. enuresis*. Bedwetting during sleep.

nodding spasm. *See* SPASMUS
NUTANS.

node (*nōd*). A swelling. *Atrio-
ventricular n.* At the base of
the interatrial septum from
which impulses pass down
the Bundle of His. *Heberden's ns.* Deformity of the
joints in the hands in arthritis. *Sinuatrial n.* The
pacemaker of the heart,
found at the opening of the
superior vena cava into the
right atrium. *N. of Ranvier.*
The constriction in the

neurilemma of a nerve fibre.

nodule (*nod-ūl*). A little knob.

non compos mentis (*non kom'-pos men'-tis*). Not sound of mind.

non-viable (*non-vī-ubl*). Unable to survive, especially as to a child of less than 28 weeks' gestation.

noradrenaline (*nor-ad-ren'-a-lēn*). Hormone of the adrenal medulla. Raises blood pressure by a general vasoconstriction so given in shock, etc.

normal (*nor'-mal*). The average or usual form.

normoblasts (*nor'-mō-blasts*). Immature nucleated red cells present in red bone marrow.

normocyte (*nor'-mō-sīt*). A normally-sized erythrocyte.

nose (*nōz*). The organ of smell and used for warming, filtering and moistening the air breathed in.

nosology (*nō-so-lo-ji*). Science of the classification of diseases.

nostalgia (*nos-tal'-ji-a*). Home sickness, or a yearning for the past.

nostrils (*nos'-trilz*). The anterior apertures of the nose.

notch (*notsh*). Indentation.

notifiable (*nō-'tif-ī-abl*). A term applied to certain cases of disease and other occurrences which must be made known to the Area Medical Officer, *e.g.* smallpox, tuberculosis, typhoid fever, dysentery, food poisoning, acute poliomyelitis, diphtheria, measles, whooping cough, etc.

noxious (*nok-si-us*). Harmful.

Nuck (*nook*). *See* CANAL OF.

nucleated (*nū'-klē-ā-ted*). With a nucleus.

nucleic acid (*nūk'-le-ik*) and its derivatives have a stimulating effect on bone marrow, producing an increase in the polymorphonuclear cells in the blood.

nucleoprotein (*nū-klē-ō-prō-tēn*). Compound of protein and nucleic acid in nuclei.

nucleus (*nū-klē-us*). Pl. **nuclei.** (1) Of cell, the spherical body containing the chromosomes. *See* CELL. (2) Of brain, demarcated mass of cell bodies, *e.g.* basal nuclei.

nucleus pulposus (*pul-pō-zus*). A pulpy mass in the centre of the intervertebral discs. May become prolapsed into the spinal canal causing pressure on the cord and spinal nerves.

nullipara (*nu-lip'-a-ra*). A woman who has never had a child.

nummulated (*num'-mū-lā-ted*). Resembling a coin; applied to a form of expectoration sometimes seen in pulmonary tuberculosis.

nutation (*nū-tā'-shon*). Involuntary nodding of the head.

nutrient (*nū'-tri-ent*). Nourishing. *N. foramen*, opening in a bone for the nourishing vessels.

nutrition (*nū-tri-shon*). Science of feeding.

nyctalopia (*nik-tal-ō'-pi-a*). A state of the eyes which causes vision to be worse at night than during the day.

nyctophobia (*nik-tō-fō'-bi-a*). Abnormal fear of darkness.

nymphae (*nim-fē*). Labia minora.

nymphomania (*nim-fō-mā'-ni-a*). Excessive sexual desire in females.

nystagmus (*nis-tag'-mus*). Involuntary oscillations of the eyeball; sometimes congenital; sometimes a symptom of brain disease, ocular affection, or lesion in the internal ear.

O

O. Chemical symbol for oxygen.

obesity (*ō-bē'-si-ti*). Excessive fatness.

objective (*ob-jek'-tiv*). (1) The object glass of a microscope. (2) Pertaining to things lying external to one's self.

O signs. Signs seen in a patient about which he may not complain.

oblique diameters of pelvis (*ō-blēk dī-am'-et-erz*). See DIAMETERS OF PELVIS.

oblique muscles (*ō-blēk mus'-lz*). The two external muscles of the eyeball, an upper and a lower. Also two large muscles of the abdominal wall, an internal and an external.

obsession (*ob-sesh'-on*). An idea of which the patient cannot rid himself. Minor obsessions are common in perfectly healthy people: but long-standing obsessions are especially frequent in the mentally ill.

obsessive compulsive neurosis (*ob-se-siv com-pul-siv nu-rō-sis*). Mental disorder in which the outstanding feature is a feeling of compulsion to act in a way which the patient realizes to be absurd.

obsolete (*ob'-sō-lēt*). No longer used.

obstetric (*ob-stet'-rik*). Pertaining to the practice of midwifery.

obstetrician (*ob-ste-tri-shon*). Doctor who practises obstetrics.

obturator (*ob-tūr-ā'-ter*). That which stops up a hole or cavity. The obturator of a sigmoidoscope, for example, is the blunt-ended rod which fills up the end of the instrument when it is introduced into the rectum, and thus prevents any scratching of the mucous membrane. The *obturator foramen* is a hole on each side of the pelvis, closed by the powerful *obturator ligament.* The *obturator muscles* are two muscles on each side in the same region, and there are also *obturator vessels* and *nerves*.

obtusion (*ob-tū'-zhon*). A blunting, as of sensitivity.

occipital (*ok-sip'-i-tal*). Relating to the back of the head.

occipito-anterior ⎱ The two
occipito-posterior ⎰ kinds of vertex presentation, according as the back of the head (occiput) is directed forwards or backwards.

occiput (*ok'-si-put*). The back of the head or skull. *See* SKULL.

occlusion (*ok-klū-zhon*). Closure.

occlusive therapy (*ok-lū-siv the-ra-pi*). The patient is encouraged to use the lazy eye by covering the good eye.

occult blood (*ok'-ult blud*). Not visible to naked eye. Term used to describe blood passed in faeces in such small amounts that no dark colour is present. This blood can only be demonstrated by the occult blood test.

Occultest. Tablets which contain reagents for the demonstration of occult blood.

occupational disease (*ok-ū-pā'-sho-nal di-zēz*). Illness induced by the patient's occupation.

occupational therapist. One who practises occupational therapy.

occupational therapy. Any occupation given to a patient to help in his recovery, both mentally and physically.

ocular (*ok'-u-lar*). Relating to the eye.

oculist (*ok'-ū-list*). An eye specialist.

oculogyric (*o-kū-lō-jī-rik*). Making the eyes roll.

oculomotor nerves (*ok-ū-lō-mō-tor*). The third pair of cranial nerves which help to move the eyeball.

Oddi, sphincter of (*o'-di sfinkter ov*). Muscular sphincter at the opening of the common bile duct into the duodenum.

odontalgia (*o-don-tal'-jia*). Toothache.

odontoid (*o-don'-toyd*). Toothlike. *O. process.* Peglike projection of second cervical vertebra.

odontolith (*o-don'-to-lith*). Calcareous matter deposited on teeth; tartar.

odontology (*o-don-to'-lo-ji*). Dentistry.

odontoma (*o-don-tō'-ma*).

Tumour arising from a tooth or a developing tooth.

oedema (*e-dē'-ma*). Abnormal amount of fluid in the tissues causing a puffy swelling. The fluid tends to collect in the dependent parts, *e.g.* oedema of the ankles.

Oedipus complex (*ēd'-i-pus*). A persistence of the normal love of a boy for his mother so that it rivals that of his father. Named after Oedipus who, according to Greek mythology, unknowingly married his mother and killed his father.

oesophageal (*ē-sof'-a-je-al*). Pertaining to the oesophagus. *O. varices*. Varicose veins in the lower part of the oesophagus resulting from hypertension in the hepatic portal system which occurs in cirrhosis of the liver.

oesophagectomy (*ē-so-fa-jek-to-mi*). Resection of the oesophagus.

oesophagitis (*ē-so-fa-jī-tis*). Inflammation of the oesophagus, especially *reflex o.*, due to hiatus hernia when stomach acid regurgitates into the lower part of the oesophagus causing damage and inflammation of the wall.

oesophagoscope (*ē-sof'-a-go-skōp*). An instrument for viewing the interior of the oesophagus.

oesophagostomy (*ē-so-fa-gos'-to-mi*). An artificial opening is made into the oesophagus.

oesophagus (*ē-sof'-a-gus*). The canal which runs from the pharynx into the stomach.

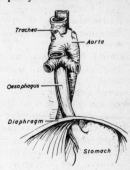

32 The oesophagus

oestradiol (*ē-strā'-dē-ol*). Hormone contained in Graafian follicles. Administered in oestrogen deficiency. *See* OESTROGENIC HORMONE.

oestrogen (*ēs-tro-jen*), or **oestrogenic substance or hormone.** Any substance, usually a steroid, capable of producing genital tract changes characteristic of the follicular phase of the menstrual cycle: an oestrogen is secreted by the ovaries. Oestrogens are also produced by the placenta during pregnancy and by the adrenal cortex. The female secondary sexual characteristics are under the influence of oestrogens.

ohm (*ōm*). Unit of electrical resistance.

oidium albicans (*oyd'-i-um*). *Syn. Candida albicans.* A microscopic fungus which is the cause of thrush. *See also* SACCHAROMYCES.

ointment. A soft application to promote healing, usually consisting of a base impregnated with some drug.

olecranon (*ō-lek'-ra-non*). The bone composing the point of the elbow. The extreme upper end of the ulna, the inner of the two bones of the forearm. (*See illustration,* p. 121.)

oleum morrhuae (*ō-lē-um mor-oo-ē*). Cod-liver oil: usual abbreviation Ol. Morrh.

oleum ricini (*ris'-ēn-i*). Castor oil: usually written Ol. Ric.

olfactory (*ol-fak'-tur-i*). Relating to the sense of smell.

oligaemia (*ol-i-gē'-mi-a*). Lack of blood.

oligo- (*ol-i'-gō*). Prefix meaning deficiency.

oligohydramnios (*ol-i-gō-hi-dram'-ni-os*). Deficiency of amniotic fluid.

oligomenorrhoea (*o-li-gō-me-nor-rēa*). Sparse menstrual flow.

oligospermia (*o-li-gō-sper-mēa*). Insufficient secretion of semen or deficiency of sperms in the semen.

oligotrophia (*ol-ig-ō-trōf'-i-a*). Lack of nourishment.

oliguria (*ol-i-gūr'-i-a*). A diminution in the amount of urine passed.

olivary body (*ol-iv-ar-i bo-di*). An oval mass of grey matter behind the anterior pyramid of the medulla oblongata.

olive oil. An oil obtained from olives. Used as a demulcent.

omentocele (*ō-men-tō-sēl*). Hernial sac containing omentum.

omentopexy (*o-men-tō-pek-si*). Fixation of the omentum.

omentum (*ō-men-tum*). A fold of the peritoneum. The *great o.* is suspended from the greater curvature of the stomach and hangs in front of the gut. The *lesser o.* passes from the lesser curvature of the stomach to the transverse fissure of the liver.

omphalitis (*om-fal-ī'-tis*). Inflammation of the umbilicus.

omphalocele (*om'-fal-ō-sēl*). An umbilical hernia.

omphaloproptosis (*om-fa-lō-prop-tō-sis*). Protrusion of the umbilicus.

oncoma (*on-kō'-ma*). A swelling or tumour.

onychia (*ō-nik'-i-a*). Inflammation of the matrix of a nail.

onychogryphosis (*o-ni-kō-gri-*

fō-sis). Bizarre overgrowth of the nails, often the nail of the big toe.

onychomycosis (*o-ni-kō-mi-kō-sis*). Infection of the nails by fungi.

oocyte (*o'-ō-sit*). An ovum before it has left the Graafian follicle.

oogenesis (*o-o-jen'-e-sis*). The production of ova in the ovary.

oophorectomy (*o-o-fo-rek-to-mi*). Removal of an ovary. *See* OVARIECTOMY.

oophoritis (*o-of-o-rī'-tis*). Inflammation of an ovary.

oophoron (*o-of'-or-on*). That portion of the ovary which produces the ova. Or the ovary itself.

oophorosalpingectomy (*sal-pin-jek-to-mi*). Removal of the ovary and its associated Fallopian tube.

opacity (*ō-pas'-i-ti*). Want of transparency, cloudiness.

opaque (*ō-pāk*). Not transparent.

opening snap. Adventitious heart sound which often precedes the mid-diastolic murmur of mitral stenosis.

ophthalmia (*of-thal'-mi-a*). Inflammation of the eye. The term is applied especially to severe inflammations of the conjunctiva. There is an acute infectious form which

occurs in epidemics, especially in schools and military camps.

ophthalmia neonatorum (*of-thal-mi-a nē-ō-nā-tor'-um*). Severe inflammation of the eyes in the newly born, due to gonorrhoeal or septic infection of the conjunctiva during the passage of the head through the vagina. When due to the gonococcus it responds to intensive treatment with penicillin, locally and by injection.

ophthalmic (*of-thal'-mik*). Pertaining to the eye.

ophthalmitis (*of-thal-mī'-tis*). Inflammation of the eye.

ophthalmologist (*of-thal-mo-lo-jist*). A surgeon specializing in diseases of the eye.

ophthalmology. The study of diseases of the eye.

ophthalmoplegia (*of-thal-mo-plē'-ji-a*). Paralysis of the muscles of the eye.

ophthalmoscope (*of-thal'-mo-skōp*). A small instrument, fitted with a lens, used to examine the interior of the eye.

ophthalmotonometer (*of-thal'-mō-tō-no-me-ter*). Instrument to measure the intra-ocular tension of the eye.

opiate (*o'-pē-āt*). An opium preparation. A hypnotic.

opisthotonos (*op-is-thot'-o-nōs*). Backward retraction of the head and lower limbs with arched back; seen in severe cases of tetanus, meningitis and in strychnine poisoning.

opium (*ō'-pi-um*). A preparation of poppy juice, much used to induce sleep and to allay pain. It contains the alkaloids, morphine, codeine, papaverine and narcotine. Its use is controlled because can cause addiction.

opponens (*op-pō'-nens*). Opposing. Applied to muscles, *e.g. opponens pollicis* which brings the thumb towards the little finger.

opsonins (*op-so'-ninz*). Chemical substances found in the blood serum that are said to prepare the bacteria for phagocytosis.

optic (*op'-tik*). Relating to the sight. *O. atrophy.* Degeneration of the optic nerve.

optic chiasma (*kī-as'-ma*). The crossing of the fibres of the optic tract.

optic disc (*op-tik di'-sk*). The point where the optic nerve enters the eye. This point is insensitive to light and is known as the blind spot.

optician (*op-ti'-shan*). Maker of optical instruments.

optics (*op'-tiks*). The study of the properties of light.

optimum (*op'-ti-mum*). The

best possible in the particular circumstances.

optometry (*op-to'-me-tri*). Measurement of visual powers.

oral (*aw'-ral*). Pertaining to the mouth.

orbicularis (*or-bik-u-la'-ris*). A name given to a muscle which encircles an orifice, *e.g. O. oris*, around the mouth.

orbit (*or'-bit*). The bony cavity in the skull which holds the eye.

orbital (*or'-bi-tal*). Pertaining to the orbit.

orchidectomy (*or-kid'-ek'-to-mi*). Removal of one or both testicles. Castration.

orchidopexy (*or-kid'-o-pek-si*). The bringing down of an imperfectly descended testicle into the scrotum and fixing it there by sutures.

orchiepididymitis (*or-ki-e-pi-di-di-mī-tis*). An inflamed epididymis and testicle.

orchis (*or'-kis*). Testicle.

orchitis (*or-kī'-tis*). Inflammation of the testicles.

organ (*or'-gan*). A part constructed to exercise a special function.

organic (*or-gan'-ik*). Relating to the organs; thus, organic disease of the heart means that the structure itself is affected. *O. chemistry.* Chemistry relating to the carbon compounds.

organism (*or'-ga-nism*). A living cell or cells.

orgasm (*or'-gazm*). Highest point of excitement in sexual intercourse.

Oriental sore (*or'-i-en-tal saw*). Delhi boil.

orientation (*or-i-ent-ā'-shon*). The location of one's position and attitude in relation to surrounding objects.

orifice (*o'-ri-fis*). An opening.

ornithosis (*or-ni-thō'-sis*). Respiratory disease of birds, transmissible to man.

oropharynx (*o-rō-fā-rinks*). That part of the throat which lies between the mouth and the oesophagus.

orphan viruses. *See* ADENOVIRUS.

orthodontics (*or-tho-don-tiks*). The correction of irregularities of the teeth.

orthopaedic (*or-thō-pē'-dik*). Surgery relating to the correction of deformities of the skeleton.

orthopnoea (*or-thop-ne'-a*). Breathlessness, the patient gaining relief only in an upright position.

orthoptics (*or-thop'-tiks*). Term applied to correcting defective vision in a squint by exercises, etc.

orthostatic. Pertaining to or caused by standing upright.

os (*os*). A bone.

os (*ōs*, but often pronounced *os*). The mouth. *External o.* The opening of the cervix into the vagina. *Internal o.* Opening of cervix into the uterine cavity.

os calcis (*kal-sis*). The bone of the heel.

oscheal (*os'-kē-al*). Pertaining to the scrotum.

oscillation (*os-si-lā'-shon*). A swinging movement.

Osgood Schlatter's disease (*osgood schla-ter*). Osteochondritis of unknown cause affecting the tibial tuberosity.

Osiander's sign. Sign appears during first three months of pregnancy when vaginal pulsation is felt.

Osler's disease (*o'-zler*). Polycythaemia.

Osler's nodes (*oz-lerz nōdz*). Small tender inflamed areas in the skin particularly in the pulp of the fingers due to small emboli; occurs in bacterial endocarditis.

osmosis (*oz-mō'-sis*). The passage of a dilute solution to a more concentrated one through a semi-permeable membrane.

osmotic fragility test. Method of determining the fragility of red blood cells.

osmotic pressure (*oz-mot'-ik*). Pressure required to prevent the passage of water by osmosis. The osmotic pressure depends on the number of solute molecules in solution.

osseous (*os'-e-us*). Like bone, bony.

ossicle (*os'-sik-al*). A small bone. Name applied to the tiny bones of the middle ear. *See* EAR.

ossification (*os-si-fi-kā'-shon*). Hardening into bone.

osteitis (*os'-tē-ī'-tis*). Inflammation of bone. *O. fibrosa*, a disease of bone caused by an adenoma of the parathyroid glands. As the result of excessive secretion calcium is absorbed from the bones into the blood.

osteitis deformans. *See* PAGET'S DISEASE.

osteoarthritis (*os-teo-ar-thrī'-tis*), or **osteoarthrosis** (*os-teo-ar-thrō-sis*). Disease due to excessive wear and tear on joint surfaces. Affecting chiefly weight-bearing joints, late in life, and resulting in pain, especially at night, deficient movement, and deformity.

osteoarthropathy (*os-tē-ō-ar-throp-ath-i*). Damage or disease affecting bones and joints.

osteoarthrotomy (*os'-tē-ō-ar-thro'-to-mi*). Excision of joint and neighbouring bone.

osteoblasts (*os'-tē-ō-blasts*). Bone cells.

osteochondritis (*os-tē-ō-kon-dri'-tis*). Combined inflammation of bone and cartilage. *O. deformans juvenilis.* A form occurring in children in which the head of the femur is affected. (Perthes' disease.) *O. dissecans.* Separation of loose bodies from the joint surface.

osteochondroma (*os-tē-ō-kon-drō'-ma*). Benign tumour derived from bone and cartilage.

osteoclastoma (*os-tē-ō-klas-tō-ma*). Tumour of osteoclasts.

osteoclasts (*os'-tē-ō-klasts*). Multinucleated cells which break down the calcified bone matrix, Remodelling of bone by the combined activity of osteoclasts and osteoblasts occurs continuously during bone growth.

osteocytes (*os-tē-ō-sīts*). Osteoblasts which have become incorporated into bone.

osteogenesis (*os'-tē-ō-jen'-e-sis*). Formation of a bone. *O. imperfecta.* Abnormally fragile bones.

osteogenic sarcoma (*os-tē-ō-je-nik sar-kō-ma*). Sarcoma derived from osteoblasts.

osteolytic (*os-tē-ō-li-tik*). Bone destroying.

osteoma (*os-tē-ō'-ma*). A bony tumour.

osteomalacia (*os-tē-ō-ma-lā'-ki-a*). Softening of bones in adults.

osteomyelitis (*os-tē-ō-mi-e-lī'-tis*). Inflammation of the marrow of bone.

osteopath (*os-tē-ō-path*). One who practises osteopathy.

osteopathy (*os-tē-op'-ath-i*). A school of thought ascribing many diseases to structural derangement of skeletal parts and treating same by manipulation of joints. Term can also mean any bone disease.

osteopetrosis (*os-tē-ō-pe-trō'-sis*). *See* MARBLE BONE DISEASE.

osteophony (*os-tē-o'-fo-ni*). Conduction of sound by bone.

osteophyte (*os'-tē-ō-fit*). A bony outgrowth or nodosity; occurs in osteoarthritis.

osteoplastic (*os-tē-ō-plas-tik*). Pertaining to the repair of bones.

osteoporosis (*os-tē-ō-po-rō'-sis*). Fragility of bones due to reabsorption of calcium.

osteosarcoma (*os-tē-ō-sar-kō'-ma*). A malignant tumour growing from a bone.

osteosclerosis (*os-tē-ō-skle-rō'-sis*). Increase in bone density.

osteotome (*os'-tē-ot-ōm*). A surgical instrument resembling a chisel and used for cutting through bones. The instrument is bevelled on both sides.

osteotomy (*os-tē-ot'-o-mi*). The operation of cutting through a bone, usually performed for the relief or cure of bony deformities.

ostium (*os'-ti-um*). An opening. The orifice of any tubular passage.

otalgia (*ō-tal'-ji-a*). Ear-ache.

otitis (*o-tī'-tis*). Inflammation of the ear. *O. externa*. Inflammation of the skin of the external ear. *O. interna*. Inflammation of the inner ear affecting the organs of balance. *O. media*. Inflammation of the middle ear.

otologist (*ō-to-lo-jist*). Ear specialist.

otology (*ō-to-lo-ji*). Study of diseases of the ear.

otophone (*ō'-to-fōn*). Ear-trumpet.

otorrhoea (*ō-tor-re'-a*). A purulent discharge from the ear.

otosclerosis (*ō-tō-skler'-ō-sis*). A chronic, progressive thickening of the ear ossicles leading to deafness.

otoscope (*ō-tos-kōp*). Auriscope.

ounce (*owns*). In fluid measure, about two tablespoonfuls; or 28·4ml. In weight, 1/16lb or 28·34g.

outlet of pelvis (*owt'-let*). The space bounded by the lower edges of the pubes, ischium, sacrum and coccyx and by the sacro-sciatic ligaments.

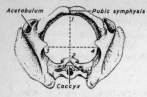

33 The pelvic outlet:
1–2 Antero-posterior diameter
3–4 Transverse diameter

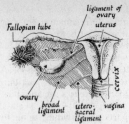

34 The left ovary and
Fallopian tube

ovarian cyst (*o-vā-ri-an sist*). Cyst of the ovary; may be developmental or associated with ovarian tumour.

ovaries (*ō'-va-rēz*). Two small oval bodies situated on either side of the uterus; the female organs in which ova are formed. They are also endocrine glands.

ovariectomy (*ō-vā-rē-ek-to-mi*). Oophorectomy. Surgical removal of ovary.

ovariotomy (*o-vā-ri-ot'-o-mi*). The operation of cutting into an ovary.

ovaritis (*ō-va-rī-tis*). *See* OOPHORITIS.

ovary. *See* OVARIES.

overcompensation. (1) Homeostasis is achieved by the body compensating for changes brought about in various circumstances. When the compensatory mechanism too far outweighs the change which it opposes, overcompensation is said to

have taken place. (2) In psychiatry applies to exaggerated compensatory behaviour, *e.g.* extreme aggressiveness in response to a feeling of inadequacy.

overdosage. Excessive concentration of a drug in the blood. This may be an accumulation from repeated doses or from too high a dose.

overextension (*ō-ver-ek-sten'-shon*). Extension beyond the normal limit, *e.g.* of a joint or muscle.

oviduct (*o'-vid-ukt*). The Fallopian tube between the ovary and the womb, conveying the ova.

ovulation (*ov-ū-lā'-shon*). The development and discharge of ova from the ovary.

ovum (*ō'-vum*). The egg cell produced in the female ovary.

oxalic acid (*ok-sal'-ik*). A poisonous acid obtained

from wood sorrel; chalk and magnesium are the antidotes.

oxaluria (*ox-al-ū'-ri-a*). A disease marked by the presence of oxalic acid crystals in the urine.

oxidation (*ok-si-dā-shon*), **oxidization** (*ok-si-dī-zā-shon*). The chemical combination of oxygen with a substance producing oxides, etc. Can also denote a reduction in the hydrogen content of a molecule, or a loss of electrons from an atom or molecule resulting in an increased ability to take up oxygen, *cf.* reduction.

oxycephaly (*ok-sē-ke-fa-li*). Abnormal development of the skull with resultant egg-shaped appearance. Most cases develop increased intracranial pressure.

oxygen (*ok'-si-jen*). A colourless, odourless gas, forming about 20 per cent of the atmosphere. It supports combustion and is indispensable to life. Inhalations are given in cases of cyanosis and shock. Applied also in the form of hydrogen peroxide to ulcers and septic wounds.

oxygen administration (*ok-si-jen ad-min-is-trā'-shon*). By (1) nasal catheters at approximately 4 litres per minute. This will raise the alveolar oxygen to approximately 30 per cent.
(2) Oxygen Tent. Rate of flow depends upon amount of disturbance for nursing care. With average care, the alveolar oxygen can be kept at 45 per cent.
(3) Mask. Rate of flow adjusted so that a little gas is left in the bag at the end of inspiration; possible to raise alveolar oxygen to 90 per cent. Humidification by moisture in the bag.

oxygen debt. If the metabolic requirement for oxygen exceeds the supply, the metabolic processes are carried on under partially anaerobic conditions until at a later time the 'oxygen debt' is repaid.

oxygenation (*ok-si-je-nā-shon*). To saturate with oxygen.

oxyhaemoglobin (*ok-si-hēm-o-glō'-bin*). Haemoglobin in which oxygen is in combination—as in the red cells of the blood.

oxyntic (*ok-sin-tik*). Term applied to cells secreting hydrochloric acid in the stomach.

oxytocics (*ok-si-tō'-siks*). Drugs used to induce labour and to promote uterine contractions, *e.g.* pituitrin.

oxytocin (*ok-si-tō'-sin*). The oxytocic hormone of the posterior lobe of the pituitary gland.

oxyuriasis (*ok'-si-ū-rī-a-sis*). Infection with oxyuris vermicularis.

oxyuris vermicularis (*ok-si-ūr'-is ver-mik-ū-la'-ris*). Threadworm found in the rectum and large intestine, especially in children.

ozaena (*o-zē-na*). Form of atrophic rhinitis.

ozone (*ō'-zōn*). O_3. An oxidizing agent sometimes used as a disinfectant.

ozonic ether (*o-zo'-nik ē'-ther*). A solution of hydrogen peroxide in ether.

P

P. Chemical symbol for phosphorus.

Pacchioni's bodies (*pak-ī-ō-nis*). Villi from the arachnoid membrane, through which drainage of the cerebrospinal fluid into the venous sinuses occurs.

pacemaker (*pās-mā-ker*). Initiator of heart impulse at sinuatrial node. An electrical stimulator can be fitted surgically.

pachy-. A prefix denoting thick.

pachydermia (*pak-i-der'-mi-a*). Thickening of the skin.

pachymeningitis (*pak-i-men-in-jī'-tis*). Inflammation of the dura mater, with thickening of the membrane.

Pacini's corpuscles (*pa-chē-nis kor'-pusls*). Specialized sensory receptors which register pressure and to some extent vibration. They are situated in the deeper connective tissues of the skin and consist of nerve endings surrounded by concentric lamellae of fibrous tissue.

pack. (1) Moistened material applied to a patient. A *cold pack* consists in wrapping the patient in a sheet wrung out in cold water; he is then enveloped in a dry blanket and mackintosh and left for thirty minutes, or the prescribed time. An *ice pack* consists in wringing out towels in ice water and applying them to the patient, perpetually changing them as they get warm A *hot pack* is sometimes applied to relieve the pain of muscle spasm, *e.g.* in poliomyelitis. The pack is first applied at 100° F and hotter packs applied subsequently until one of 130° F is tolerated. *Warm packs* wrung out in saline, etc., are used in operations, to cover or secure organs. Packs or swabs used in the theatre should either be attached by large rings or clamps or labelled with a radio-opaque band. (2) The dressing and/or instruments required for a sterile procedure, sterilised in a paper container.

paediatrician (*pē-dē-a-tri-shon*). Specialist in diseases of children.

paediatrics (*pē-dē-at-riks*). The science or study of diseases of children.

Paget's disease. (1) Of bone, osteitis deformans, is a disorder of unknown cause which usually affects a number of bones to a greater or lesser extent. Clinical features are pain, tendency to pathological fractures and hyperdynamic circulation. (2) Of nipple. Eczema of the nipple associated with underlying duct carcinoma of the breast.

painter's colic (*pānt-erz kol-ik*). Lead poisoning.

palate (*pal'-āt*). The roof of the mouth.

palatoplegia (*pa-la-tō-plē-ji-a*). Paralysis of soft palate.

palliative (*pal'-i-a-tiv*). A medicine which relieves but does not cure.

pallidectomy (*pal-li-dek-to-mi*). Operation used in Parkinson's disease to decrease the activity of part of the lentiform nucleus in the base of the brain.

pallidotomy (*pa-li-do-to-mi*). Operation performed to relieve tremor in Parkinson's disease. Fibres from the cerebral cortex are severed.

pallor (*pal'-or*). Paleness.

palm (*parm*). The hollow or flexor surface of the hand.

palmar (*pal'-mar*). Pertaining to the palm of the hand.

palpation (*pal-pā'-shon*). Examination by the hand.

palpebra (*pal-pe'-bra*). The eyelid.

palpitation (*pal-pi-tā'-shon*). Rapid throbbing of the heart, producing consciousness of the heart's action.

palsy (*pawl'-zi*). Paralysis. *See* ERB'S PARALYSIS.

pan. A prefix signifying all, total.

panacea (*pan-a-sē'-a*). A medicine which is claimed or advertised to cure all diseases.

panarthritis (*pan-ar-thrī-tis*). Generalized inflammation of joint structures.

pancarditis (*pan-kar-dī-tis*). Generalized inflammation of the heart.

pancreas (*pan'-krē-as*). Sweetbread. A gland situated in the mesentery in relation to the duodenum and crossing the mid-line of the body. It secretes an alkaline mixture of digestive enzymes through the pancreatic duct into the duodenum when stimulated by the hormone *secretin*. It also contains groups of cells which secrete insulin into the blood. *See* LANGERHANS, ISLETS OF.

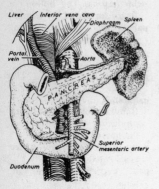

Liver — Inferior vena cava — Diaphragm — Spleen — Portal vein — Aorta — PANCREAS — Superior mesenteric artery — Duodenum

35 The pancreas

pancreatectomy (*pan-krē-a-tek'-to-mi*). Excision of pancreas.

pancreatitis (*pan'-krē-a-ti'-tis*). Inflammation of the pancreas.

pandemic (*pan-dem'-ik*). A widely spread epidemic.

panhypopituitarism (*pan-hī-pō-pi-tū-i-ta-rism*). Simmonds' disease. Deficient secretion of all of the anterior pituitary hormones with additional secondary reduction in production of hormones by the thyroid and adrenal cortex.

panhysterectomy (*his-te-rek'-to-mi*). Total removal of the uterus.

pannus (*pan'-nus*). Vascularization of the cornea; in joints the replacement of cartilage by granulation tissue.

panophthalmia, panophthalmitis (*pan-of-thal-mī'-tis*). Generalized inflammation of the eyeball.

panotitis (*pan-o-tī'-tis*). Inflammation of the middle and internal ear.

Papanicolaou stain (*pa-pa-ni-kō-law*). Stain frequently employed for the examination of vaginal smears.

papilla (*pa-pil'-la*), plu. **papillae.** (1) A small nipple-shaped eminence. (2) The optic disc. *Circumvallate papillae.* These are found at the root of the tongue. *Filiform papillae.* The common *P.* of the tongue and found at its tip. *Fungiform papillae* are the broad *P.* of the tongue.

papillitis (*pap-pil-ī'-tis*). Inflammation of the optic disc.

papilloedema (*pap-il-e-dē'-ma*). Oedema of the optic disc indicative of raised intracranial pressure.

papilloma (*pap-il-lō'-ma*). Benign neoplasm of epithelial cells.

papule (*pap'-ūl*). A small solid pimple.

papyraceus (*pap-i-rā'-shus*). *See* FETUS PAPYRACEUS.

para (*pa'-ra*). Prefix meaning beside or near.

para-aminobenzoic acid (*pa-ra-a-mī-nō-ben-zō-ik*). A bacterial growth factor antagonized by the sulphanilamides.

para-aortic (*pa-ra-ā-or'-tik*). Near the aorta.

paracentesis (*par-a-sen-tē'-sis*). Withdrawing fluid from the body cavity. *See* ASPIRATION.

paracusis (*par-a-kū'-sis*). Disordered hearing.

paradoxical breathing. Part of the lung inflates during expiration and vice versa.

paraesthesia (*par-es-thēz'-i-a*). Disorder of sensation, such as tingling and pins and needles.

paraffin. Any hydrocarbon of the methane series. Liquid paraffin is refined petroleum. Soft paraffin is used as a lubricating jelly. Hard paraffin is paraffin wax. *P. gauze dressing.* Gauze impregnated with soft yellow paraffin jelly; used for burns and wounds.

paraformaldehyde (*pa-ra-for-mal-di-hīd*). Used to fumigate closed spaces, also for sterilization of catheters and instruments when kept in an air-tight container filled with paraformaldehyde.

paralysis (*par-al'-i-sis*). Loss of power of movement or of sensation. Usually due to a lesion in the nervous system. *Spastic p.* is due to a lesion of upper motor neurones. *Flaccid p.* is the result of an injury to lower motor neurones. *Infantile paralysis* is another name for poliomyelitis.

paralysis agitans (*aj'-it-anz*). *See* PARKINSON'S DISEASE.

paralytic ileus (*pa-ra-li-tik ī-lē-us*). Intestinal obstruction due to paralysis of the muscles of peristalsis, often caused by peritonitis. *See* ILEUS.

paramedian (*pa-ra-mē'-di-an*). Close to the middle.

paramedical (*pa-ra-me'-di-kal*). Allied to medicine.

parametritis (*pa-ra-met-rī-tis*). Inflammation of the parametrium. Also called *pelvic cellulitis*.

parametrium (*pa-ra-mēt-rium*). The connective tissue around the uterus, chiefly found round large vessels and between the layers of the broad ligament.

paramnesia (*par-am-nē'-si-a*). False memory; usually memory of events which did not occur in the connection related.

paramyotonia congenita (*pa-ra-mī-ō-tō-ni-a kon-jen-i-ta*). Form of myotonia congenita with tonic spasm esp. of face. It is aggravated by cold.

paranoia (*par-a-noy'-a*). Delusions of persecution.

paranoid (*pa-ra-noyd*). Relating to paranoia.

paraphimosis (*pa-ra-fi-mō'-sis*). Retraction of the prepuce behind the glans penis with inability to restore it to the natural position.

paraplegia (*par-a-plē'-ji-a*). Paralysis of both lower limbs or both upper limbs.

parasite (*par-a-sīt*). Any living thing which lives on or in another organism.

parasiticide (*pa-ra-sī'-ti-sīd*). Substance lethal to parasites.

parasympathetic system (*pa-ra-sim-pa-the-tik sis-tem*). Part of the autonomic nervous system acting in opposition to the sympathetic system, *e.g.* parasympathetic action causes constriction of the pupil, stimulation of the gut, etc.

parathormone (*para-thor'-mōn*). The hormone of the parathyroid glands.

parathyroid (*para-thī'-royd*). Small endocrine glands which control calcium and phosphate metabolism. They are usually four in number and they are situated in the vicinity of the thyroid gland.

paratyphoid (*pa-ra-tī'-foyd*). An infectious disease resembling typhoid fever and caused by an organism not identical with but closely allied to the bacillus of typhoid.

paravertebral (*pa-ra-ver'-te-bral*). To one side of the spinal column.

parenchyma (*par-en'-kī-ma*). The functional part of an organ.

parenteral treatment (*pa-ren-te-ral'*). Therapy by drugs given by routes other than the alimentary tract.

paresis (*par'-ēs-is*). A partial paralysis.

parietal (*pa-rī'-e-tal*). The two bones which form the crown and sides of the cranium. *See* SKULL and FONTANELLE.

parietes (*pa-rī-e-tēz*). The walls of any cavity of the body.

parity (*pa'-ri-ti*). The number of children a woman has borne.

Parkinson's disease (*par'-kin-sonz*), also called paralysis agitans. A chronic disease of later life, showing tremors, rigidity of joints and muscles, a mask-like expression and walking with a tendency to fall forwards.

paronychia (*par-o-nik'-i-a*). Whitlow; inflammation and abscess at the end of a finger near the nail.

paroophoron (*par-o-of'-or-on*). *See* PAROVARIUM.

parosmia (*pa-ros-mi-a*). Perverted sense of smell.

parotid (*par-ot'-id*). Near the ear; applied to a salivary gland under the ear. (*See illustration.*)

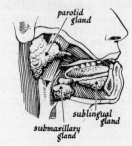

36 The parotid gland

parotitis (*par-o-tī'-tis*). Inflammation of the parotid gland. (1) Mumps. (2) Spread of infection from a septic mouth.

parovarium (*pa-ro-vā'-rium*). A vestigial structure in the broad ligaments of the uterus which occasionally gives origin to small cysts in this region.

paroxysm (*par'-oks-izm*). A sudden temporary attack.

paroxysmal nocturnal dyspnoea (*pa-rok-sis-mal nok-ter-nal dis-ne-a*). Attacks of breathlessness occurring at night due to pulmonary oedema resulting from left ventricular failure.

paroxysmal tachycardia (*pa-rok-sis-mal ta-ki-kar-di-a*). Is due to the regular and rapid discharge of impulses from ectopic focus in the atrial walls of the heart. The focus thus replaces the sinuatrial node as the cardiac pacemaker and drives the heart at a rate of about 180 beats per minute. Attacks may last anything from a minute to several days.

parrot disease (*pa'-rot*). Psittacosis.

parturient (*par-tū'-ri-ent*). In the condition of giving or being just about to give birth to a child. The *parturient canal* is the passage traversed by the fetus during birth, from the brim of the pelvis to the vulva.

parturition (*par-tū-rish'-un*). The act of giving birth to a child.

Paschen bodies (*pash-en*). Minute bodies containing the virus of smallpox.

passive. Submissive. Not active or spontaneous. *P. immunity. See* IMMUNITY. *Passive movements* are performed on a patient's joints by a physiotherapist to increase the mobility, prevent contractures and to improve the circulation.

Pasteurella (*pas-te-re-la*). Group of bacilli causing

bubonic and pneumonic plague. Carried by rats to man.

pasteurization (*pas'-tur-ī-zā-shon*). Method of sterilization of fluids introduced by Pasteur which involves heating for 30 minutes at 70° C.

patella (*pa-tel'-la*). The kneecap. A sesamoid bone in front of the knee joint.

patellar bursae (*ber'-sē*). The bursae around the patella. Inflammation of the prepatellar bursa used to be called housemaid's knee, as it occurs after much kneeling.

patellectomy (*pa-tel-lek-to-mi*). Operation to excise the patella.

patent (*pā'-tent*). Open. *P. ductus arteriosus.* Failure of the ductus arteriosus to close at birth. *P. foramen ovale.* Failure of closure of the foramen ovale.

pathogenesis (*pa-thō-jen'-e-sis*). The origin and progress of disease.

pathogenic (*path-ō-jen-ik*). Capable of causing disease.

pathognomonic (*pa-tho-nō-mon'-ik*). Characteristic of, or peculiar to, a particular disease.

pathological (*pa-tho-loj'-i-kal*). Relating to pathology. Morbid, abnormal.

pathology (*pa-thol'-o-ji*). The study of disease, particularly regarding the changes in the tissues resulting from disease.

patulous (*pat'-ū-lus*). Open wide.

Paul-Bunnell test (*porl-boo-nel*). A serological test for glandular fever (infective mononucleosis).

Paul's tube (*pawls tūb*). Glass drainage tube used to drain the bowel.

Pearson bed. Special bed for nursing fractures.

peau d'orange (*pō dor-anj'*). Orange-skin appearance of skin overlying carcinoma of the breast which is caused by obstruction to superficial lymphatics.

pectin (*pek'-tin*). A polysaccharide found in fruit.

pectoral (*pek'-tor-al*). Relating to the chest. *P. muscles* are on the anterior surface of chest.

pectus (*pek'-tus*). The thorax, chest.

pediatrics (*pē'-di-at'-riks*). See PAEDIATRICS.

pedicle (*ped'-ē-kl*). The stalk of an organ or tumour containing blood vessels.

pedicle needle. An instrument for passing a ligature round the pedicle of a tumour.

pediculosis (*ped-ik-ū-lō'-sis*). Infestation with lice.

pediculus (*pe-dik'-ū-lus*). The louse, a parasite infesting the hair and skin. *P. capitis* infests the head; *P. corporis*, the body and clothing; *P. pubis*, the pubic hair. These three varieties are different in shape and size.

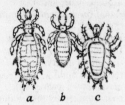

a b c

37 Pediculus (magnified):
A = Capitis B = Corporis
C = Pubis

pedunculated (*ped-ung'-kū-lā-ted*). Possessing a pedicle.

Pel-Ebstein's fever (*pel-eb-stīns*). A regularly remitting fever which sometimes occurs in Hodgkin's disease.

pellagra (*pe-lah-gra*). A nutritional disease especially prevalent in southern Europe and in the southern United States of America. It is marked in the initial stages by recurring redness and exfoliation—resembling sunburn —of the hands and face. There may be glossitis, diarrhoea and peripheral neuritis, and mental changes. The anti-pellagra factor is vitamin B_6.

pellet (*pel-let*). A small pill, esp. those used as implants.

pellicle (*pel'-le-kl*). A thin skin or membrane.

pelvic (*pel'-vik*). Relating to the pelvis.

pelvic cellulitis (*sel-ū-lī-tis*). *See* PARAMETRITIS.

pelvic exenteration. Operauve removal of organ from pelvis.

pelvimetry (*pel-vi-me-tri*). Measurement of pelvic dimensions.

pelvis (*pel'-vis*). The bony cavity composed of the hips and the lower bones of the spine and holding the bowels, bladder and organs of generation.

pemphigus (*pem'-fi-gus*). Disease characterized by the formation of large blisters on the skin and mucous membranes. *P. neonatorum* is a misnomer. It is an acute staphylococcal impetigo occurring in newborn infants.

pendulous (*pen'-dū-lus*). Hanging down.

penetration (*pen-et-rā'-shon*). Entering into a surface. Focal depths of a microscope.

penicillinase (*pe-ni-si-li-nās*). Enzyme found in penicillin-resistant organisms. It inactivates penicillin.

penis (*pē'-nis*). The male organ of coition containing the urethra.

pentagastrin (*pen-ta-gas-trin*). A gastric acid stimulant used to test the secretion of the stomach.

peppermint (*pep'-per-mint*). Carminative and stimulant. O1. menth. pip. on a lump of sugar or Aqua menth. pip.

pepsin (*pep'-sin*). An enzyme which breaks down proteins in acid solution to form peptides (*peptidase*). It is secreted in the stomach with hydrochloric acid.

peptic (*pep'-tik*). Pertaining to digestion. *P. ulcer*, a gastric, duodenal, or gastrojejunal ulcer.

peptone (*pep-tōn*). Compound formed during breakdown of protein.

perception (*per-sep-shon*). An awareness. Receiving impressions through the senses.

percolation (*per-kol-ā'-shon*). The passage of a liquid through a solid but porous substance. Liquid extracts are made in this way. The drug is coarsely powdered, packed into a cylindrical vessel and the solvent trickles slowly through.

percussion (*per-kush'-on*). Striking upon the body, the sound heard being helpful in diagnosis. The note emitted is resonant or dull according to the conditions of the organ underneath.

perforation (*per-fo-rā'-shon*). A hole in an organ caused by disease or injury. The act of perforating.

peri- (*per-i*). Prefix signifying around, near, about.

perianal (*pe-ri-ā'-nal*). Around the anus.

periarteritis (*pe-ri-ar-ter-ī-tis*). Inflammation of the outer coat of an artery.

periarteritis nodosa. A disease of unknown cause which is characterized by the production of multiple nodules in the connective tissues surrounding the smaller arteries. The symptoms and signs associated with this disorder depend on the distribution of the lesions.

periarthritis (*pe-ri-ar-thri'-tis*). Inflammation of the tissues round a joint.

pericardial (*pe-ri-kar-dē-ai*). Pertaining to the pericardium.

pericardial adhesions. Fibrosis of the pericardium which may follow pericarditis in which the two layers of the pericardium become stuck together.

pericardiotomy (*pe-ri-kar-de-o-to-mi*). An opening made into the pericardium.

pericarditis (*per-i-kar-di'-tis*). Inflammation of the pericardium; apt to follow on cases of acute rheumatism, typhoid, Bright's disease, pneumonia or pyaemia.

pericardium (*per-i-kar'-di-um*). The membranous sac which holds the heart. *Adherent p.* Rheumatic carditis is often followed by an adherent pericardium, especially after a pericarditis. This condition interferes with the free action of the heart.

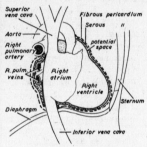

38 The pericardium

perichondritis (*per-i-kon-drī'-tis*). Inflammation of perichondrium.

perichondrium (*per-i-kon'-drē-um*). The membranous covering of a cartilage.

pericolitis (*pe-ri-kol-ī-tis*). Inflammation round the colon.

pericolpitis or **paracolpitis** (*per-i-kol-pī'-tis*). Inflammation of the structures around the vagina.

pericranium (*per-i-krān'-i-um*). The membrane covering the bones of the skull.

perilymph (*pe-ri-limf*). Clear fluid in the osseous labyrinth of the ear.

perimeter (*pe-ri-me-ter*). (1) Circumference, outer boundary of a given area. (2) Instrument for measuring field of vision.

perimetritis (*per-i-me-trī'-tis*). Inflammation of the peritoneum covering the uterus.

perimetry (*pe-ri-me-tri*). Measurement of visual field.

perinatal mortality rate (*pe-ri-nā'-tal*). The number of stillbirths and deaths in the first week of life of babies weighing more than 1,000g at birth per 1,000 births.

perineal (*pe-ri-nē-al*). Pertaining to the perineum. *P. body.* Wedge-shaped muscular body which forms the focus of the pelvic floor.

perineoplasty (*pe-rin-e-ō-plas-ti*). Perineorrhaphy.

perineorrhaphy (*per-i-ne-or'-raf-hē*). Operation for repairing a perineum ruptured during labour.

perinephric (*pe-ri-nef-rik*). Round about the kidney. *P. abscess*, a collection of pus in the tissues round the kidney.

perineum (*per-i-nē'-um*). The region of the pelvic floor, anterior to the anus.

perineurium *(pe-ri-nū-rē-um)*. A sheath investigating a bundle of nerve fibres.

periodontal membrane. Ligament attaching the tooth to the walls of its socket. *P. disease*. Abnormalities of the supporting structures of the teeth.

periosteal *(pe-ri-os'-te-al)*. Pertaining to periosteum. *P. sarcoma*, sarcoma growing from periosteum.

periosteal elevator *(per-i-os'-tē-al)*. *See* RUGINE.

periosteotome *(pe-rē-os-tē-o-tōm)*. Knife used to incise the periosteum.

periosteum *(per-i-os'-tē-um)*. The membrane covering a bone.

periostitis *(per-ē-os-tī-tis)*. Inflammation of the periosteum.

peripheral *(pe-rif'-er-al)*. Relating to the circumference or outer surface. *P. neuritis*. Inflammation of the peripheral nerves.

periproctitis *(pe-ri-prok-tī'-tis)*. Inflammation of tissue around the rectum or anus.

perisalpingitis *(pe-ri-sal-pin-ji'-tis)*. Inflammation of peritoneum covering the uterine tube.

peristalsis *(per-ē-stal'-sis)*. The contractions and movements of the alimentary tract forcing on the contents.

peritomy *(pe-rit'-om-i)*. Incision of the conjunctiva near the margin of the cornea for the cure of pannus.

peritoneal *(pe-ri-tō-nē-al)*. Pertaining to peritoneum.

peritoneum *(per-i-to-nē'-um)*. The membrane or sac which surrounds the intestines and most other abdominal viscera, and which also lines the abdominal cavity. It secretes a serous fluid which prevents friction.

peritonitis *(per-i-to-nī'-tis)*. Inflammation of the peritoneum. *General p.* Generalized infection of the peritoneal cavity. *Pelvic p.*, of the pelvic peritoneum. *Tuberculous p.* Infection of the peritoneum by tubercles either deposited by bloodstream, or as a spread from tuberculous Fallopian tubes, or from tuberculous ulceration of the bowel. There are two types: (1) *Plastic*, where many adhesions are present and whole bowel may be matted together; (2) *Ascitic*, when abdomen is greatly distended with fluid.

peritonsillar abscess *(pe-ri-ton-sil-a)*. *See* QUINSY.

perityphlitis *(pe-ri-tif-lī-tis)*. Inflammation of the peritoneum around the caecum and appendix.

periurethral (*pe-ri-ūr-ēth'-ral*). Around the urethra.

permanent teeth (*per-'manent*). Teeth of the second dentition. *See* TEETH.

permanganate of potash (*perman'-gan-āt of pot'-ash*). Antiseptic and disinfectant. Care should be employed in its use, as it is poisonous in crystal state.

permeable (*per'-me-abl*). Capable of being penetrated.

pernicious (*per-nish'-us*). Tending to a fatal issue. *P. anaemia.* Anaemia resulting from cyanocobalamin (vitamin B_{12}) deficiency.

pernicious vomiting. *See* VOMITING OF PREGNANCY.

pernio (*per-nē-ō*). A chilblain.

peroneal (*pe-rō-nē-al*). Pertaining to the fibula.

peroral (*per-aw-ral*). Through the mouth.

peroxide of hydrogen. *See* HYDROGEN PEROXIDE.

perseveration (*per-sev-e-rā'-shon*). A recurring idea, feeling or way of action from which the patient finds it difficult to escape.

personality (*per-so-na-li-ti*). The make-up of a person with all his individual characteristics, both inherited and acquired.

perspiration (*per-spi-rā-shon*). Sweat, which is excreted through the pores of the skin.

Perthes' disease (*per-thās*). *See* OSTEOCHONDRITIS.

pertussis (*per-tus'-sis*). Whooping cough; an infectious spasmodic cough, common in childhood. The cough ends with a whoop and sometimes causes an attack of vomiting. The disease runs its course in four to eight weeks' time. A serious disease in young children who may be vaccinated against it. Caused by haemophilus pertussis.

perversion (*per-ver'-shon*). Turned away from the normal course. *Sexual p.*, aberrations of normal sexual behaviour.

pes (*pāz*). The foot. *Pes cavus*, a greatly exaggerated longitudinal arch of the foot, with deformity of the toes. *Pes planus*, flat foot.

pessary (*pes'-sar-i*). (1) An instrument placed in the vagina to prevent or remedy malpositions of the uterus or vaginal prolapse. The Hodge or the ring pessary are often used, usually made of plastic. Patients wearing a pessary should be seen and examined by a doctor every three months. (2) A medicated suppository for insertion into the vagina.

pesticide (*pes-ti-sīd*). Term used to describe a substance that kills harmful or disease carrying insects or organisms.

pestilence (*pes-ti-lens*). Virulent infectious epidemic disease.

petechiae (*pe-te'-chi-ē*). Small red spots on the skin formed by effusion of blood.

petit mal. *See* EPILEPSY.

Petri dish (*pet-ri*). A small flat glass dish used in bacteriological laboratories for the culture of micro-organisms.

petrous (*pet'-rus*). Stony; a term given to a hard part of the temporal bone.

Peyer's patches (*pā'-yerz pa'-ches*). Small glands situated on the surface of the ileum and jejunum. Seat of ulceration in typhoid and paratyphoid fever.

pH. Scale of values denoting the hydrogen ion concentration of solutions and thus their alkalinity or acidity. Values below 7 are acid and those above 7 are alkaline.

phaeochromocyte (*fē'-ō-krō-mō-sit*). One of two cell types present in the adrenal medulla and in the sympathetic ganglion.

phaeochromocytoma (*fē-ō-krō-mō-si-tō'-ma*). Tumour of phaeochromocytes usually arising in the adrenal medulla and producing hypertension, hyperglycaemia and irregularity of cardiac rhythm.

phage typing (*fāj tī-ping*).

Method of identifying bacteria which depends on their sensitivity to lysis by bacteriophase viruses.

phagocytes (*fag'-ō-sītz*). The polymorphonuclear white cells of the blood, so called from their property of being able to ingest and destroy micro-organisms of disease which may be circulating in the blood or attacking the tissues.

phagocytosis (*fag-ō-sī-tō'-sis*). The process of enveloping and absorbing a hostile germ by a phagocyte.

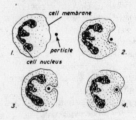

39 Phagocytosis

phalanges (*fal-an'-jēz*). The small bones of the fingers and toes.

phallus (*fa'-lus*). The penis.

phantasy (*fan'-ta-si*). *See* FANTASY.

phantom limb (*fan'-tom lim*). Sensation often experienced by patient, after an amputation, that the limb is still there.

pharmaceutical (*far-ma-sū'-tik-al*). Pertaining to drugs.

pharmacology (*far-ma-kol'-o-ji*). A study of drug action.

Pharmacopoeia (*far-ma-ko-pē'-a*). An authorized handbook of drugs. *British P.* has a legal status.

pharmacy (*far'-ma-sē*). (1) The science of preparing and mixing medicines or drugs. (2) The place where drugs are prepared and distributed.

pharyngeal (*far-in'-je-al*). Pertaining to the pharynx. *P. pouch.* Diverticulum in the wall of the pharynx which may form between the two portions of the inferior constrictor muscle of the pharynx.

pharyngectomy (*fa-rin-jek'-to-mi*). Excision of part of the pharynx.

pharyngismus (*far-in-jiz'-mus*). Spasm of the pharynx.

pharyngitis (*far-in-jī'-tis*). Inflammation of the pharynx.

pharyngotympanic tube (*fa-rin-gō-tim-pa'-nik tūb*). Eustachian tube, running from the pharynx to the middle ear.

pharynx (*far'-inks*). The musculo-membranous sac at the back of the mouth leading to the oesophagus and to the larynx.

phenylalanine (*fē-nil-al-a-nĕn*). Essential amino-acid.

phenylketonuria (*fē-nil-kē-tō-nū'-ri-a*). Genetically determined error of metabolism in which there is an inability of the liver to convert phenylalanine to tyrosine. Instead phenylalanine is broken down to phenyl-pyruvic acid which is excreted in the urine. There is associated mental deficiency.

phial (*fī-al*). A glass capsule or container.

phimosis (*fī-mō'-sis*). Contraction of the orifice of the prepuce; usually treated by the operation of circumcision.

phlebectomy (*fleb-ek'-to-mi*). Excision of a vein.

phlebitis (*fle-bī'-tis*). Inflammation of a vein, most commonly caused by the invasion of its coats by micro-organisms. Associated with thrombosis, or coagulation of the blood in the vein.

phlebolith (*fleb'-ō-lith*). Calcified venous thrombus.

phlebothrombosis. Thrombosis in veins, particularly the veins of the legs, due to prolonged haemostasis.

Phlebotomus (*fle-bo-to-mus*). Genus of small flies bringing disease such as kala-azar.

phlebotomy (*fle-bot'-o-mi*). Bleeding a patient by opening a vein. Venesection.

phlegm (*flem*). Sputum.

Abnormal secretion of mucus from respiratory tract, the result of inflammation.

phlegmasia (*fleg-mā-zi-a*). Inflammation. *P. alba dolens*, white leg; a form of phlebitis occurring sometimes after labour. The leg becomes swollen, white and tense, and is very painful.

phlegmatic (*fleg-mat'-ik*). Sluggish, dull.

phlyctenule (*flik-ten-ūl*). Red pimples met with on surface of eye. *Phlyctenular conjunctivitis*, a form of disease when phlyctenules appear upon white of eye near the cornea, each becoming the centre of a small inflamed patch. They then rupture, forming a small ulcer which readily heals. *Phlyctenular keratitis*, when cornea is similarly affected.

phobia (*fō'-bi-ah*). Abnormal fear, *e.g.* cancerophobia, claustrophobia.

phonation (*fō-nā'-shon*). The utterance of vocal sounds.

phonetic. Relating to the voice.

phonocardiograph (*fō-nō-kar'-dē-ō-graf*). Instrument recording heart sounds.

phosphatase (*fos-fa-tāz*). Enzyme concerned in phosphate metabolism.

phosphate (*fos'-fāt*). A salt of phosphoric acid. A compound of phosphoric acid and a base.

phosphaturia (*fos-fat-ū'-ri-a*). Excess of phosphates in the urine.

phospholipid (*fos-fō-li-pid*). Lipids containing phosphates, *e.g.* lecithin. They are particularly concerned in living systems with forming membranes.

phosphonecrosis (*fos-fō-ne-krō'-sis*). Necrosis of the jaw, caused by inhaling phosphorus; occurs in certain trades, such as matchmaking, but is rare.

phosphorus (*fos'-for-us*). Poisonous non-metallic element the salts of which are used as 'nerve tonics'.

photalgia (*fō-tal-ji-a*). Pain caused by exposure to light.

photobiology (*fō-tō-bī-ol-o-ji*). The study of the effect of light on animal life.

photochemical (*fō-tō-ke-mi-kal*). Chemical changes caused by exposure to light.

photophobia (*fō-tō-fō'-bi-a*). Abnormal intolerance of light, a symptom of inflammation of the eyes.

photosensitization *fō-tō-sen-si-tī-zā-shon*). Tendency of tissues to react abnormally to light usually as the result of the presence in the tissues of certain chemicals which magnify the damaging effect of the incident radiation.

phrenic (*fren'-ik*). (1) Relating to the diaphragm. (2) Relating to the mind.

phrynoderma (*frī-no-der-ma*). Follicular keratosis as occurs, for example, in vitamin A deficiency.

Phthirus pubis (*fthī-rus pū-bis*). The pubic louse.

phthisis (*thī'-sis*). Consumption; tubercular disease of the lungs.

physic (*fiz'-ik*). (1) The art of medicine. (2) Any medicinal preparation.

physician (*fi-si-shan*). Qualified medical practitioner.

physicist (*fis'-i-sist*). An expert in the science of physics.

physics (*fi-siks*). Sciences concerned with properties and interaction of matter and energy.

physiological saline (*fi-si-ō-lo-ji-kal sā-līn*). A 0·9 per cent solution of sodium chloride in water. Also known as normal saline.

physiology (*fiz-ē-ol'-o-ji*). The study of processes occurring in living systems.

physiotherapy (*fis-ē-ō-ther-api*). Therapy by physical means, *i.e.* heat, light, electricity, massage, and exercises.

physique (*fiz-ēk*). The form and constitution of the body.

pia mater (*pē-a mā-ter*). The fine membrane surrounding the brain and spinal cord. The inner layer of meninges.

pica (*pi'-ka*). Morbid appetite. Craving for unnatural articles of food.

Pick's disease (*piks dis-ēz*). (1) Disorder affecting serous membranes resulting in effusions in the peritoneum, pericardium and pleura. The cause is unknown. (2) Presenile dementia due to cerebral atrophy.

picric acid (*pik-rik as-id*). A yellow powder. 1 per cent sol. in water is used for burns. 1 per cent sol. in spirit used as an antiseptic for the skin. Idiosyncrasy to the drug is not uncommon.

pigment (*pig'-ment*). An organic colouring matter. Abnormal pigmentation of the skin occurs in certain diseases, *e.g.* Addison's disease.

piles (*pī-lz*). Enlarged veins about the anus; haemorrhoids.

pilonidal (*pī-lō-nē-dal*). Containing hair as in some cysts. *P. sinus.* Sinus containing hairs which may form in anal cleft and become infected, resulting in an abscess.

pilosis (*pī-lō-sis*). Abnormal growth of hair.

pilula (*pil-ū-la*). A pill; abbreviation, *pil.*

pineal body (*pī'-ne-al bo-di*). The so-called 'third eye'.

Develops from outgrowths of the forebrain, part of which forms an eye-like structure in the lamprey. In man it is a gland-like structure whose function is not determined.

pinguecula (*pin-gwe-kū-la*). Small yellow patch of connective tissue on conjunctiva occurring in old age.

pink disease. Infantile acrodynia. A form of polyneuritis with particular involvement of the autonomic nervous system thought to be due to sensitivity to mercury from calomel containing teething powder.

pink-eye (*pink'-ī*). Infectious conjunctivitis.

pinna (*pin'-na*). The outspread part of the ear.

pint (*pīnt*). Twenty fluid ounces.

pipette (*pi-pet'*). A small graduated glass tube for taking up liquids.

pisiform (*pēs'-i-form*). Pea shaped; applied to a bone of the wrist.

pitting. Pits are formed in the skin on pressure, as in oedema.

pituitary gland (*pit-ū'-it-a-ri*). Endocrine gland in the base of the skull; there are two lobes separated by a cleft. The *anterior lobe* secretes thyrotropic hormone (TSH), corticotrophic hormone (ACTH), gonadotrophic hormones (FSH, LH), growth hormone (GH) and prolactin. The *posterior lobe* secretes antidiuretic hormone (ADH) and oxytocin.

pityriasis rosea (*pi-ti-rī-a-sis rō-sē-a*). Skin disease characterized by scaly, erythematous macula eruption. Thought to be caused by a virus related to the measles virus.

placebo (*pla-sē'-bō*). Medicine given to please the patient, but which is generally inactive. May be given in a drug trial in order to exclude the psychological effect of the drug.

placenta (*pla-sen'-ta*). The after-birth; a circular flesh-like substance through which the mother's blood nourishes the fetus; it is expelled from the womb after the birth of the child.

placenta praevia (*prē-vē-a*). The placenta attached partially or totally to the lower uterine segment.

plague (*plāg*). An acute epidemic infectious disease caused by Pasteurella pestis derived from infected rats and transmitted to man by fleas.

plantar (*plan-tar*). Relating to the sole of the foot. *P. response*. Reflex movement

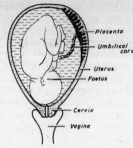

Placenta
Umbilical cord
Uterus
Foetus
Cervix
Vagina

40 The placenta

of toes when the sole of the
foot is stroked.

plasma (*plaz'-ma*). The liquid in
which the corpuscles of the
blood are suspended.

plasmodium malariae (*plas-mo-di-um ma-lā-ri-ē*). Organism causing quartan malaria.

plaster (*pla'-ster*). Adhesive
tape used for keeping dressings in position or for applying extension to a limb.

plaster of Paris. Used for preparing bandages, in making
splints to immobilize part of
the body.

plastic surgery. Restoration of
tissue to its normal shape and
appearance by operative
means.

platelets (*plāt'-lets*). Blood cells
concerned with the clotting
of blood. Normally number
200,000–500,000 per mm³.

platinum (*pla-ti-num*). A
silver-white metal of which

containers are made for
radium.

Platyhelminthes (*pla-ti-hel-min-thes*). Genus of flat-bodied worms.

pleocytosis (*plē-ō-sī-tō-sis*).
Increase of lymphocytes in
cerebrospinal fluid.

pleomorphism (*plē-ō-mor-fism*). Occurring in more than
one form as with a crystal.

plethora (*pleth'-o-ra*). Unhealthy repletion. An excess
of blood.

pleura (*plū'-ra*). A thin membrane which covers each lung
and lines the inner surface of
the thoracic cavity.

pleural rub (*plū-ral rub*). A
squeaking sound produced
by friction between the layers
of the pleura.

pleurisy (*plū'-ri-si*). Inflammation of the pleura. There are
three kinds: dry, with effusion, and empyema or purulent pleurisy.

pleurodynia (*plū-ro-din'-i-a*).
Pain in the side, ordinarily in
the intercostal muscles.

plexor (*plek-sor*). Small hammer used in testing deep
reflexes, etc.

plexus (*pleks'-us*). A network of
vessels or nerves.

plica (*pli'-ka*). A fold.

plicate (*pli'-kāt*). Folded.

plumbism (*plum'-bizm*). Lead-poisoning.

plumbum. *See* LEAD.

Plummer-Vinson syndrome (*sin'-drōm'*). Dysphagia occurring in patients with severe nutritional iron-deficiency anaemia.

pneumatocele (*nū-ma-tō-sēl*). A swelling containing air or gas.

pneumaturia (*nū-mă-tū-ri-ā*). Diagnostic feature of vesico-intestinal fistula. Air is passed through the urethra.

pneumococcal (*nū-mō-kok'-kal*). Pertaining to the pneumococcus.

pneumococcus (*nū-mō-kok'-us*). A bacterium which causes pneumonia. *See* BAC-TERIA.

pneumoconiosis (*nū-mō-kō-ni'-ō-sis*). Fibrosis of the lungs caused by working in an atmosphere full of powdered grit and stone.

pneumomycosis (*nū-mō-mī-kō'-sis*). Fungus disease of the lungs.

pneumonectomy (*nū-mo-nek'-to-mi*). Surgical removal of a lung.

pneumonia (*nū-mō'-ni-a*). An infective disease characterized by inflammation of the lungs. Double pneumonia, both lungs are diseased. *Hypostatic p.* is caused by lack of movement in a debilitated patient. May occur after operation or in the aged. *Lobar p.*, affecting one or more lobes of the lung.

Lobular p., *see* BRONCHO-PNEUMONIA.

pneumonitis (*nū-mo-nī-tis*). Inflammation of the lung.

pneumoperitoneum (*nū-mō-pe-ri-to-nē'-um*). Air in the peritoneal cavity.

pneumothorax (*nū-mō-tho'-raks*). Air in the pleural space. *Spontaneous p.* due to rupture of one of the air passages which may lead to a rise in pressure inside the chest (*tension pneumothorax*) and difficulty in breathing. *Artificial pneumothorax.* Air is introduced into the chest through a needle or incision.

pock (*pok*). A pustule or the scar left by it.

podalic version (*pod-al'-ik ver-shon*). A turning round of the fetus in utero, so that the breech presents in delivery.

poikilocytosis (*poy'-ki-lō-sī-tō-sis*). Variation in the form of the red blood cells.

poison (*poy'-son*). A substance deleterious to the body if absorbed in toxic concentrations. The term is usually reserved for substances which are toxic in low concentrations, *e.g.* cyanide.

polar bodies. Two small structures formed after mitotic division of the primary oocyte.

poliomyelitis (*pōliō-mī-e-lī'-tis*). Acute virus infection causing degeneration of the anterior horn cells of the spinal cord and consequent paralysis of the appropriate muscles.

Politzer's bag (*po-lit'-serz*). An india-rubber bag with long tube and nozzle. Used for inflating the middle ear through the nose and Eustachian tube.

pollution (*po-lū'-shon*). The act of rendering impure.

poly- (*poli*). A prefix denoting much or many.

polyarteritis nodosa (*po-li-ar-te-rī-tis no-dō-sa*). *See* PERIARTERITIS NODOSA.

polyarthritis (*po-li-ar-thrī-tis*). Inflammation of many joints.

Polya's operation (*pol-yus op-e-rā-shon*). Operation for duodenal ulcer in which the stump of the stomach is anastomosed to the side of the jejenum.

polycystic (*pol-i-sis'-tik*). Composed of many cysts.

polycythaemia (*pol'-i-sūt-hē'-mi-a*). (1) *Primary polycythaemia*. Excessive (neoplastic) production of erythropoietic cells. (2) *Secondary polycythaemia*. Increase in the number of red blood cells in the blood due to stimulation of the bone marrow, *e.g.* by anoxia at high altitudes or due to respiratory disease.

polydactyly (*pol-i-dak'-ti-li*). The presence of supernumerary fingers or toes.

polydipsia (*po-li-dip-si-a*). Abnormal thirst.

polyglandular (*pol-i-glan'-dū-lar*). Pertaining to several glands.

polyhedral (*pol-i-hē'-dral*). Having many surfaces.

polymorphonuclear (*pol-i-mor-fō-nū'-kle-ar*). Having nuclei of various shapes. Name given to the most numerous form of white blood cells, of which there are normally about 70 per cent of total. These are the chief phagocytes, and therefore they are increased in number in the presence of pus.

polymyositis (*po-li-mī-ō-sī-tis*). Weakness and wasting of muscles due to inflammation of unknown aetiology.

polyneuritis (*po-li-nū-rī'-tis*). Multiple neuritis.

polyopia (*pol-i-ō'-pi-a*). Seeing multiple images of the same object.

polyosteotic fibrous dysplasia (*po-li-o-stē-o-tik fī-brus dis-plā-si-a*). Albright's syndrome. A congenital disorder characterized by widespread osteitis fibrosa, segmental hyperpigmentation of the skin and, in girls, precocious sexual development.

polypeptide (*pol-i-pep'-tīd*). A

complex compound of several amino-acids.

polypoid (*po-li-poyd*). Like a polypus.

polypus (*pol'-i-pus*). A small simple tumour occurring in the ear, nose, uterus or rectum.

polysaccharides (*pol-i-sak'-ar-īdz*). A group of carbohydrates which contain three or more molecules of simple carbohydrates combined with each other, *e.g.* starch, glycogen.

polyuria (*pol-i-ū'-ri-a*). Excessive flow of urine.

polyvalent (*po-li-vā-lent*). As applied to sera, meaning those which are active against many different strains of the same micro-organisms.

pompholyx (*pom'-fo-liks*). A dermatitis with vesicles. A vesicular eruption occurring on the palms and soles. Probably a form of eczema.

pons Varolii (*ponz va-rō'-li-ē*). That portion of the base of the brain which connects together the medulla oblongata, cerebrum and cerebellum. *See* BRAIN.

pontine (*pon-tīn*). Pertaining to the pons.

popliteal (*pop-li-te'-al*). Pertaining to the popliteal space, the area behind the knee.

pore (*por*). A minute passage in the skin for perspiration; an opening between the molecules of a body.

porphyria (*por-fī'-ri-a*). Rare metabolic disturbance which may cause mental damage in young children. There are convulsions, delirium, polyneuritis, etc.

porphyrins (*por'-fi-rins*). Pyrrole derivatives produced in the metabolism of haemoglobin.

portal hypertension (*por-tal hi-per-ten-shon*). Hypertension in the hepatic portal system usually resulting from cirrhosis of the liver.

portal vein (*por'-tal vān*). The vein which conveys to the liver the blood circulating through the gastro-intestinal system and spleen.

position (*po-si'-shon*). Attitude or posture.

positive pressure ventilation. Air is pushed into the lungs either by manual method such as the Holger Nielsen or by a mechanical device.

posset (*pos'-set*). In infant feeding, regurgitation of a feed.

post (*pōst*). Behind or after.

postclimacteric (*post-klī-mak-te-rik*). After the menopause.

postencephalitis (*pōst-en-ke-fa-lī-tis*). Condition which may remain after encephalitis.

posterior chamber of eye (*pō-stēr'-i-or chām'-ber*). Small space lying behind iris and the lens and containing aqueous humour.

postganglionic (*pŏst-gan-gli-o-nik*). Behind a ganglion.

posthumous (*pos'-tū-mus*). After death; a posthumous child is one born after the father's death.

postmature (*pŏst-ma-tūr*). Infant born after the expected date of delivery.

post mortem (*pŏst mor'-tem*). The opening and examining of a dead body.

post-natal (*nā-tal*). Following birth.

postoperative (*pŏst-o'-per-ā-tiv*). After operation.

post-partum (*par'-tum*). After labour. *Post-partum haemorrhage* is excessive vaginal bleeding occurring either immediately after the birth of the baby (primary), or within a few days (secondary).

postprandial (*pŏst-pran-di-al*). After a meal.

postural (*pos'-tū-ral*). Pertaining to posture. (1) *P. treatment* by means of posture; thus the 'knee-elbow' posture is sometimes useful in treating retroversion of the gravid uterus, or in prolapse of the umbilical cord during labour. (2) *P. drainage*; the positions used to drain the various parts of the lungs. (3) *P. hypotension*. Excessively

low blood pressure induced by standing upright. A side-effect of some drugs given for hypertension.

post-vaccinal (*pŏst-vak-si-ni-al*). Occurring after vaccination.

potassium (*po-tas'-sē-um*). A metallic element present in living cells and essential to life.

potential (*pō-ten'-shal*). Capable of action.

Pott's disease (*po'tz diz-ēz'*). Tuberculous disease of the spine, usually in children.

Pott's fracture (*frak'-tūr*). Fracture of the ankle with or without displacement of the joint mortice. Treatment dependent on the degree of injury.

pouch of Douglas (*dug'-las*). *See* DOUGLAS'S POUCH.

poultice (*pōl'-tis*). Soft and moist applications generally containing heat and applied to relieve pain, *e.g.* kaolin. Starch poultices (cold) may be used in certain skin conditions.

Poupart's ligament (*poo-parz'*). The ligament of the groin, stretching between the anterior superior spine of the ilium and the os pubis.

p.r. Per rectum—Examination made with one finger in the rectum, by which information can be obtained of the condition of the rectum and adjacent structures.

pre- (*prē*). Prefix meaning before.

precancerous (*prē-kan'-se-rus*). A state before a cancer has arisen but which may become cancerous.

precipate labour (*pre-sip'-it-āt*). Labour which is concluded in a time very much shorter than the average.

precipitation (*pre-sip-i-tā-shon*). The process of separating solids from the liquids which hold them in solution, by the application of heat or cold, or the addition of chemicals.

precipitins (*pre-sip'-it-ins*). Protective substances in the blood which kill bacteria by 'precipitating' their protein content.

precordium (*prē-kor'-dium*). The area of the chest over the heart.

precursor (*prē-ker'-sor*). Forerunner.

predigestion (*prē-di-jes-chon*). Food is partially digested artificially before it is eaten as with a junket when rennet has curdled the milk.

predisposed (*prē-dis-pōsd*). Susceptible.

pre-eclampsia (*prē-e-klamp'-si-a*). Antenatal state before eclampsia develops and when it can still be prevented.

There are proteinuria, raised blood pressure and swelling of the ankles. *See* ECLAMPSIA.

prefrontal (*pre-frun'-tal*). Lying in the anterior part of frontal lobe of the brain. *P. leucotomy. See* LEUCOTOMY.

pregnancy (*preg'-nan-si*). The state of being with child. Usual period 280 days. *See also* ECTOPIC GESTATION.

premature labour (*prē'-ma-tūr*). Labour resulting in birth of premature baby, i.e. one weighing 2,500g or less.

premedication (*prē-me-di-kā'-shon*). Drug given as a narcotic before a general anaesthetic.

premenstrual (*prē-men-stroo-al*). Before menstruation. *P. tension syndrome.* Syndrome consisting of tension, anxiety, aches, depression and often accident-proneness which occurs for a few days before menstrual period in some women. It is thought to be hormonal in origin.

premolar (*prē-mō-la*). The two bicuspid teeth in each jaw which lie between the canine and the molars. *See* TEETH.

premonitory (*prē-mon'-it-ori*). Giving warning beforehand.

prenatal (*prē-nā'-tal*). Prior to birth, during the period of pregnancy.

preparalytic (*prē-pa-ra-li-tik*).

State before paralysis has occurred.

prepuce (*pre'-pūs*). Loose skin covering the glans penis: foreskin.

presbyopia (*pres-bi-ō'-pi-a*). Long-sightedness due to inability to make lens of the eye convex by contraction of the ciliary muscles, *i.e.* failure of adaptation of the lens.

prescription (*pre-skrip'-shon*). A formula written by the physician to the dispenser. Consists of the heading, usually the symbol R meaning 'take', the names and quantities of the ingredients, the directions to the dispenser, the directions to the patient, the date and the signature.

presentation (*prez-en-tā'-shon*). The part of the fetus which first engages or tends to engage in the pelvis is said *to present*, and the description of this part is the presentation.

pressor (*pres'-sor*). Substance causing blood pressure to rise.

pressure areas (*pre-shor ā-rē-us*). Parts of the body where the bone is near the skin surface and where a pressure sore is likely to occur if there is prolonged pressure owing to diminished blood supply to these parts.

pressure points. Points at which pressure may be applied to check haemorrhage. *See* illustration, p. 160.

presystole (*prē-sis'-to-li*). Period in the cardiac cycle before systole.

priapism (*prī-a-pism*). Persistent erection of the penis.

prickle cells (*pri-kl*). Epidermal cells furnished with radiating processes which connect with similar cells. *P. layer*, the lowest stratum of the epidermis.

prickly heat. Miliaria papillosa.

primary focus (*fō-kus*). First site of infection in tuberculosis. Healing usually takes place uneventfully.

primary lesion. Original lesion from which others may arise.

primary sore. Initial site of infection in syphilis.

primigravida (*prī-mi-gra-vi-da*). A woman pregnant for the first time.

primipara (*prī-mip'-a-ra*). A woman who has borne one child.

primordial (*prī-mor'-dial*). Pertaining to the beginning.

probe (*prōb*). A slender rod, sometimes of silver, used for exploring wounds.

process (*prō'-ses*). A prolongation or eminence of a part.

procidentia (*pro-sid-en'-shi-ah*). Prolapse. A falling down.

proctalgia (*prok-tal'-ji-a*). Pain about the rectum.

proctectomy (*prok-tek'-to-mi*). Excision of rectum.

proctitis (*prok-tī'-tis*). Inflammation of the rectum.

proctocele (*prok'-to-sēl*). Prolapsed rectum.

proctoclysis (*prok-to-klī-sis*). Introduction into the rectum of fluid for absorption.

proctorrhaphy (*prok-to-ra-fi*). Suturing of the rectum.

proctoscope (*prok'-tō-skōp*). An instrument for viewing the interior of the rectum.

prodromal period (*prō-drō'-mal*). The period that elapses in an infectious disease between the appearance of the first symptoms and the development of the rash, *e.g.* in smallpox, 3 days.

progeria (*prō-jē'-ri-a*). A condition in which premature senility is combined with infantilism.

progesterone (*prō-jes'-ter-ōn*). The hormone of the corpus luteum which causes secretory changes in the uterine mucous membrane in pregnancy and during the menstrual cycle.

progestogen (*prō-jes-tō-jen*). Substance having similar action to progesterone.

proglottis (*prō'-glo-tis*). Segment of tapeworm.

prognosis (*prog-nō'-sis*). The considered opinion as to the course of a disease.

progressive muscular atrophy. Loss of power and wasting of muscles. Degenerative changes are found in the motor cells of the brain and anterior horns of the spinal cord.

projection (*pro-jek'-shon*). Painful thoughts, feelings and motives are relieved by transferring them on to someone else, *e.g.* blaming one's own mistake on to another.

prolactin (*prō-lak'-tin*). Milk-producing hormone of the anterior lobe of the pituitary.

prolan (*prō'-lan*). The original name given to the secretion of the anterior lobe of the pituitary gland. *Prolan A* stimulates the Graafian follicle to ripen, and the production of oestrin. This is now called the follicle stimulating hormone or FSH. *Prolan B* stimulates the formation of the corpus luteum and the secretion of progesterone. This is now called luteinizing hormone or LH.

prolapse (*prō'-laps*). Sinking or falling down, *e.g.* prolapse of uterus, rectum, umbilical cord.

prolapsed intervertebral disc (*prō-lapst in-ter-ver-te-bral disk*). Slipped disc due to prolapse of the central part of the cartilaginous intervertebral disc. *See* NUCLEUS PULPOSUS.

proliferation (*prō-lif-er-ā-shon*). Reproduction. Cell-genesis.

promontory (*prom'-on-to-ri*). A projecting part. An eminence.

pronation (*pro-nā'-shon*). Downward turning of the palm of the hand.

prone. Lying with the face downwards.

propensity (*prō-pen-si-ti*). Inclination or tendency.

prophylactic (*prō-fi-lak'-tik*). Tending to prevent disease.

proprietary drug (*prop-rī'-et-a-ri*). A remedy with a registered trade name.

proprioceptor (*prō-pri-ō-sep-tor*). Sensory end organ which detects changes in position, *e.g.* of muscles or joints or fluid in the balancing apparatus of the inner ear.

proptosis oculi (*prop-tō'-sis ok'-ū-lē*). Protrusion of eyeballs.

prostate (*pros-tāt*). A gland associated with the male reproductive system. Its size and secretion are under the influence of androgens. Its function is not clear but it appears to supply supportive substances to the sper-matozoa in the seminal vesicle.

prostatectomy (*pros-tat-ek'-to-mi*). Operation of removing the prostate gland. The operation may be suprapubic when the bladder is first incised, or retropubic (*see* MILLIN'S PROSTATECTOMY) or transurethral.

prostatic (*pros-ta'-tik*). Pertaining to the prostate.

prostatitis (*pros-ta-tī'-tis*). Inflammation of the prostate gland.

prosthesis (*pros-thē'-sis*). The replacement of an absent limb or organ by an artificial apparatus.

prostration (*pros-trā'-shon*). Extreme exhaustion.

protein (*prō'-tēn*). Very complex organic compound made up of a large number of amino-acids which are synthesized by living systems. There are 20 different amino-acids commonly found in proteins and these are arranged in different sequences which give the specific characteristics to the proteins.

proteinuria (*pro-ti-nū-ri-a*). Protein in the urine.

proteolysis (*pro-te-ol'-is-is*). The change of proteins into peptones.

prothrombin (*prō-throm'-bin*). The substance which when activated by thrombokinase in the presence of calcium ions becomes thrombin.

protoplasm (*prō'-tō-plasm*). The living jelly-like substance which forms the main part of a cell. It is made up chiefly of water, proteins, and inorganic salts.

prototype (*prō'-tō-tīp*). The original form from which others are copied.

protozoa (*prō-tō-sō'-a*). A class of unicellular organisms, forming the lowest division of the animal kingdom, *e.g.* an amoeba.

proud flesh (*prow'd*). Excessive granulation tissue in a wound.

provitamin (*prō-vi'-ta-min*). A precursor of a vitamin, *e.g.* ergosterol.

proximal (*prok'-si-mal*). Nearest to the centre.

prurigo (*pru-rī'-go*). A skin disease marked by irritating papules.

pruritus (*pru-rī'-tus*). Itching.

prussic acid (*prus-sik as'-id*). Hydrocyanic acid. Violent poison found in bitter almonds and laurel leaves.

pseudarthrosis (*sū-dar-thrō'-sis*). A false joint.

pseudo (*sū'-dō*). A prefix meaning false or spurious.

pseudo-angina (*sū-dō-an-jī-na*). A neurotic disease resembling angina pectoris.

pseudocyesis (*sū-dō-sī'-ē-sis*). Changes mimicking pregnancy but without a fetus.

pseudohermaphrodite (*sū-dō-her-ma-frō-dīt*). The external sex organs are of different sexual type to the sex glands.

pseudoplegia (*sū-dō-plē'-ji-a*). Hysterical paralysis.

pseudopodium (*sū-dō'-pō'-di-um*). Temporary protrusion of cell serving as method of locomotion and phagocytosis.

psittacosis (*sit-a-kō'-sis*). A virus disease found in parrots and other birds which is communicable to man. It manifests itself as an atypical pneumonia, which may be successfully treated with antibiotics.

psoas (*sō'-as*). A large muscle attached above to the lumbar vertebrae and below to the femur. It flexes the femur on the trunk. *P. abscess. See* ABSCESS.

psoriasis (*so-rī'-a-sis*). Genetically determined abnormality of keratinization producing skin lesions consisting of raised, red, scaly areas.

psyche (*si'-ki*). The mind.

psychiatric social worker (*sī-ki-a-trik' sō-shal wer-ker*). One who works under a psychiatrist to rehabilitate mentally ill people.

psychiatrist (*si-kī'-a-trist*). A doctor who specializes in psychiatry.

psychiatry (*sī-kī-at'-ri*). The study and treatment of mental disorders.

psychical (*sī'-ki-kal*). Relating to the mind.

psycho-analysis (*sī-kō-an-al'-is-is*). A method of treatment, based upon the theories of Freud, tracing nervous conditions to their antecedent causes.

psychodynamics (*sī-kō-dī-na-miks*). Science of mental processes.

psychogenic (*sī-kō-je'-nik*). Originating in the mind.

psychologist (*sī-ko'-lo-jist*). One who studies psychology but is not a doctor of medicine.

psychology (*sī-ko'-lo-ji*). The study of the mind.

psychoneurosis (*sī-kō-nū-rō'-sis*). A functional mental disease.

psychopath (*sī-ko-path*). A mentally deranged person.

psychopathology (*sī-kō-pa-tho-lo-ji*). Study of the mechanism of mental disorders.

psychosis (*sī-kō'-sis*). A severe mental disorder. (Plu. psychoses.)

psychosomatic (*si-kō-sō-ma'-tik*). Relating to mind and body.

psychotherapeutics, psychotherapy (*sī-kō-the-ra-pū'-tiks, sī-kō-ther'-a-pi*). Treatment of the mind. A term which includes any treatment for functional nervous disorders, *e.g.* by hypnotism, suggestion, psycho-analysis, etc.

psychotic (*sī-ko'-tik*). Relating to a psychosis.

pterygium (*te-rij'-ēum*). Mucous membrane growing on the conjunctiva and tending to grow on to the cornea.

pterygoid (*te-ri-goyd*). Wing-shaped.

pterion (*te'-rē-on*). The point of junction of the frontal, parietal, temporal and sphenoidal bones.

ptomaine (*tō-mān*). Poisonous amines from bacterial decomposition of animal or vegetable matter.

ptosis (*tō'-sis*). Drooping of the upper eyelid.

ptyalin (*tī'-a-lin*). An enzyme which is present in saliva. It has the power of digesting starch. Now called salivary amylase.

ptyalism (*tī'-a-lizm*). Excessive flow of saliva.

puberty (*pū'-ber-ti*). The point in development when the reproductive organs become active.

pubes (*pū'-bēz*). The two pubic bones. Also applied to the area above the bones.

pubiotomy (*pū-bē-ot'-o-mi*).

Cutting the pubis; an operation sometimes performed to enlarge a contracted pelvis and so facilitate delivery.

pudenda (*pū-den'-da*). The external genital organs.

pudendal block (*pū-den-dal blok*). Method of anaesthesia in second stage of labour by injecting pudendal nerves transvaginally.

puerperal (*pū-er'-per-al*). Relating to the six weeks following childbirth.

puerperal fever. A continued fever following labour, and due to infection.

puerperal insanity (*pū-er'-peral in-san'-i-ti*). Mental disorder following childbirth. A rare occurrence.

puerperium (*pū-er-pē-rē-um*). The period after a confinement until the uterus is involuted.

Pulex irritans (*pū-leks i'-ritans*). Common flea. *See* FLEA.

pulmonary (*pul'-mun-a-ri*). Relating to the lungs. *P. stenosis.* Narrowing of the pulmonary valve of the heart. *P. valve.* The valve at the exit of the right ventricle into the pulmonary artery.

pulp (*pulp*). The interior, fleshy part of vegetable or animal tissue.

pulsation (*pul-sā'-shon*). Beat-ing of the heart, or of the blood in the arteries.

pulse (*puls*). Can be felt where an artery crosses a bone. It is usually taken at the wrist with three fingers on the radial artery. The pulse in health beats about 120 to the minute in infants; 80 in children: 60 to 70 in adults. *See* DICROTIC PULSE and CORRIGAN'S PULSE.

pulsus alternans (*pul-sus orlter-nans*). The pulse is alternately strong and weak though regular in time.

pulvis (*pul'-vis*). A powder.

punctate (*punk'-tāt*). Dotted.

puncture (*punk'-tūr*). To make a hole with a sharp instrument.

pupa (*pū'-pa*). Second stage of insect development following the larval stage.

pupil (*pū'-pil*). The orifice in the centre of the iris.

pupillary (*pū-pil'-a-ri*). Pertaining to the pupil.

purgative (*per'-ja-tiv*). A medicine for causing evacuation of the bowels.

purine (*pū'-rin*). A protein substance from which may be derived a series of compounds including uric acid.

purine diet, low (*pū'rin*). Prescribed for gout.

Purkinje cells (*per-kin-ji sels*). Nerve cells found in the cortex of the cerebellum.

purpura (*per'-pū-ra*). Red or purple spots or patches due to haemorrhages into the skin. May be a symptom of severe illnesses such as bacterial endocarditis, cerebrospinal meningitis. *P. haemorrhagica*. A severe form with diminished number of blood platelets.

purulent (*pu'-rū-lent*). Pus-like.

pus. Matter. Consists of dead leucocytes, dead bacteria, cell debris and tissue fluid.

pustula maligna (*pus'-tū-la mal-ig-na*). Anthrax.

pustulation (*pus-tū-lā-shon*). The formation of pustules.

pustule (*pus'-tūl*). A pimple containing pus.

putrefaction (*pū-tre-fak'-shon*). The rotting away of animal matter. Decomposition advanced to an offensive stage.

p.v. Abbreviation for *per vaginam*. Examination of the pelvic organs by inspection or palpation through the vagina.

pyaemia (*pī-ē-mi-a*). The circulation of septic emboli in the blood stream causing multiple abscesses.

pyarthrosis (*pī-ar-thrō'-sis*). Suppuration in a joint.

pyelitis (*pī-e-lī'-tis*). Inflammation of the pelvis of the kidney. The organism is usually the bacillus coli communis. Now thought that it always includes renal substance and therefore is pyelonephritis.

pyelography (*pī-el-og'-raf-i*). The method to demonstrate kidneys, ureters and bladder, following intravenous injection of contrast medium opaque to x-rays. *Retrograde p.* The method to demonstrate kidneys and ureters following introduction of ureteric catheter into which contrast medium is injected.

pyelolithotomy (*pī-e-lō-li-tho'-tō-mi*). Operation to remove a stone from the renal pelvis.

pyelonephritis (*pī-el-ō-nef-rī'-tis*). Inflammation of the kidney and its pelvis.

pyknic (*pik-nik*). One of Kretschmer's types, fat and jolly.

pylorectomy (*pī-lo-rek'-tom-i*). Removal of the pyloric end of the stomach.

pyloric stenosis (*pī-lo'-rik sten-ō'-sis*). Narrowing of the pylorus. (1) A condition found in infants, more commonly male than female. It is not apparently present at birth and is usually noted after the age of ten days. Projectile vomiting after all feeds, constipation, wasting, are the chief symptoms, while on examination visible peristalsis may be present and a hard tumour to the right of the umbilicus may be felt. Condition is supposed to be due to muscular spasm and consequent hypertrophy of muscle surrounding the pylorus, so preventing the passage of food. The stomach is always dilated. The condition can be treated in its early stages by gastric lavage, and small and frequent feeds; but once a tumour is felt, it is best to open the abdomen and divide hypertrophied muscle (Ramstedt's operation). (2) In adults when it is usually due to a gastric ulcer, or to a growth.

pyloroplasty (*pī-lo'rō-plas'-ti*). Operation for widening the contracted pylorus.

pylorus (*pī-lor'-us*). Region of the junction between the stomach and the duodenum. There is a thickening of the circular muscle at this point which acts as a sphincter allowing the passage of food out of the stomach.

pyocolpos (*pī-o-kol'-pos*). Pus retained in the vagina.

pyoderma (*pī-ō-der'-ma*). Any septic skin lesion.

pyogenic (*pī-ō-jen'-ik*). Producing, forming pus.

pyometra (*pī-ō-mē'-tra*). Pus retained in the uterus.

pyonephrosis (*pī-ō-nef-rō'-sis*). Pus in the kidney.

pyopericardium (*pī-ō-per-i-*
kar'-di-um). Pus in the pericardium.

pyopneumothorax (*pī-ō-nū'-mō-thor'-ax*). Pus and air in the pleural cavity.

pyorrhoea (*pī-ō-rē'-a*). A flow of pus. Generally used as meaning the same as *pyorrhoea alveolaris*, a condition in which pus oozes out from the gums around the roots of the teeth. This is also known as Rigg's disease.

pyosalpinx (*pī-ō-sal-pinks*). Abscess in a Fallopian tube.

pyramid (*pi'-ra-mid*). Elevation on the medulla oblongata caused by the pyramidal tract.

pyramidal (*pi-ram'-id-al*). Shaped like a pyramid. *P. cells.* Cells in the cerebral cortex giving out impulses to voluntary muscles. *P. system.* Tracts in the brain and spinal cord transmitting impulses from the pyramidal cells.

pyrexia (*pī-reks'-i-a*). Fever. Elevation of the body temperature. *Intermittent p.*, temperature high at night, below normal in the morning. *Remittent p.*, temperature high at night, down in the morning, but never reaching normal. *Continuous p.*, with a variation of less than one degree Celsius.

pyridoxin (*pi-ri-dok'-sin*). Vitamin B$_6$ or adermin.

pyrosis (*pī-rō'sis*). A burning pain in the stomach with eructation; heart-burn.

pyroxylin (*pi-rok'-si-lin*). A substance prepared by the action of sulphuric and nitric acids on cotton wool. Very inflammable. Is the basis of collodion.

pyuria (*pī-ū'-ri-a*). Pus in the urine.

Q

'Q' fever. Also called Queensland fever. An acute disease resembling pneumonia and caused by Rickettsia burneti.

quack (*kwak*). One who pretends to knowledge or skill which he does not possess.

quadriceps (*kwod'-ri-seps*). Four-headed: name given to four separate muscles, covering the front of the thigh, which are all inserted into the tubercle of the tibia, and extend the knee.

quadriplegia (*kwo-dri-plē-ji-a*). Paralysis of both legs and arms. *See* TETRAPLEGIA.

quadruple vaccine (*kwo-droo-pl vak-sēn*). Vaccine immunizing against tetanus, diphtheria, whooping cough and poliomyelitis.

quarantine (*kwo-ron-tēn*). A period of separation of infected persons or contacts from others, necessary to prevent the spread of disease.

quartan (*kwor'-tan*). An intermittent fever rising and falling in period of 72 hours.

quaternary ammonium compounds (*kwa-ter-na-ri*). Bactericides such as cetrimide, benzalkonium and domiphen.

Queckenstedt's test (*kwek-en-stetz*). To elicit the presence of spinal block, *e.g.* tumour. A lumbar puncture is performed. If the manometer shows no increase of intraspinal pressure when the jugular veins are pressed there is spinal block.

quickening (*kwik'-ning*). The first perception of movement of the fetus in the womb, usually felt by the mother at the end of the fourth month.

quiescent (*kwē-es-sent*). Not active. Dormant.

quinism (*kwi-nizm*). *See* CINCHONISM.

quinsy (*kwin'-zi*). A peritonsillar abscess, situated immediately outside the capsule of the tonsil. *See* TONSILLITIS.

quintan (*kwin'-tan*). Remittent fever, which recurs every fifth day.

quotidian (*kwo-tid'-ē-an*). Recurring daily. Intermittent malarial fever.

quotient (*kwō'-shent*). Result

obtained by dividing one quantity by another. *See also* INTELLIGENCE QUOTIENT.

R

rabid (*ra-bid*). Having rabies.

rabies (*rā'-bēz*). A specific infective disease: affects dogs chiefly, but may be transferred to human beings. *See* HYDROPHOBIA.

racemose (*ras'-e-mōs*). Resembling a bunch of grapes. *R. glands*, having the cells arranged in saccules with numerous ducts leading to a main duct, *e.g.* Salivary glands.

rachis (*rak'-is*). The spine.

rachitic (*rak-it'-ik*). Due to rickets. A *rachitic flat pelvis* is a deformity of the pelvis due to rickets during childhood.

rachitis (*ra-ki'-tis*). *See* RICKETS.

rad. A unit of measurement for energy absorbed by tissue exposed to x or gamma radiation.

radial (*rā'-dē-al*). Relating to the radius.

radiation (*rā-di-ā'-shon*). Emanation of energy from a source. The usual form is that of *photons* which according to their frequency of emission are known as radio waves, light, x-rays, gamma rays, etc. Subatomic particles such as *electrons*, *neutrons*,

protons, and *positrons*, *mesons* and many subnuclear particles may also be radiated.

radiation sickness. Diarrhoea and vomiting resulting from radiation.

radical (*rad'-i-kal*). That which goes to the root; thus radical treatment aims at an absolute cure, not a palliation.

radioactive fallout (*rā-di-ō-ak-tiv fawl-owt*). Radioactive isotopes distributed in the atmosphere as the result of atomic explosions. Constitutes a biological hazard as isotopes give off damaging radiations.

radioactive isotopes (*rā-dē-ō-ak'-tiv ī-sō-tōps'*). Varieties of chemical elements which exhibit radioactivity.

radioactivity (*rā'-di-ō-ak-tiv'-i-ti*). A radioactive substance is one which emits spontaneously some form of radiation, and which in course of time by spontaneous disintegration becomes converted into another substance. *See* RADIUM.

radiobiology (*rā-di-ō-bī-ol-o-ji*). Science studying the results of radiation on living tissue.

radiocarbon (*rā-di-ō-kar-bon*). Radioactive isotope of carbon.

radiographer (*rā-dē-og'-raf-er*).

Person trained to take x-rays.

radiography (*rā-di-og'-ra-fi*). Science of examination by means of x-rays.

radiologist (*rā-di-ol'-oj-ist*). A doctor who has made a special study of radiology.

radiology (*rā-di-ol'-o-ji*). The study of diagnosis by means of radiography.

radiosensitive (*rā-di-ō-sen-si-tiv*). Term applied to a structure, especially a tumour, responsive to radiotherapy.

Radiostoleum (*rā-di-ō-stōl'-e-um*). Brand of vitamin A and D solution. An anti-rachitic preparation.

radiotherapy (*rā-di-ō-the'-ra-pi*). The treatment of disease by radium, x-rays or other radioactive substances.

radium (*rā-di-um*). A disintegration product of uranium. It belongs to the group of radioactive elements; when isolated it is a white metal, but for medical purposes it is used as a compound, *i.e.* radium bromide for the production of radon, and radium sulphate for use in needles, plaques, etc. Radium disintegrates slowly, reaching half-strength in 1,690 years. Radium is a valuable therapeutic agent, and is used chiefly to destroy malignant growths.

radium rays (*rā'-di-um rāz*). The rays emitted by radium are of three types, *i.e.* alpha, beta, and gamma rays.

radius (*rā'-di-us*). The outer bone of the forearm, from the elbow to the wrist. *See* SKELETON.

radon (*rā-don*). Radioactive gas derived from radium. *R. seeds.* Sealed containers of radon.

râle (*rahl*). Slight rattling sound heard in the air passages upon auscultation.

Ramstedt's operation (*ram'-stet*). *See* PYLORIC STENOSIS.

ramus (*rā-mus*), (plu. **rami**). A branch; thus *ramus abdominalis*, branch from lumbar artery to abdominal walls. The term is also applied to branches of nerves.

ranula (*ran'-ū-la*). Cyst of mucous gland.

raphe (*rā'-fē*). Fibrous junction between muscles.

rapport (*ra-paw*). A good relationship between two people.

rarefaction (*rā-re-fak'-shon*). The process of becoming less dense.

rash. Skin eruption.

raspatory (*ras'-pa-tor-i*). A blunt instrument for dissecting tissues.

rat-bite fever (*rat'-bīt*). Disease which occurs in China and Japan. It is conveyed by the bite of an infected rat. The organism is known as the spirillum minus.

rationalization (*ra-shon-al-ī-zā'-shon*). A justification to oneself of one's action or behaviour. The explanation is based on unconscious or instinctive motives.

raucous (*raw'-kus*). Hoarse.

ray fungus. The organism which causes actinomycosis.

Raynaud's disease (*rā-nō'*). Recurring vascular spasm of the extremities. The fingers become cold and white. Occasionally dry gangrene occurs.

reaction (*rē-ak'-shon*). Response to stimulus.

reagent (*rē-ā'-jent*). An agent taking part in a reaction.

recalcitrant (*rē-kal-si-trant*). Resistant, esp. of a disease to its treatment.

recall (*re-kawl*). Bringing back a memory.

receptaculum chyli (*re-sep-tak'-ū-lum kil'-ē*). The lower expanded portion of the thoracic duct.

receptor (*re-sep'-ter*). Sensory nerve ending.

recessive (*re-ses'-siv*). (1) Tending to disappear. (2) An inherited characteristic which does not appear in the next generation if the dominant gene is present.

recipient (*re-si-pē-ent*). The person receiving blood by a transfusion.

Recklinghausen's disease (*rek'-ling-how-sen*). *See* VON RECKLINGHAUSEN'S DISEASE.

recrudescence (*re-krü-des'-sens*). Return of symptoms.

rectal. Relating to the rectum.

rectified spirit. *See* ALCOHOL.

rectocele (*rek'-tō-sēl*). Prolapse of posterior vaginal wall. Strictly the term applies to any herniation of the rectum.

rectopexy (*rek-tō-pek'-si*). Surgical procedure to fix a prolapsed rectum.

rectoscope (*rek'-tō-skōp*). Proctoscope.

rectosigmoidectomy (*rek-tō-sig-moy-dek'-to-mi*). Operation to excise the rectum and the sigmoid colon.

rectovesical (*rek-tō-ve-sī'-kal*). Of the rectum and bladder.

rectum (*rek'-tum*). The lower part of the large intestine from the colon to the anal canal. *See* BOWEL.

rectus (*rek'-tus*). Straight; applied to certain muscles. *R. abdominis*. Two external abdominal muscles one each side of mid-line running from pubic bone to ensiform cartilage and the fifth, sixth and seventh ribs. It is enclosed in a strong sheath. There are also four short muscles of the eye, external, internal, superior and inferior rectus.

R. femoris, muscle on the front of the thigh, one of the four forming the quadriceps extensor.

recumbent (*re-kum'-bent*). Lying down.

recuperate (*re-kū'-pe-rāt*). To get better.

recurrent (*re-ku'-rent*). Returning again after an interval. *R. laryngeal nerve*, supplying vocal cords. If cut or compressed by a tumour loss of voice results.

red blood cell. These are the blood cells which contain haemoglobin (*erythrocytes*). There are about 5,000,000 in each ml of blood and they carry nearly all the oxygen required by the body cells. Red blood cells are formed in the bone marrow, normally at a rate of about one million a second, and are notable for the absence of a nucleus in the mature state. They do not divide and have a lifetime of about 120 days when they are destroyed in the spleen.

red lotion (*red lō'-shon*). Astringent, contains sulphate of zinc.

reduction (*re-duk'-shon*). (1) Replacing to a normal position, *e.g.* after fracture, dislocation or hernia. (2) In chemistry, the addition of electrons to the reduced substance.

reef knot (*rēf not*). It does not slip; the ends lie parallel.

referred pain (*re-ferd'*). Pain felt at a point quite different from the position of the affected part.

reflex (*rē-fleks*). Simplest form of nervous behaviour whereby a stimulus produces an almost instantaneous response due to an inborn nerve pathway, the *reflex arc*.

reflux (*rē-fluks*). Flowing back, *e.g.* oesophageal reflux is the flow of stomach acid into the oesophagus.

refraction (*rē-frak'-shon*). The bending of light rays as they pass from one medium to another. This bending is an essential part of the process by which the image of an object is focussed on the retina of the eye. Errors of refraction are caused when the eyeball is too short or too long from before backwards which prevents the rays of light from converging on the retina. Spectacles will correct the error.

refractory (*rē-frak'-to-ri*). Stubborn; not amenable to treatment.

refrigeration (*re-fri-je-rā'-shon*). The cooling of part of the body to reduce its metabolic requirements or to anaesthetize a part.

regeneration (*rē-je-ne-rā'-shon*).

Renewal of damaged tissue such as regenerating nerve fibres.

regimen (*rej'-i-men*). A rule of diet or of hygiene, or of life.

regional ileitis (*rē-jo-nal ī-lē-ī-tis*). See CROHN'S DISEASE.

regression (*rē-gre'-shon*). Reverting to a more primitive stage. In psychology, reverting to childlike behaviour as is often seen in illness.

regurgitation (*re-ger-ji-tā'-shon*). Flowing back. A backward flow of blood through defective valves. Also used when fluid taken by the mouth regurgitates through the nose. This occurs with paralysis of the pharynx or soft palate, and may be one of the complications of diphtheria. See MITRAL VALVE.

rehabilitation (*rē-ha-bi-li-tā-shon*). Fitting a patient to take his place in the world again, *e.g.* rehabilitation of an amputee.

Reiter protein complement fixation test (*rī-ter*). One of the three screening tests for syphilis. The other two tests are the WR and the Kahn test.

Reiter's syndrome (*rī-ters sin-drōm*). Urethritis combined with arthritis and conjunctivitis.

relapse (*re-laps'*). A return of disease after convalescence has once begun.

relapsing fever (*re-lap'-sing*). Famine fever. A tropical disease caused by spirochaetes of the genus Borrelia.

relaxant (*re-lak-sant*). Applied to drug used to relax muscle tone.

relaxation (*rē-lak-sā-shon*). Reduction of muscle tone.

relaxin (*re-lak-sin*). Ovarian secretion which softens the cervix and ligaments at childbirth.

remission (*re-mi'-shon*). Period when a disease subsides and shows no symptoms.

remittent (*re-mit'-tent*). Returning at regular intervals; applied to certain fevers. *R. pyrexia.* See PYREXIA.

renal (*rē'-nal*). Relating to the kidney. *R. calculus.* Stone in the kidney. *R. threshold see* THRESHOLD.

renin (*re-nin*). Enzyme produced by the kidneys which may cause hypertension when there is a poor blood supply to the kidneys.

rennin (*ren'-nin*). A milk-curdling enzyme present in the gastric juice.

repression (*rē-pre-shon*). Psychiatric term when the individual keeps painful memories away from consciousness thus distorting reality for him.

resection (*re-sek'-shon*). A complete removal.

resectoscope (*rē-sek-to-skōp*). Instrument to view and remove pieces of tissue in transurethral prostatectomy.

reserpine (*re-ser'-pin*). An alkaloid from rauwolfia. The drug is a sedative which lowers blood pressure and slows the heart.

residual (*re-zi'-dū-al*). That which is left. *R. air*, that remaining in the lungs after forced expiration. *R. urine*, that left in the bladder after the organ has apparently been emptied naturally, measured by catheterization.

resistance (*re-zis'-tans*). The degree of opposition to an action.

resolution (*rez-ol-ū'-shon*). (1) A resolve. (2) Absorption—as for instance when an inflammatory tumour or exudate disappears without suppurating. This term is also applied to the process whereby the lung returns to normal after an attack of pneumonia.

resonance (*rez'-o-nanz*). Increase of sound by reverberation, applied to voice sounds in auscultation.

resorption (*re-sorp-shon*). Absorption of secreted matter.

respiration (*re-spi-rā'-shon*). Breathing. Rate should be in infants 50 to the minute, in children 36, in adults 16. *Inverted r.* The pause is after inspiration instead of after expiration; noticed in babies with broncho-pneumonia.

respirator (*res'-pi-rā-tor*). (1) Appliance worn over the mouth and nose to prevent the inhalation of poisonous gas. (2) Apparatus used to assist the muscles of respiration when paralysed, *e.g.* in poliomyelitis. There is a variety of types of these respirators.

respiratory distress syndrome. *See* HYALINE MEMBRANE.

resuscitation (*re-sus-si-tā'-shon*). Reviving those who are apparently dead.

retardation (*re-tar-dā'-shon*). A slowing down of activity; backwardness.

retching (*retsh'-ing*). Ineffectual efforts to vomit.

retention (*rē-ten'-shon*). A holding back. Inability to void urine.

reticular (*ret-ik'-ū-lah*). Resembling a network. Applied to tissue.

reticulocyte (*re-ti'-kū-lō-sīt*). Immature erythrocyte found in blood regeneration.

reticulocytosis (*re-ti-kū-lō-sī-tō'-sis*). Excessive reticulocytes found in the blood stream.

reticulo-endothelial system (*re-ti-kū-lō- en-dō-thē'-lē-al sis-tem*). Special endothelial cells which are phagocytic and are found in spleen, lymph glands, liver and bone marrow. These cells aid in the destruction of red cells and form bilirubin from haemoglobin.

reticuloses (*re-ti-kū-lō-sis*). A group of neoplastic disorders affecting the reticulo-endothelial tissue and causing lymph node and splenic enlargement, *e.g.* Hodgkin's disease, lymphosarcoma.

retina (*ret'-i-na*). The delicate inner coat of the eye between choroid and vitreous humour which is sensitive to light. It is the termination of the optic nerve upon which objects are focussed. *See* EYE.

retinal (*ret'-i-nal*). Pertaining to the retina.

retinitis (*ret-in-ī-tis*). Inflammation of the retina.

retinoblastoma (*re-ti-nō-bla-stō'-ma*). Tumour arising from germ cells in the retina.

retinopathy (*re-ti-no-pa-thi*). Pathological lesion affecting the retina, *e.g.* diabetic retinopathy, hypertensive retinopathy.

retractile (*re-trak-tīl*). That which can be drawn back.

retraction (*re-trak'-shon*). Shortening, drawing back-ward. The process whereby the muscular fibres of the uterus remain permanently shortened to a slight degree after each contraction or labour pain; by this process the uterus when empty does not require to continue in a state of active contraction in order to maintain its lessened bulk and for the prevention of haemorrhage. The *retraction* ring, or *Bandl's* ring, is a ridge, which can sometimes be felt on the uterus above the pubes in cases of prolonged or obstructed labour. Its appearance is an indication for immediate completion of labour by artificial means.

retractor (*re-trak'-ter*). Instrument used to withdraw structures obscuring the field of operation.

retro- (*re-trō*). Prefix denoting backwards.

retrobulbar (*re-trō-bul'-ba*). Behind the globe of the eye.

retrocaecal (*re-trō-sē'-kal*). Behind the caecum.

retroflexion (*re-trō-flek'-shon*). A bending back, as of the body of the uterus on the cervix.

retrograde pyelography (*ret'-rō-grād-pī-el-og'-ra-fi*). *See* PYELOGRAPHY.

retrogression (*rē-trō-gre-shon*). Moving backwards.

retrolental fibroplasia (*re-trō-len'-tal fi-brō-plā-sē-a*). The posterior part of the capsule of the lens of the eye becomes fibrosed and blindness may result. Found in premature babies who have been given too much oxygen.

retro-ocular (*re-trō-o-kū-la*). Posterior to the eye.

retroperitoneal (*re-trō-pe-rit-on-ē-al*). Behind the posterior layer of the peritoneum.

retropharyngeal (*re'-trō-far-in-jē'-al*). Behind the pharynx. *R. abscess*, a collection of pus behind the wall of the pharynx and anterior to the cervical vertebrae. An acute abscess may develop from inflammation of two glands near mid-line, a chronic one from cervical caries.

retropubic (*re-trō-pū-bik*). Behind the pubis. *R. prostatectomy. See* MILLIN'S PROSTATECTOMY.

retrospection (*re-trō-spek'-shon*). Looking back into the past.

retrosternal (*re-trō-ster'-nal*). Behind the sternum.

retroversion (*re-trō-ver'-shon*). A turning backwards. The uterus is normally turned considerably forwards, that is, the cervix is directed towards the lower end of the sacrum and the fundus towards the suprapubic region. Any deviation from this in the backward direction is termed retroversion. *Retroversion of the gravid uterus* may prevent the enlarging uterus from rising out of the pelvis.

retroverted gravid uterus (*retrō-ver'-ted gra-vid ū'-te-rus*). *See* RETROVERSION.

Reverdin's needle (*rev-er-dinz nē'-dl*). A long handle with a curved needle at right angles. Used for deep work in pelvis. Needle is inserted beneath tissue required to be tied, threaded, then withdrawn, leaving ligature *in situ*. It can thus be tied.

rhagades (*rag'-ad-ēz*). A crack or fissure of skin causing pain; a term especially used of radiating scars at angle of mouth due to congenital syphilis.

Rhesus (Rh) factor (*rē'-sus*). *See* BLOOD GROUPING.

rheumatic (*rū-ma'-tik*). Pertaining to rheumatism. *R. fever*. Acute rheumatic fever is a disorder affecting connective tissue, particularly that of the heart and the joints. The cause is considered to be an allergic reaction to toxins from haemolytic streptococcus (Lancefield group A). *R. heart disease.* Chronic rheumatic heart disease is the result of severe damage and deformation of the heart due to rheumatic fever.

rheumatism (*ru-ma-tizm*). General term covering diverse conditions which have in common rather ill-defined pains of the muscles and joints.

rheumatoid (*rū-ma-toyd'*). Similar to rheumatism.

rheumatoid arthritis (*rū-ma-toyd arth-rī'-tis*). A subacute or chronic form of arthritis. Gross changes occur in the joints leading to deformity and ankylosis.

rheumatologist (*ru-ma-to'-lo-jist*). One who studies rheumatic disease.

rhinitis (*rī-nī-tis*). Inflammation of the nose.

rhinoplasty (*rī-nō-plas'-ti*). Making a false nose.

rhinorrhoea (*rī-no-re'-a*). Discharge from the nose.

rhinoscope (*rī'-no-skōp*). Nasal speculum.

rhizodontropy (*rī-zō-don-tro-pi*). Dental term for crowning the root of a tooth.

rhizotomy (*rī-zo'-to-mi*). Division of spinal nerve roots.

rhodopsin (*rō-dop'-sin*). Visual purple contained in the retina.

rhonchus (*rong'-kus*). A rattling bronchial sound heard on auscultation.

rhythm (*ri'-thum*). Movement following a definite pattern. The *Alpha r.* is the normal pattern recorded by electro-encephalogram of changes in electrical potential. The *Beta r.* is the rhythm recorded occasionally from the front of the brain.

riboflavin (*ri-bō-flā'-vin*). Part of vitamin B complex.

ribonuclease (*rī-bō-nū-klē-ās*). Enzyme which degrades RNA.

ribonucleic acid (*rī-bō-nū-klā-ik a-sid*). Chemical substance in animal cells. It is concerned in synthesis of protein.

ribs. Long lateral bones enclosing the chest. The upper seven ribs on each side join the sternum by separate cartilages, and are called true ribs, the lower five ribs being termed false ribs. Of the latter, the upper three pairs are attached to the sternum by a common cartilage on each side; while the lower two ribs on each side are not attached to the sternum at all, and are therefore called floating ribs.

rice-water stools (*rīs-waw-ter stoolz*). Stools of cholera which look like water in which rice has been boiled.

Richter's hernia (*rik-ters her'-nē-a*). Hernia which involves only a portion of the lumen of the intestine.

ricinoleic acid (*rī'-sin-ō-le-ik*). The unsaturated fatty acid of castor oil.

rickets (*ri'-ketz*). Disease of childhood due to a diet lacking in vitamin D and lack of fresh air and sunshine. The child is fat but flabby, irritable: delay in walking and teething, profuse sweats, head large, anterior fontanelle open at 2 years, bossing of frontal bones, pigeon breast, beading of ribs, enlargement of epiphyses, deformities of long bones, enlarged abdomen, tendency to bronchitis and gastroenteritis. *See* VITAMINS.

Rickettsia (*ri-ket-sē-a*). Microorganisms responsible for typhus and similar infections.

Rigg's disease (*rigz*). *See* PYORRHOEA.

rigor (*rī'-gor*). Sudden feeling of cold accompanied by shivering which raises the body temperature above normal. Due to disorder of thermoregulatory centre of the brain caused by toxins, etc.

rigor mortis (*rī'-gor mor'-tis*). The stiffening of the body after death.

rima (*rī'-ma*). A fissure; thus *rima glottidis*, slit between vocal cords.

Ringer's solution (*rin-gers so-lū'-shon*). Physiological saline which includes, in addition to sodium, potassium, calcium, magnesium and some other ions normally present in extracellular fluid.

ring pessaries (*ring pes'-a-riz*). *See* PESSARY.

ringworm (*ring'-werm*). Also called tinea, fungus infection or dermatophytosis. Infection of the skin, hair or nails by various kinds of fungi. Some forms of ringworm as *microsporon audouini* only affect man; *tinea verrucosum* affects cattle but may be passed on to man, affecting the scalp. *Microsporon felinum* affects dogs and cats and man secondarily. In body ringworm, *tinea circinata*, there are spreading rings with blistery or scaling edges; in *tinea pedis* or athlete's foot, the skin between and behind the toes is specially affected; *onychomycosis* is ringworm of the nails usually caused by trychophyton rubrum. Ringworm of the scalp may be caused by *microsporon audouini* or infection from cattle, dogs or cats. There are circular patches of dull colour. The hairs in the infected areas break off just above the scalp. Diagnosis is made with Wood's light and also microscope. Modern treatment is a course of griseofulvin by mouth for at least six weeks.

Rinne's test (*rin-ners*). A vibrating tuning-fork is placed on the mastoid process until no longer heard, then quickly put in front of the meatus; normally the vibration is still heard. The test is negative when obstruction exists in the external or middle ear.

Ripple mattress. Apparatus designed to reduce the incidence of pressure sore by rhythmically shifting weight of the patient from one area to the other by means of pumping air into linear compartments causing the mattress to 'ripple'.

risus sardonicus (*rē-sus sardo'-ni-kus*). A convulsive grin, symptomatic of tetanus.

RNA. *See* RIBONUCLEIC ACID.

rodent ulcer (*rō'-dent ul'-ser*). Basal cell carcinoma of skin.

rods. Retinal organs giving night vision.

Romberg's sign (*rom'-bergz sīn*). Inability to stand erect when the eyes are closed and the feet placed together; seen in tabes dorsalis.

Röntgen rays (*rern-shen*). X-rays. *See* RADIATION.

Röntgen unit. Unit of radiation defined as the quantity of radiation necessary to produce 1 electrostatic unit of charge (1 e.s.u.) in 1 ml of dry air under standard pressure and temperature conditions. This is not a satisfactory unit for estimating the biological effects of radiation and a number of alternative units have been introduced.

rosacea (*rō-zā'-se-a*). Vasculomotor disturbance affecting the face with associated hyperplasia of the sebaceous glands.

roseola (*rō-zē-ō'-la*). A rose-coloured rash.

rotation (*rō-tā'-shon*). Twisting. Applied to the twisting of the head upon the shoulders of the fetus as it passes down the birth canal and follows its curves.

rotators (*rō-tā'-tors*). Muscles which cause circular movement.

roughage (*ru'-fij*). Cellulose part of food which gives bulk and aids peristalsis.

round ligaments (*row'nd liga-ments*). Two thin cords passing from the uterus through the broad ligaments, and terminating in the canals of Nuck in the inguinal regions. When these are shortened for retroverted uterus, this is called Mackendrodt's operation.

287 **RYL**

roundworm. *See* ASCARIS LUM-
BRICOIDES.

Rovsing's sign (*rōv-sings sīn*).
In appendicitis, pressure
in the left iliac fossa will
cause pain in the right iliac
fossa.

RPCFT. Reiter protein complement fixation test.

rubefacients (*ru-be-fā'-sē-ents*).
Mild irritants which cause
redness of the skin.

rubella (*roo-bel'-la*). Also
called German measles. A
mild infectious disease
caused by a virus. Incubation
period 14–20 days, infectiv-
ity less than measles. There
may be slight catarrh and
fever and swelling of suboc-
cipital glands. The rash
begins on the face and
spreads to the body and fades
quickly. Complications are
few but if a woman has
the disease during the first
four months of pregnancy,
she may have a deformed
child.

rugae (*roo-jē*). Wrinkles or
creases.

rugine (*rū-jēn*). Instrument for
elevating the periosteum.

rugose (*rū'-jōs*). Wrinkled.

rumination (*roo'-min-a'-shon*).
Act analogous to chewing the
cud. Infant brings up some of
feed and plays with it in
mouth. Considered to have a
psychological basis.

rupia (*roo'-pi-a*). A skin disease
with crusts due to tertiary
syphilis.

rupture (*rup'-tūr*). A bursting.
In popular language a rup-
ture means a hernia. In obstetric practice *rupture of the
perineum* is not uncommon
as a result of labour, especially in primiparae; *rupture of
the uterus* is a rare event due
to unrelieved obstructed
labour, or more rarely still to
unskilful attempts at delivery
by the use of instruments;
rupture of the membranes is
the normal sequence of full
dilatation of the cervix in
labour, and marks the commencement of the second
stage. *Rupture of a tubular
extra-uterine pregnancy* may
result in severe internal
haemorrhage and would
require immediate opera-
tion.

Russell traction (*ru'-sel trak-
shon*). Method to reduce a
fractured femur. There is an
upward pull to a Balkan
beam from a sling beneath
the knee and from the lower
part of the leg a longitudinal
pull towards the foot of the
bed. The resultant direction
of the pull helps to straighten
the femur.

Ryle's tube (*rīls tūb*). Narrow
bore rubber tube, slightly
weighted, used for giving a

test meal or aspirating the stomach.

S

Sabin's vaccine (*sā-bins vak-sēn*). One of the poliomyelitis vaccines. It is taken orally.

sac. A small pouch, such as a hernial sac.

saccharin (*sak'-ka-rin*). An intensely sweet substance used as a substitute for sugar. It has no food value.

Saccharomyces (*sak-a-rō-mī'-sez*). A group of fungi including yeasts. One is the cause of thrush.

sacculated (*sak'-ū-la-ted*). Bagged, or pursed out.

sacral (*sā-kral*). Pertaining to the sacrum. *S. analgesia, see* CAUDAL ANALGESIA. *S. canal.* This passes through the sacrum and contains the cauda equina.

sacro-iliac synchondrosis or **joint** (*sak-ro-i-li-ak sin-kon-drō-sis*). The articulation between the sacrum and the hip bone. Normally there is no movement at this joint. During pregnancy the joint becomes more movable and this, to a slight extent, facilitates the birth of the child.

sacro-anterior, sacrolateral and **sacroposterior.** These terms indicate positions of breech presentations.

sacrococcygeal joint (*sā-krō-kok-si-jē-al joynt*). The joint between the sacrum and coccyx. When the baby is delivered there is a backward movement of the coccyx.

sacrum (*sā'-krum*). A wedge-shaped bone consisting of five fused vertebrae. They form the posterior wall of the pelvic cavity.

saddle-nose (*sa-dle-nōs*). A flattened bridge of the nose.

sadism (*sā-dism*). A sexual perversion in which pleasure is derived from inflicting cruelty upon another.

sagittal (*saj'-it-tal*). In the median plane. *S. section.* Section made by cutting through a specimen from top to bottom so that there are equal right and left halves. *S. suture*, the suture between the parietal bones.

St. Vitus' dance (*vī'-tus*). Chorea.

sal. A salt.

salicylate (*sa-li-si-lāt*). A salt of salicylic acid, *e.g. sodium salicylate* used in rheumatism. It relieves pain and reduces the temperature. *Methyl salicylate* (chief constituent of oil of wintergreen) is applied to painful joints.

salicylic acid (*sal-i-sil'-ik as'id*). An antiseptic used on the skin. *See* SALICYLATE.

Acetyl-salicylic acid is aspirin.

saline (*sā'-lĭn*). Containing salt. *Normal saline solution* is 0·91 per cent. This is isotonic with the blood. Sterile saline is given intravenously or subcutaneously.

saliva (*sa-lī'-va*). The secretion of the salivary glands.

salivary glands (*sal-ī'-va-ri*). Three pairs of glands. The sublingual and submaxillary situated in the floor of the mouth; the parotid above the angle of the lower jaw. *See* PAROTID.

salivation (*sal-i-vā'-shon*). The act of secretion of saliva.

Salk vaccine (*salk vak-sēn*). One of the vaccines given to protect against poliomyelitis. It contains dead virus.

Salmonella (*sal-mon-el'-la*). Group of bacilli; common cause of food poisoning in England.

salpingectomy (*sal-pin-jek'-tō-mi*). Removal of one or both Fallopian tubes.

salpingitis (*sal-pin-ji'-tis*). Inflammation of a tube, usually applied to the Fallopian tubes.

salpingocyesis (*sal-ping-gō-sī-ē'-sis*). Tubal pregnancy.

salpingography (*sal-pin-gō-gra-fi*). Examination of the Fallopian tubes by x-rays.

salpingo-oophorectomy (*salpin'-go-oo-for-ek'-to-mi*). The surgical removal of Fallopian tubes and ovaries.

salpingostomy (*sal-pin-gos'-to-mi*). Opening artificially a Fallopian tube whose aperture has been closed by inflammation or previous surgery.

salpinx (*sal'-pinks*). A tube, either Eustachian or Fallopian.

salt (*sor'lt*). Substance formed by the combination of a base with an acid, *e.g.* sodium chloride (common salt) is formed by the union of sodium hydroxide and hydrochloric acid.

saltpetre (*sawlt-pē'-tr*). Nitrate of potassium.

sanatorium (*san-at-or'-ium*). Any institution for convalescent patients can technically be called a sanatorium; but until recently indicated an institution for the open-air treatment of tuberculosis.

sandfly fever (*sand-flī fē'ver*). Tropical disease due to infection by organism transmitted by sandfly bites.

sanguine (*san-gwin*). (1) Full-blooded. (2) Hopeful.

sanguineous (*san-gwin'-e-us*). Bloodstained. Containing blood.

sanitary (*sa-ni-ta-ri*). Pertaining to health.

sanitation (*san-i-tā'-shon*). The use of methods conducive to the public health.

sanity (*sa-ni-ti*). Being of sound mind.

saphena varix (*sa-fē-na vā-riks*). Saccular enlargement of the termination of the long saphenous vein often without obvious varicose veins.

saphenous nerve. Large branch of the femoral nerve.

saphenous opening (*saf-ē'-nus*). Just below groin near inner side of thigh where superficial saphenous vein passes deep to enter femoral vein.

saphenous veins (*sa-fē-nus vāns*). Superficial leg veins. *Long s.v.* begins on the foot and extends to the groin. *Short s.v.* joins the popliteal vein at the knee.

sapo. Soap. *S. mollis.* Soft soap.

saponify (*sa-po'-nifī*). To make into a soap.

saprophytes (*sap'-rō-fīts*). Organisms that exist only in dead matter.

Sarcina (*sar'-sin-a*). A genus of Schizomycetes which form rectangular bundles as they divide; usually non-pathogenic.

sarcoidosis (*sar-koy-dō'-sis*). A systemic granulomatous disease of unknown cause, the lesions being histologically similar to tuberculosis follicles. Affects lymph nodes, lungs, liver, spleen, skin, eyes, parotid glands and phalanges.

sarcoid reaction. Histological change resembling sarcoidosis but seen in individual organs only.

sarcolemma (*sar-kō-lem'-ma*). The membrane which covers each fibril of muscle.

sarcology (*sar-kol'-o-ji*). Anatomy of the soft tissues as distinguished from osteology.

sarcoma (*sar-kō'-ma*). A malignant tumour composed of embryonic connective tissue. Spread is by way of the blood-stream, and metastases are found in lungs, brain, and other organs.

Sarcoptes scabiei (*sar-kop'-tēz skā-bē-ā-ē*). The itch mite or insect causing scabies. It burrows into the skin where it lays its eggs which hatch out. The 'burrows' often terminate in a papule on the skin. The disease is treated with benzyl benzoate.

sartorius (*sar-tor'-ē-us*). The long ribbon-shaped muscle of the front of the thigh.

saturation (*sat-ū-rā'-shon*). A solution in which no more of the solute can be dissolved.

scab. An incrustation formed over a wound.

scabies (*skā'-bēz*). A contagious skin disease due to a parasitic insect, the acarus scabiei or Sarcoptes scabiei.

scald (*skawld*). Burn caused by hot fluids.

scalenus anterior syndrome (*ska-lē-nus an-tā-ri-or sin'-drōm*). Characterized by pain in the arm and tingling of the fingers with loss of power and muscle wasting due to compression of the lower fibres of the brachial plexus by the scalenus anterior muscle.

scale (*skāl*). The horny epidermis the skin sheds.

scalp (*skal'-p*). The skin covering the cranium.

scalpel (*skal'-pel*). A straight knife with convex edge, used in dissecting and surgery.

scanning speech. *See* STACCATO or SCANNING SPEECH.

scaphoid (*skāf'-oyd*). Boat-shaped. The name of a bone of the carpus and of the tarsus.

scapula (*skap'-ū-la*). The shoulder blade.

scar (*skar*). The connective fibrous tissue found after any wound has healed.

scarification (*skar-i-fi-kā'-shon*). Shallow incisions just penetrating the epidermis. A technique used in vaccination.

scarlatina (*skar-la-tē'-na*). Scarlet fever; an infectious fever. There is a widespread erythematous rash produced by a toxin released by haemolytic streptococci.

Scarpa's triangle (*skar'-pas trī-angle*). The femoral triangle bounded by Poupart's ligament, the adductor longus and sartorius.

SCAT. Sheep cell agglutination test. A serum test for rheumatoid arthritis.

Scheuermann's disease (*shoy'-er-mans*). Vertebral osteochondritis found in adolescents. It affects the two rings of cartilage and bone around the margin of both superior and inferior surfaces of the vertebral body. The condition does not cause general ill-health.

Schick test (*shik*). A test for antibody in the patient's blood to the Klebs-Loeffler bacillus which causes diphtheria. A minute amount of diphtheria toxin (and protein) is injected into the patient's left forearm. If there is antitoxin in the patient's blood the toxin will be neutralized and there will be no reaction. If the patient's blood has little or no anti-toxin, there will be an area of redness on the skin 1 cm in diameter, within 24 hours, reaching its height in four days. This patient is susceptible to diphtheria. A control solution containing protein and inactive toxin is injected into the right arm. If there is a protein reaction or false reaction, this reaches its height in 24 hours and then fades.

schistosomiasis (*skis-tō-so-mī-a-sis*). *See* BILHARZIA.

schizoid temperament (*skit-zoyd*). One that is reticent and aloof.

Schizomycetes (*skiz-o-mī-sē'-tēz*). A group of fungi which includes the yeasts.

schizophrenia (*skit-zō-frē-ni-a*). Term used for a group of mental disorders characterized by a progressive loss of emotional stability, judgement and contact with reality.

Schlatter's disease (*shla'-ters*). Osteochondritis of the anterior tubercle of the tibia. Also called Osgood-Schlatter's disease.

Schlemm's canal (*shlem*). Lymphatic channel leading to a venous plexus at the root of the ciliary body of the eye. It allows the intraocular fluid (aqueous humour) to drain. Failure to do so results in raised hydrostatic pressure in the anterior chamber of the eye (glaucoma).

Schultz-Charlton reaction (*shootz-charl'-ton*). Test to confirm scarlet fever. Antitoxin is injected into the skin where the rash is bright red. If the disease is present, there is a blanching ring round the injection site in about 18 hours.

Schwann substance (*shwon sub-stans*). White sheath of nerve fibre.

sciatica (*sī-at'-ik-a*). Neuralgia of the sciatic nerve—the large nerve of the thigh. It may be caused by pressure on the nerves in the spinal canal or the pelvis.

scirrhous (*ski'-rus*). Hard and fibrous.

scissor-leg deformity (*si-zer-leg di-for'-mi-ti*). Deformity due to exaggerated tone in the adductor muscles usually resulting from cerebral damage.

sclera (*sklē-ra*). The opaque outer coat of the eyeball, forming five-sixths of the globe of the eye, the remaining one-sixth being formed by the cornea. *See* EYE.

scleritis (*skle-rī'-tis*). An inflamed sclera.

scleroderma (*sklēr-ō-der'-ma*). A collagen disease affecting the dermis causing contracture and deformities of joints and widespread systemic effects.

sclerosis (*skler-ō'-sis*). Hardening. *See also* DISSEMINATED SCLEROSIS.

sclerotic (*skle-rot'-ik*). Pertaining to the sclera.

sclerotomy (*skler-ot'-to-mi*). An operation on the sclerotic coat of the eye, for the relief of glaucoma.

scolex (*skō'-leks*). Head of a tapeworm.

scoliosis (*skō-li-ō'-sis*). Lateral curvature of the spine.

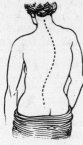

41 Scoliosis

scorbutus (*skor-bū-tus*). Scurvy.

scotoma (*sko-tō'-ma*). A blind spot in the field of vision.

'screening' (*skrēn'-ing*). Radiological examination by means of a fluorescent screen.

scrofuloderma (*skro-fū-lō-der'-ma*). Tuberculous condition of the skin.

scrotocele (*skrō'-tō-sēl*). Hernia in the scrotum.

scrotum (*skrō'-tum*). The bag which holds the testicles.

scurf (*skerf*). Dandruff. Scales from the epidermis of the scalp.

scurvy (*sker'-vi*). A rare deficiency disease, due to an extremely low intake of vitamin C. *See* VITAMINS. Characterized by swelling of the gums, haemorrhages into skin and subcutaneous tissues, and from mucous membranes, and by anaemia. *Infantile s.* A type of the above occurring in infancy, characterized by subperiosteal haemorrhages and anaemia. Due to same cause.

scybala (*sib'-a-la*). Faeces passed as hard dry masses.

sebaceous (*se-bā'-shus*). Fatty, secreting oily matter, *S. glands,* of skin, secrete fatty material called sebum. *S. cysts,* dilatation of one of these glands, due to blocking of its opening on to the skin. Cyst is filled with sebum.

seborrhoea (*seb-o-rē'-a*). Excessive secretion of the sebaceous glands.

sebum (*sē'-bum*). The fat of the skin, secreted by the sebaceous glands.

secondary areola (*a-rē-o-la*). A peculiar pigmentation of the skin often seen on the breast around the nipple during pregnancy. *See* AREOLA.

secondary disease. A disease consequent on another disease already active.

secondary haemorrhage (*hem-o-ráj*). *See* HAEMORRHAGE.

secondary uterine inertia (*sek-on-da-ri ū'-te-rin in-er'-sha*). *See* INERTIA OF UTERUS.

second intention (*in-ten-shon*). The healing of a wound by means of granulation, and the growing of new skin. Takes longer than healing by first intention.

second stage (of labour) (*stāj*). From complete dilatation of the cervix, usually associated with rupture of the membranes, to the complete expulsion of the child. During this stage, which lasts normally two to four hours in primigravidae, and up to one hour in multiparae, the pains are very severe, and the uterine contractions are assisted by those of the abdominal muscles. This is the stage for which anaesthetics are often given. *See also* LABOUR.

secretin (*se-krē'-tin*). A hormone formed in the mucous membrane of the duodenum. It is carried by the blood to the pancreas, exciting it to activity. It also stimulates the secretion of bile.

secretion (*se-krē'-shon*). The active production, filtering or extrusion of material from cells. Gland cells have specialized secretory activity.

section (*sek-shon*). Usually applied to thin slices of tissue cut for microscopical examination.

sedative (*sed'-a-tiv*). Drug allaying excitement or pain, *e.g.* morphia and barbiturates.

sedimentation rate (*se-di-men-tā-shon rāt*). *See* ESR.

segment (*seg'-ment*). A small piece; section; a subdivision.

segregation (*se-gre-gā'-shon*). A setting apart. Isolation.

sella turcica (*ter'-si-ka*). Pituitary fossa of the sphenoid bone.

semen (*sē'-men*). The secretion of the testicles mixed with that of the seminal vesicles and prostate.

semi (*se'-mi*). Half.

semicircular canals (*sem-i-ser'-kū-la can-als'*). Three canals of the internal ear, the sense organs of equilibrium or balance. *See* EAR.

semilunar cartilages (*sem-i-lū-na kar'-til-āj-es*). Menisci. Two crescentic cartilages, an internal and an external, lying in the knee joint between the femur and tibia. These may be torn and displaced, giving rise to pain and deformity and fluid in the knee joint. Usually removed by operation.

seminal (*sem'-in-al*). Relating to the semen. *S. vesicles.* Two small structures in the male genito-urinary system which secrete part of the seminal fluid.

senescence (*se-nes-sens*). Growing old.

Sengstaken tube (*seng-sta-ken tūb*). Oesophageal tube used to compress bleeding varices.

senility (*se-nil'-i-ti*). Degenerative changes due to advanced age.

sensible (*sen'-si-bl*). That which the senses perceive.

sensitive (*sen'-si-tiv*). Able to react to a stimulus.

sensitization (*sen-si-tī-zā-shon*). Act of producing an immunological state in which there is a disproportionate reaction to a substance which normally acts as an antigen.

sensory nerves (*sen'-sor-i*). Afferent nerves carrying sensory information to the central nervous system. *Cf.* motor nerves.

sepsis (*sep'-sis*). The condition of being infected by pyogenic bacteria.

septic (*sep'-tik*). Pertaining to sepsis.

septicaemia (*sep-ti-sēm-i-a*). The circulation and multiplication of micro-organisms in the blood; a very serious condition.

septum (*sep'-tum*). The division between two cavities; such as *septum ventriculorum*, which separates the right

ventricle of the heart from the left.

sequelae (*se-kwe'-lē*). Morbid conditions remaining after, and consequent on, some former illness.

sequestrectomy (*se-kwes-trek'-to-mi*). Operation to remove sequestrum.

sequestrum (*se-kwes'-trum*). A fragment of dead bone.

serosa (*se-rō'-sa*). A serous membrane. Serous membranes line the large lymph spaces, *e.g.* pleural, pericardial, peritoneal cavities.

serositis (*se-rō-sī'-tis*). An inflamed serous membrane.

serotonin (*se-rō-tō-nin*). Amine found in blood platelets, the intestines and brain substance. Mono-amine oxidase inactivates it.

serpiginous (*ser-pij'-in-us*). Serpent-like in shape.

serrated (*se-rā-ted*). With a saw-like edge.

serum (*sēr'-um*). (1) The fluid part of the blood, after clot and cells have been removed. (2) Fluid used for providing passive immunity against infection. The serum is taken from an animal which has been rendered immune against a certain pathogenic micro-organism, and which therefore must contain a large quantity of antibodies to that micro-organism. The best known are the anti-diphtheritic and the anti-tetanic sera. The antibodies contained in the injected serum combine chemically with the disease toxins, rendering the latter harmless. *S. sickness*. Late reaction to serum injections, arising eight to ten days after. *Symptoms*: Oedema, urticarial rash, joint pains, slight temperature.

sesamoid bones (*ses-a-moyd*). Small foci of bone formation in the tendons of muscles. The patella is the largest.

sessile (*ses'-īl*). Having no stem (applied to tumours).

sex (*seks*). State of being male or female. *S.-linked*. Characteristics not inherited equally by both sexes.

Sheehan's syndrome (*shē-hans sin-drom*). Panhypopituitarism resulting from thrombosis of the pituitary blood supply occurring in association with post-partum haemorrhage.

Shiga's bacillus (*shē-gus ba-si-lus*). The Shigella dysenteriae. A cause of dysentery, especially in the Far East.

shin-bone. The tibia. *See* SKELETON, p. 299.

shingles. *See* HERPES.

shock. General depression of the vital functions. Most common after haemorrhage, severe injuries, or operations or in toxaemic states. The essential factor in shock is a deficiency in the volume of blood in active circulation. Primary or neurogenic shock is seen where the injury is severe and the patient under the influence of pain. Secondary shock is due to the absorption of toxic substances, including histamine, which damage the walls of the capillaries. The capillaries dilate and a good deal of blood stagnates there, and the blood pressure is lowered. *Symptoms*: Pulse, short, quick and rising in rate; respiration, shallow, quick, irregular; face, blanched; nose, pinched and cold; skin, pale, cold and clammy; temperature, subnormal. *Treatment*: Warmth, gradually applied; posture, raise end of bed so that blood may flow to brain. *Stimulants*: Coramine, noradrenaline. If there is pain, morphia is ordered. Administration of fluid is most essential to give the heart something further to work on. Blood, plasma or saline are given by the appropriate route.

short circuit (*shawt ser-kit*). Anastomosis between gut or blood vessels which allows the contents to by-pass a section of the normal pathway.

short-sighted (*shawt-sī-ted*). Myopic.

shoulder presentation (*shōl'-der*). A form of transverse lie which must be converted into breech or vertex before delivery is possible.

show (*shō*). Popular term for the discharge of slightly blood-stained mucus common at the beginning of labour.

sialectasis (*si-a-lek-ta-sis*). Dilatation of salivary gland due to obstruction to the flow of saliva.

sialogogue (*si-al'-o-gog*). A medicine causing increased salivation, *e.g.* pilocarpine, mercury.

sialolith (*sī-al-ō-lith*). A salivary calculus.

sibilus (*sib'-il-us*). A hissing sound heard on auscultation of the chest during respiration in bronchitis, etc.

sibling (*sib'-ling*). One of two or more children of the same parents.

sickle-cell anaemia (*sikl-sel a-nē-mi-a*). Hereditary anaemia found sometimes in negroes. The red blood cells become sickle-shaped or crescentic.

siderosis (*si-de-rō-sis*). (1) Inhalation of iron particles caus-

ing pneumoconiosis. (2) Excess of iron in the blood.

sight (*sīt*). The power of seeing.

sigmoid (*sig'-moyd*). Like the Greek letter ς applied especially to a bend in the pelvic colon just before it becomes the rectum.

sigmoidoscope (*sig-moyd'-os-cōp*). An instrument for viewing the interior of the rectum and sigmoid flexure of the colon.

sigmoidostomy (*sig-moy-dos-to-mi*). Opening into the sigmoid colon.

sign (*sīn*). An indication of the presence of disease.

signatura (*sig-na-tū'-ra*). A label.

silicones (*si-li-kōns*). Water-repellent organic compounds.

silicosis (*sil-i-kō'-sis*). Lung disease due to the inhalation of very fine particles of silica which irritate the lungs causing fibrotic changes.

silkworm gut (*silk'-werm gut*). A suture material much used by surgeons for sewing up abdominal wounds. It is very strong, not absorbed, and can be sterilized by boiling.

silver nitrate (*sil'-ver nī'-trāt*). When solid this substance constitutes *lunar caustic*: used to destroy excess granulation tissue; it burns the skin and stains it dark brown or

black. In weak solution it is
used as an antiseptic.

Simmonds' disease (*sim-mons
di-sēz*). *See* PANHYPOPITUITAR-
ISM.

simple fracture. *See* FRACTURE.

Sims' position. The patient lies
in the semi-prone position,
across the bed. The buttocks
are brought to the edge of the
bed. The right knee is flexed
more than the left. Used for
vaginal examination.

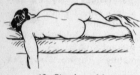

42 Sims' position

Sims' speculum (*spek-ū-lum*).
Vaginal speculum.

sinciput (*sin'-si-put*). The upper
fore part of the head.

sinew (*sin'-nū*). A tendon uniting a muscle to a bone.

sinuatrial node (*sī-nu-ā'-tri-al
nōd*). Cells found in the heart
at the junction of the superior
vena cava and the right
atrium. The node is the
pacemaker of the heart.

sinus (*sī'-nus*). (1) A passage
leading from an abscess, or
some inner part, to an external opening. (2) A dilated
channel for venous blood,
e.g. Lateral s., a large venous
channel on inner side of the

skull. It passes near the mastoid antrum and empties
itself into the jugular vein.
(3) Air sinuses, hollow
cavities in the skull bones
which communicate with the
nose. They are the frontal,
maxillary, ethmoidal and
sphenoidal sinuses.

sinus arrhythmia (*sī-nus
a-rith-mi-a*). Irregular cardiac rhythm due to the controlling effect of the vagus on
the sinuatrial node. The heart
rate increases on inspiration
and slows during expiration.

sinusitis (*sī-nu-sī-tis*). Inflammation of a sinus, especially
one of the air sinuses of the
bones of the skull.

sinusoid (*sī-nu-soyd*). Like a
sinus. Channels for small
blood vessels as found in
the liver, suprarenal glands,
etc.

siphonage (*sī-fo-nij*). The
method of drawing fluid from
one vessel to another by
means of a bent tube and the
use of atmospheric pressure.

Sjögren's syndrome (*sher-grens
sin-drōm*). Keratoconjunc-
tivitis and dry mouth usually
in postmenopausal women.

skatole (*skā-tōl*). A nitrogenous
product of protein digestion
found in the faeces.

skeleton (*skel'-e-ton*). The bony
framework of the body. (*See
illustration*, p. 299.)

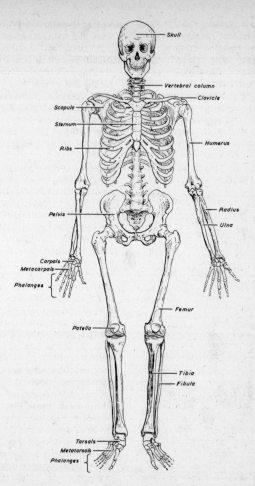

Skull

Vertebral column

Clavicle

Scapula

Sternum

Ribs

Humerus

Pelvis

Radius

Ulna

Carpals

Metacarpals

Phalanges

Femur

Patella

Tibia

Fibula

Tarsals

Metatarsals

Phalanges

43 The skeleton

Skene's glands (*skēns*). These open into posterior wall of the female urethra, just within the orifice; almost always infected in acute gonorrhoea.

skin. The outer covering of the body consisting of epidermis and its appendages (hair, sweat glands) supported by specialized dermal connective tissue.

skull. The bony framework of the head.

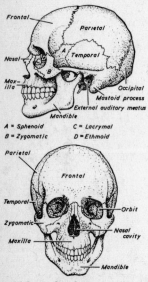

A = Sphenoid   C = Lacrymal
B = Zygomatic   D = Ethmoid

*44 Lateral and anterior views
   of the skull*

sleeping sickness. Tropical disease due to a trypanosome. The tsetse fly carries the organisms which are transferred to healthy individuals by the bite of the fly.

sleepy sickness. Encephalitis lethargica. A form of viral encephalitis.

slough (*sluf*). Dead matter, thrown off by gangrene or ulcers.

smallpox (*smawl-poks*). A highly infectious disease caused by a virus. Incubation period 12–14 days. There is high temperature, headache, backache and cough, Rash appears on the fourth day and the temperature falls, but rises again and pustulation occurs and the patient becomes very ill. *The main differences between smallpox and chickenpox* are that in smallpox the prodromal illness is much more severe. The smallpox rash is centrifugal (moves away from the centre), whereas the chickenpox rash is centripetal (seeking the centre). The pustules in smallpox take 6–8 days to mature, whereas in chickenpox from a few hours to a day or two. The smallpox rash lies deep in the skin compared to the superficial one of chickenpox. Recent vaccination usually protects against smallpox which is also known as variola.

smear (*smare*). Material for examination or culture which is spread on a slide or culture medium.

smegma (*smeg'-ma*). Thick white secretion forming under the prepuce.

Smith-Petersen nail (*smith-pē-ter-sen nāl*). Inserted to fix the two fragments of bone in a fracture of the neck of the femur.

Snellen's test types (*snel'-lens*). A chart showing letters of different size and used for testing vision. The patient sits at a distance of six metres from it. If only the large top letter can be seen the patient's vision is termed 6/60, *i.e.* he can see at 6 metres what the normal eye can see at a distance of 60 metres.

snow (*snō*). *See* CARBON DI-OXIDE.

snow blindness (*blī'-nd-ness*). Ophthalmia with photophobia caused by the glare from snow.

snuffles (*snufls*). Occurs in babies with congenital syphilis, due to changes in the mucous membrane of the nose.

sodium (*sō'-di-um*). A metallic element; the salts of which

form an important part of animal tissue.

sodium chloride (*sō'-di-um klaw'-rīd*). Common salt. It is found in the body and maintains the osmotic tension of the blood. Given in infusions with dextrose for fluid replacement in dehydration.

soft sore (*so-ft sor'*). A venereal sore not due to syphilis. Also known as *chancroid*, and *non-infecting sore*. The infecting organism is Ducrey's bacillus.

solar plexus (*sō-la plek'-sus*). A plexus of nerves and ganglia in the upper region of the abdomen.

soleus (*so'-le-us*). A muscle in the calf of the leg.

solution (*so-loo'-shon*). A liquid containing a solid which has been dissolved in it.

solvent (*sol'-vent*). A liquid able to dissolve another substance (solute).

somatic (*so-ma'-tik*). Pertaining to the body.

somnambulism (*som-nam'-bū-lizm*). Walking and carrying out other activities whilst asleep. There is dissociation which may be hysterical.

Sonne dysentery (*son-ni dis'-en-te-ri*). A type of bacillary dysentery, common in Britain. There is abdominal pain, diarrhoea and vomiting. The disease is usually slight except in infants and debilitated persons. The fluid intake must be adequate to prevent dehydration. Sulphonamides and antibiotics may be used.

soporific (*so-po-rif'-ik*). An agent which induces sleep, *e.g.* chloral.

sordes (*sor-dēz*). Brown crusts about the lips and teeth of a feverish patient which should be removed during routine oral toilet.

souffle (*soofl*). A soft blowing sound. During late pregnancy the *funic souffle* can sometimes be heard by auscultation of the maternal abdomen, a sound synchronous with the fetal heart and supposed to be produced in the umbilical cord. The *uterine souffle* is a blowing murmur heard over the uterus due to pulsations in the maternal arteries.

sound (*sownd*). A probe-like instrument used for exploring cavities such as the uterus, bladder, etc.

Southey's tubes (*sow-thēz*). Small perforated metal tubes, used to drain oedematous tissue.

Soxhlet bottle. An upright bottle used in infant feeding.

Spalding's sign (*sporl-dings sīn*). Sign of fetal death. There is overlapping of the skull bones on x-ray.

spasm (*spazm*). (1) Sudden convulsive involuntary movement. (2) Sudden contraction of a muscle or muscles, especially of the unstriped muscle coats of arteries, intestines, heart, bronchi, etc. The effect of such spasm depends on the part affected: thus asthma is believed to be due to spasm of the muscular coats of the smaller bronchi; and renal colic is due to spasm of the muscle coat of the ureter.

spasmolytic (*spaz-mo-li'-tik*). Substance which relieves spasm.

spasmus nutans (*spaz-mus nū-tanz*). A condition known as nodding spasm in babies, in which the head is continually nodding or turning from side to side.

spastic (*spas'-tik*). (1) In a state of spasm. (2) Popular term for cerebral palsy. In patients with this disease the muscles are often spastic, *i.e.* hypertonic, and there is excessive neuromuscular excitability.

spasticity (*spas-tis'-i-ti*). The condition of being spastic. Occurs in an upper motor neurone lesion.

spatula (*spat'-ū-la*). (1) A flat, flexible, blunt knife, used for spreading ointments and poultices. (2) A tongue depressor.

species (*spē-sēz*). A group of organisms having many of the same characteristics. In natural history various species form a genus or class of animals.

specific (*spe-sif'-ik*). Applied to a medicine or treatment, it means the particular remedy for a certain disease; *S. disease*, due to a distinct specific micro-organism which causes that disease alone` (term sometimes applied to venereal disease).

specific gravity (*spe-sif-ik gra'-vi-ti*). By this is meant the ratio between the weight of a substance and the weight of an equal volume of water, the latter being taken, as a matter of convenience, to be 1·000, formerly written as 1000. The specific gravity of a liquid depends on the amount of solid in solution.

spectroscope (*spek'-tro-skōp*). An instrument for the production and examination of spectra in luminous bodies.

spectrum (*spek'-trum*). The band of colours formed when rays of white light are passed through a prism.

speculum (*spek'-ū-lum*). A polished instrument for examining the interior cavities of the body, especi-ally the vagina, the rectum, the ear, and the nose.

speech (*spē-tch*). The power of speaking; conveying a meaning by vocal sounds.

speech centre. The parts of the brain controlling speech.

speech therapist (*spē-tch the'-ra-pist*). One trained to treat defects and disorders of language, voice and speech.

Spencer-Wells forceps. The usual forceps for haemostasis during operations.

sperm (*sper'm*). Semen.

spermatic cord (*sper-mat'-ik*). Composed of arteries, veins. lymphatics and nerves, and the vas deferens (the duct of the testicle); it suspends the testicle from the abdomen.

spermatocele (*sper-ma-tō-sēl*). A retention cyst from some part of the epididymis.

spermatozoa (*sper-ma-tō-zō'-a*). The male generative cells; minute cells found in the semen, which are possessed of the power of self-propulsion by means of a flagellum, and which can fertilize the ovum, or female germ cell.

spermicide (*sper-mi-sīd*). Substance destroying spermatozoa.

sphenoid (*sfē-'noyd*). Wedge-shaped. The name of one of the bones forming the base of the skull.

sphenoidal (*sfen-oy'-dal*). Pertaining to the sphenoid bone.

sphincter (*sfink'-tur*). A circular muscle which contracts the orifice of an organ.

sphincterotomy (*sfink-te-ro'-to-mi*). Division of sphincter muscles.

sphygmocardiograph (*sfig-mō-kar'-dē-ō-graf*). Apparatus recording both pulse and heart beats.

sphygmograph (*sfig'-mō-graf*). An instrument affixed to the wrist, which moves with the beat of the pulse and registers the rate and character of the beats.

sphygmomanometer (*sfig-mō-ma-no'-m'e-ter*). An instrument for measuring the arterial tension (or blood pressure) of the circulation.

spica (*spī'-ka*). A spiral bandage done with a roller in a series of figure eights. Most used for the shoulder, groin, thumb, and great toe.

spicule (*spi-kūl*). Fragment of bone.

spigot (*spi'-got*). Conical peg closing a tube.

spina bifida (*spī-na bi-fid-er*). A congenital malformation of the spine due to the neural arch of one or more vertebrae failing to fuse in the midline. The vertebral canal is exposed at this site and may herniate through the open-

ing. *See* MENINGOCELE. The defect most commonly occurs in the lumbo-sacral region.

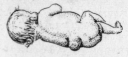

45 Spina bifida—meningocele

spinal column (*spi'-nal ko'-lum*). The backbone. It is composed of seven cervical, twelve thoracic and five lumbar vertebrae and the sacrum with its five fused vertebrae and the coccyx or tailbone.

spinal cord (*spī'-nal kord*). The portion of the central nervous system within the spine. It is composed of nerve cells and bundles of nerve fibres connecting the various levels of the spinal cord with the brain. Thirty-one pairs of spinal nerves form the peripheral nervous system of the trunk and limbs. *See also* NERVE ROOT.

spinal curvature (*spī-nal ker'-va-tūr*). The *normal* curvature of the spine is divided into primary curvature (giving an ape-like stooping posture) and secondary curvatures (cervical and lumbar). For abnormal spinal curvature *see* SCOLIOSIS, KYPHOSIS, LORDOSIS.

spine (*spīn*). The backbone or spinal column.

spirillum (*spi-ril'-lum*). Corkscrew-shaped bacteria.

spirochaete (*spī-ro-kēt*). Elongated spiral bacteria which move by flexions of the body. Parasitic spirochaetes cause syphilis and Weil's disease.

spirochaetaemia (*spī-rō-kē-tē-mi-a*). The presence of spirochaetes in the blood.

spirograph (*spī'-rō-grarf*). Instrument for recording respirations.

spirometer (*spi-rom'-e-ter*). An instrument for measuring the capacity of the lungs.

splanchnic (*splank'-nik*). Pertaining to the viscera. *S. nerves.* Group of sympathetic nerve fibres which supply the viscera.

splanchnicectomy (*splank-ni-sek'-to-mi*). Surgical removal of the splanchnic ganglia and transection of the splanchnic nerves.

splanchnology (*splank-no'-lo-ji*). The study of the viscera.

splay foot (*splā*). Flatfoot. Pes planus.

spleen (*splēn*). A mass of lymphoid tissue situated in the mesentery of the abdomen. Unlike the lymph nodes, the spleen acts as a filtration organ for blood. The spleen forms an important part of the reticulo-endothelial system, and is the generative centre of the formation of many lymphocytes. The spleen is largely responsible for the removal of red blood cells at the end of their life-span.

splenectomy (*splen-ek'-to-mi*). Removal of the spleen.

splenic anaemia (*a-nē'-mi-a*). Banti's syndrome. It is characterized by anaemia and splenomegaly associated with portal hypertension due to hepatic cirrhosis.

splenic flexure (*splen'-ik flek'-cher*). Bend of the colon on the left side, near the spleen.

spleniculus (*sple-ni'-kū-lus*). A second little spleen.

splenitis (*splen-ī'-tis*). Inflammation of the spleen.

splenomegaly (*sple-nō-me'-ga-li*). An enlarged spleen.

'splinter' haemorrhages (*splinter he-mo-rā-jes*). Bleeding from the longitudinal capillaries in the nail bed giving the appearance of splinters under the nail. Characteristically occur in subacute bacterial endocarditis.

splints (*splin'-tz*). Used to immobilize a limb in the case of fracture, disease or deformity. They are now made chiefly of plaster of Paris, metal, rarely of wood, and the limb is slung on pieces of material attached to sides of splints. The aim is to immobilize the limb as required, at the same time allowing as much movement as possible.

spondyle (*spon'-dīl*). A vertebra.

spondylitis (*spon-di-lī'-tis*). Inflammation of a vertebra or vertebrae. *Ankylosing s.* Condition of unknown origin occurring characteristically in young men. There is ossification of spinal ligaments with ankylosis of the cervical and sacro-iliac joints.

spondylolisthesis (*spon-di-lō-lis-thē'-sis*). The vertebral arch of the fifth lumbar vertebra gives way so that the body of the affected vertebra becomes displaced.

spondylosis (*spon-di-lō'-sis*). Degenerative changes in the intervertebral discs with peripheral ossification. Known as 'osteo-arthritis of spine'.

spontaneous fracture (*spon-tā'-ne-us frak'-tūr*). Fracture due to disease affecting the bone, either from abnormal development or rarefaction of the bone from other causes.

spontaneous version (*spon-tā'-nē-us ver'-shon*). The unaided conversion of a transverse lie into a cephalic or podalic one.

sporadic (*spo-rad'-ik*). A disease which is not epidemic, but occurs in one or two isolated cases in a district.

spore (*spaw*). Reproductive body which gives rise to a new individual organism. Produced by protozoa, fungi and bacteria, spores can survive in unfavourable conditions. Important spore-forming bacteria are Clostridium welchii and Clostridium botulinum.

sporotrichosis (*spo-rō-tri-kō'-sis*). Disease due to a fungoid organism causing subcutaneous abscesses.

spotted fever (*spo'-ted*). Cerebrospinal meningitis.

sprain (*sprān*). Severe strain of a joint without fracture or dislocation, but with swelling and often with effusion into joint.

Sprengel's deformity (*spreng'-els de-for'-mi-ti*). Congenital upward displacement of the scapula.

sprue (*sproo*). A disease of tropical climates which causes inflammation of the mucous membrane of the alimentary canal, characterized by soreness of tongue and mouth, chronic diarrhoea, wasting and anaemia.

spurious pains (*spū'-rē-us*). False labour pains, leading to no result, and sometimes occurring several days before confinement.

sputum (*spū'-tum*). Expectorated matter. Different types are: *Mucoid*, occurs in the early stage of irritation. *Muco-purulent* develops at a later stage, pus is mixed with mucus. *Rusty*, tenacious sputum occurs in lobar pneumonia. Copious foul smelling sputum occurs in bronchiectasis. *Frothy sputum* occurs in oedema of the lung. Separate pellets or nummular sputum occurs in pulmonary tuberculosis. It may be streaked with blood.

squamous (*skwā'-mus*). Scaly.

squint (*skwīnt*). See STRABISMUS.

stable (*stā'-bl*). Not moving, fixed. *Stable current*. Steady application of an electrode to a part.

staccato or **scanning speech** (*stak-ar'-tō*). Hesitation between syllables, and when the sound comes it comes explosively. It is a type of inco-ordination, and occurs in cerebellar lesions and disseminated sclerosis.

Stacke's operation (*staks*). Operation used in chronic infection to join the middle ear with that of the mastoid cells.

stages of labour. See LABOUR.

stain (*stān*). Dye used to colour

tissues before microscopical examination, or to produce certain reactions.

stamina (*sta'-min-a*). Vigour. Staying power.

Stanford-Binet test (*Stan-ford-Bi-nā*). A test of intelligence.

stapedius (*sta-pē'-di-us*). A muscle of the middle ear.

stapes (*stā'-pēz*). One of the three ossicles of the middle ear; stirrup-shaped. See EAR.

Staphylococcus (*staf-i-lō-kok'-us*). Genus of Gram-positive bacteria which grow in clusters when cultured. Many staphylococci are commensals on the skin. Some are serious pathogens and several strains have evolved which are insensitive to penicillin and other antibiotics.

staphyloma (*staf-i-lō'-ma*). Any protrusion of the sclerotic or corneal coats of the eyeball due to inflammation.

staphylorrhaphy (*sta-fi-lor'-ra-fi*). Operation to suture cleft soft palate.

starch (*star'-ch*). Polysaccharous carbohydrate. It can be obtained from maize, rice, wheat and potato. *S. poultice*. Used to remove scabs, especially in impetigo. Two tablespoonfuls of starch powder and one teaspoonful of boric acid powder are mixed with one pint of water brought to the boil whilst stirring. The mixture is spread on old linen.

Starr valve. Form of artificial heart valve.

stasis (*stā'-sis*). Standing still. Most commonly used for arrest of the circulation of either blood or lymph, but also for intestinal stasis, a holding up of the contents of the bowel.

status asthmaticus (*stā-tus as-thma'-ti-kus*). Severe attack of asthma unrelieved by usual medications.

status epilepticus (*stāt'-us ep-il-ep'-ti-kus*). A condition in which a series of epileptic fits occur in rapid succession.

status lymphaticus (*stāt'-us lim-fat'-i-kus*). A rare and fatal condition in which death is sudden and thought in some cases to be due to a persistent thymus gland.

steam tent. Erected around a bed to provide a moist atmosphere. Screens and a sheet or blanket are used. Steam is directed inside from a bronchitis kettle. Temperature of tent, 70°F (21°C).

steapsin (*stē-ap'-sin*). Lipase.

steatoma (*stē-at-ō'-ma*). A fatty encysted tumour. A sebaceous cyst.

steatorrhoea (*ste-at-or-ē'-ah*). The passage of excessive fat in the stools. Thought to be due to pancreatic deficiency, or deficiency of bile, or inability on the part of the lacteals to absorb fat. Sometimes produced by allergy to protein in wheat flour. A diet without fat and wheat gluten is given.

steatosis (*stē-at-ō'-sis*). Fatty degeneration.

Stegomyia (*steg'-ō-mi'-ē-a*). A variety of mosquito which acts as the carrier of the parasite of yellow fever from a patient to a healthy individual.

Stein-Leventhal syndrome (*stīn-le-ven-thal sin'-drōm*). Sterility, uterine hypoplasia, masculinization and polycystic ovaries.

Steinmann's pin (*stīn'-marn*). A fixation pin inserted through a bone in order to apply extension in the case of fractures. *See* EXTENSION.

stellate ganglion (*stel-lāt gan'-glē-on*). Star-shaped sympathetic ganglion situated in the neck.

stenosis (*ste-nō'-sis*). Contraction of a canal or an orifice.

Stensen's duct (*sten'-sens dukt*). The duct of the parotid salivary gland. Its opening is opposite the upper first molar tooth.

stercobilin (*ster-kō-bī'-lin*). The colouring matter of the faeces. It is derived from bile pigment.

stercolith (*ster'-kō-lith*). Small hard mass of faeces. Faecolith.

stereognosis (*ste-rē-og-nō'-sis*). Recognition of the form of bodies by handling them.

sterile (*ste'-rīl*). Barren; unable to have children. In *surgical practice*, sterile means entirely free from micro-organisms of all kinds, a result brought about by heat or by the use of chemicals.

sterility (*ste-ril'-it-i*). The condition of being sterile.

sterilization (*ster-il-ī-zā'-shon*). (1) Made incapable of progeny, e.g. by removal of ovaries, tying the Fallopian tubes, hysterectomy or, in the male, castration, tying the vas deferens. (2) Rendering free of micro-organisms.

sternal puncture (*ster-nal pungk'-cher*). Technique employed to obtain sample of red bone marrow for investigation. A needle is inserted into the sternum under local anaesthesia and a small amount of marrow aspirated.

sterno-mastoid muscle (*sternō-mas'-toyd mus-l*). Muscle of neck, running from the inner end of clavicle and upper border of sternum to behind the ear. *See* TORTICOLLIS.

sternum (*ster'-num*). The breastbone.

steroids (*ste'-royds*). Group of compounds including cholesterol, most of the hormones, bile salts and the precursors of vitamin D in the skin. However, the term is often used for the corticosteroids only, which are the hormones of the adrenal cortex.

stertor (*ster'-tor*). Snoring type of respiration.

stethoscope (*steth'-o-skōp*). Instrument for listening to sounds, e.g. heart sounds, respiratory sounds. The *binaural* stethoscope has two flexible ends, to apply to the ears of the listener.

Stevens-Johnson syndrome (*stē-vens-jon-son sin'-drōm*). Severe form of erythema multiforme in which mucous membranes may be extensively involved.

sthenic (*sthen'ik*). Robust.

stigma (*stig'-ma*) (plu. **stigmata**). Mark on the skin. Also any permanent conditions indicative of some constitutional peculiarity.

stilette (*sti-let'*). A probe.

stillborn (*stil'-born*). Dead when born.

Still's disease. A form of rheumatoid arthritis occurring in children. The syndrome is characterized by polyarthritis, lymphadenopathy, splenomegaly, calcification of the cornea and formation of cataract.

stimulant (*stim'-ū-lant*). That which causes temporary increase in the output of the vital energy.

stimulus (*sti'-mū-lus*). An agent provoking activity.

stitch (*stich*). (1) Suture. (2) Pain in the side due to spasm of the diaphragm.

Stokes-Adams' syndrome (*sin'-drōm*). Syncope due to cerebral hypoxia resulting from heart block.

stoma (*stō'-ma*). (1) The mouth. (2) An opening onto the skin, e.g. colostomy; *s. nurse* one who undergoes further training in care of patients with stomas.

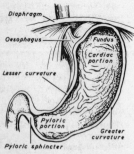

46 Section through the stomach

stomach (*stum'-ak*). The dilated portion of the intestinal canal into which the food passes from the oesophagus, and where it undergoes partial digestion.

stomach pump (*stum'-ak pum'p*). A thick rubber tube, at least 18 inches long, attached to a glass receptacle which has a rubber bulb inserted into its neck by means of which a vacuum is created in the glass flask. Used to aspirate the contents of the stomach.

stomatitis (*stom-a-tī'-tis*). Inflammation of the mouth.

stone (*stōn*). (1) A measure of weight, 14 pounds. (2) A concretion.

stools (*stū'ls*). Discharge of faeces from the bowels. *See* MOTIONS.

strabismus (*stra-biz'-mus*). Squint; *divergent* when the eye turns out; *convergent* when it turns in.

strabotomy (*stra-bot'-o-mi*). Operation to remedy squinting.

strain (*strān*). (1) To filter. (2) Condition resulting from unsuitable use of a part.

strangulated (*strang'-gū-lāted*). Constricted, so that the blood-supply is cut off. *See* HERNIA.

strangury (*stran'-gu-ri*). Painful passage of urine. Usually the result of disease of the bladder, urethra, broad ligament, etc. but occasionally occurs after labour.

strapping (*strap'-ping*). Material used to bind up injuries.

stratified (*strat'-if-īd*). In layers.

stratum (*stra'-tum*). A layer.

streptococcus (*strep-to-ko-kus*). Gram-positive bacteria which grow in chains. Pathogenic cocci produce toxins responsible for scarlet fever and acute glomerulo-nephritis.

Streptothrix (*strep'-to-thriks*). Filamentous bacteria.

stress incontinence. Incontinence of urine or faeces when the intra-abdominal pressure is raised as in coughing or sneezing.

striae (*stri-ē*). Scars on the abdomen and thighs due to stretching of the dermis during rapid expansion of the abdomen. Frequently seen in association with pregnancy.

striae gravidarum (*strī'-ē gravid-ar'-um*). The numerous marks which develop on the skin of the abdomen in the later months of pregnancy. They never quite disappear. Striae are due to the stretching of the skin, and are seen also in any condition of *rapid* enlargement of the abdomen, and also sometimes on the thighs of boys who are growing very rapidly. They are thought to be associated with increased activity of the suprarenal cortex. Syn. LINEAE ALBICANTES.

striated muscle (*strī-ā-ted musel*). Striped voluntary muscle, *cf. smooth muscle.*

stricture (*strikt'-ūr*). Contraction. Usually applied to the urethra, with consequent inability to pass urine.

stridor (*strī'-dor*). A harsh sound during breathing, caused by obstruction to the passage of air.

stroke (*strōk*). Cerebrovascular accident. *See also* HEAT-STROKE.

stroma (*strō'-ma*). The connective tissue.

stupe (*stūp*). A fomentation sprinkled with a counter-irritant, *e.g.* turpentine. *See* FOMENTATIONS.

stupor (*stū'-por*). State of unconsciousness.

Sturge-Weber syndrome (*sterj-we-ber sin'-drōm*). Syndrome characterized by capillary naevus on the face in the distribution of the fifth cranial nerve. Associated with angiomas of the cerebral cortex which may cause focal epilepsy, hemiparesis and mental deficiency.

stye (*stī*). Hordeolum. Inflammation of sebaceous gland of eyelash.

stylet (*sti-let'*). *See* STILETTE.

styptic (*stip'-tik*). Agent applied to arrest bleeding; astringent, *e.g.* adrenaline.

Stypven (*stĭp-ven*). Local haemostatic containing Russell's viper venom.

styrax (*stī'raks*). Storax: a constituent of Tinct. Benzoin Co.

sub. A prefix denoting beneath or under.

subacute (*sub-a-kūt*). Fairly severe.

subacute bacterial endocarditis (*sub-a-kūt bak-tā-ri-al endō-kar-dī-tis*). Bacterial colonization of defective heart valves with consequent bacteraemia and distribution of septic emboli throughout the body.

subacute combined degeneration of the cord. Degeneration of the posterior and lateral columns of the spinal cord due to vitamin B_{12} deficiency.

subarachnoid haemorrhage (*sub-a-rak-noyd he-mo-rāg*). Haemorrhage into the subarachnoid space.

subarachnoid space (*sub-ar-ak-noyd'*). The space between the arachnoid membrane and the pia matter. It contains cerebrospinal fluid.

subclavian (*sub-klā'-vē-an*). Under the clavicle: thus the subclavian artery and vein are vessels passing under the clavicle.

subclinical (*sub-kli'-ni-kal*). Without any obvious signs of the disease.

subconscious (*sub-kon'-shus*). The part of the mind outside an individual's awareness, but able to affect the way of acting or thinking.

subcutaneous (*sub-kū-tā'-ne-us*). Under the skin.

subinvolution (*sub-in-vō-lū'-shon*). Failure of the lately pregnant uterus to regain the normal unimpregnated size within the usual time (six weeks) of delivery.

subjacent (*sub-jā'-sent*). Lying below.

subjective (*sub-jek'-tiv*). Internal: pertaining to one's self.

sublimation (*sub-li-mā'-shon*). (1) The process of vaporizing and condensing a solid substance without melting it; (2) 'shunting off' the energy from an impulse or urge from the subconscious by changing its character and aiming at something more attainable.

subliminal (*sub-li'-mi-nal*). Beneath the threshold of consciousness.

sublingual (*sub-ling'-gwal*). Under the tongue.

subluxation (*sub-luks-ā'-shon*). Sprain and partial dislocation.

submaxillary (*sub'-mak-sil'-*

ari). Under the lower jaw. *S. glands*. One of the three pairs of salivary glands.

submucous (*sub-mū'-kus*). Under a mucous membrane; a uterine fibroid is submucous when it projects into the cavity of the uterus.

subnormal (*sub-nor'-mal*). Below normal.

subphrenic (*sub-fren'-ik*). Under the diaphragm. *S. abscess*, a collection of pus beneath the diaphragm.

substrate (*sub-strāt*). Compound on which an enzyme acts.

subtotal hysterectomy (*sub-tō'-tal his-to-rek'-to-mi*). The removal of the uterus, excluding the cervix.

succenturiate placenta (*suk-sen-tūr'-i-āt pla-sen'-ta*). An accessory placenta.

succus entericus (*suk'-us en-te'-rik-us*). The digestive juice secreted by the glands in the small intestine.

succussion (*suk-kush'-on*). Sound made on shaking a patient if fluid is present in a hollow cavity.

sudamina (*su-dam'-ēn-a*). Sweat rash.

Sudol (*sū-dol*). A phenol preparation having the same wide range of bactericidal power as Lysol, but with reduced necrotic action on the skin.

sudorific (*sū-do-rif'-ik*). An agent causing perspiration.

suffused (*su-fūz'-d*). Congested.

suggestibility (*su-jes'-ti-bi-li-ti*). A state when the patient readily accepts other people's ideas and influences.

suicide (*soo-'i-sīd*). The person who kills himself by intent.

sulcus (*sul'-kus*). A furrow.

sulphate (*sul'-fāt*). A salt of sulphuric acid, *e.g.* atropine sulphate.

sulphuric acid (*sul-fūr'-ik*). Vitriol. A poison; some of the antidotes are limewater, potash water, oil and milk.

sunstroke (*sun'-strōk*). *See* HEATSTROKE.

superciliary (*su-per-sil'-ya-ri*). Having to do with the eyebrows.

supercilium (*su-per-sil'-i-um*). The eyebrow.

superego (*soo'-per-e-go*). Term used in psychology for the part of the subconscious, founded on early experiences, which acts as a sort of conscience and sets forth standards and ideals. The superego can cause feelings of guilt and anxiety.

superfecundation (*su-per-fe-kun-dā'-shon*). The fertilization of two ova discharged by two distinct acts of insemination effected at a short interval.

superior (*soo-pār'-i-or*). Above. The upper of two organs.

supination (*su-pi-nā'-shon*). Turning the palm of the hand upwards.

supine (*sū'-pīn*). Lying face upwards; in the case of the forearm, having the palm uppermost.

supplemental air (*sup-lē-ment'-al ā-er*). That part of the residual air of the lung which after the tidal air has been expelled may be driven out by forced respiration.

suppository (*sup-pōz'-i-to-ri*). Rectally administered cones containing a medicament in a base which is soluble at body temperature.

suppression (*sup-presh'-on*). (1) Failure to secrete or when some activity is prevented. (2) In psychology, the voluntary dismissal from the mind of painful or unsuitable urges.

suppuration (*sup-pū-rā'-shon*). The formation of pus.

supra-orbital (*sū-pra-or'-bi-tal*). Above the orbit.

suprapubic (*sū-pra-pū-bik*). Above the pubes.

suprarenal (*sū-pra-rē'-nal*). Above the kidney. *S. glands*, two small ductless glands situated above the kidney and secreting adrenaline and corticosteroids.

sural (*sū'-ral*). Relating to the calf of the leg.

surface (*ser'-fes*). The outer part. *S. markings*. Lines drawn on the skin to show the position of structures beneath it.

surgery (*ser'-je-ri*). The part of medicine concerned with diseases needing treatment by operation. (2) A physician or surgeon's consulting room.

surgical (*ser'-ji-kal*). Pertaining to surgery. *S. kidney*. Pyelitis or diffuse suppuration in the kidney. *S. neck*. Narrow part of the humerus, below the tuberosities.

susceptible (*su-sep'-tibl*). Liable to, *e.g.* infection.

suspension (*sus-pen-shon*). (1) Hanging. (2) Particles in water which are not dissolved by it. *See* VENTROSUSPENSION.

suspensory bandage (*sus-pen'-so-ri ban-dāj*). A bandage to support the testicles.

sutures (*soo'-tūrs*). (1) Silk, thread, catgut, nylon, etc., used to sew a wound. (2) The union of flat bones by their margins, *e.g.* bones of the skull.

swabs (*swobz*). Small pieces of wool, gauze over wool, or gauze only, used for cleaning wounds and for removing blood at operations.

sweat (*swet*). Perspiration. The

fluid secreted on to the skin by the sweat glands.

sycosis (*sī-kō'-sis*). Inflammation of the hair follicles, especially of the beard and whiskers.

symbiosis (*sim-bī-ō'-sis*). The living together of two organisms, whose mutual association is necessary to each, although neither is parasitic on the other.

symblepharon (*sim-blef'-a-ron*). Adhesion of the eyelids to the eyeball.

Syme's amputation (*simz*). Amputation at the ankle joint.

sympathectomy (*sim-path-ek'-to-mi'*). Surgical transection of sympathetic nerves usually with excision of part of the sympathetic chain.

sympathetic system (*sim-pa-thet'-ik*). A nerve system consisting of a chain of ganglia beside the spine supplying nerves to the heart, blood-vessels and other internal viscera.

symphysiotomy (*sim'-fiz-ē-ot'-o-mi*). The operation of dividing the symphysis pubis (of the mother) so as to facilitate delivery in certain cases of contracted pelvis.

symphysis (*sim'-fi-sis*). Growing of bones together. The *symphysis pubis* is the bony mass bounding the front

of the pelvis, at the lower end of the abdomen. *See* PELVIS.

symptom (*simp'-tum*). A noticeable change in the body and its functions, evidence of disease. Usually meaning the change complained of by the patient.

symptomatology (*simp'-tō-ma-to'-lo-ji*). A study of the symptoms of disease.

synapse (*sī-naps*). Region where nerve cells communicate. There is no continuity between the neurons and impulses are transmitted from one nerve cell to another by the passage of chemical messengers which stimulate the post-synaptic nerve cell.

synarthrosis (*sin-ar-thrō-sis*). Immovable union of bones, *e.g.* the cranial bones.

synchondrosis (*sin-kon-drō'-sis*). A joint whose surfaces are united by cartilage.

synchysis (*sin'-ki-sis*). Softening of the vitreous humour of the eye. *S. scintillans*. Bright particles found in the vitreous humour.

synclitism (*sin'-klit-ism*). Descent of the fetal head through the pelvis with its planes parallel to those of the pelvis.

syncope (*sin'-kō-pē*). Fainting.

syndactyly (*sin-dak'-ti-li*). Webbed fingers or toes.

syndesmitis (*sin-des-mī'-tis*) Inflammation of ligaments.

syndrome (*sin'-drōm*). Collection of symptoms and signs which form a recognizable pattern of disease.

synechia (*sin-ek'-i-a*). Adhesion of the iris to the cornea, or to the crystalline lens.

synergy (*si'-ner-ji*). The working together of two or more agents.

Synkavit (*sin'-ka-vit*). A vitamin K analogue.

synonyms (*sin'-ō-nims*). Different words having the same meaning.

synostosis (*sīn-os-tō'-sis*). Abnormal osseous union of bones.

synovectomy (*sī-nō-vek'-tō-mi*). Operation to remove synovial membrane.

synovial fluid (*sī-nō-vi-al flū-id*). The liquid which lubricates the joints.

synovial membrane (*sī-nō'-vial mem'-brān*). That lining a joint cavity but not covering the articular surfaces.

synovitis (*sī-nō-vī'-tis*). Inflammation of the synovial membrane of a joint.

synthesis (*sin'-the-sis*). The building up of complex substances by the union and interaction of simpler materials.

synthetic (*sin-thet'-ik*). Pertaining to synthesis. Artificial.

syphilide (*sif'-il-id*). Lesion of the skin due to syphilis. May be papular, macular, squamous, etc.

syphilis (*sif'-i-lis*). A venereal disease. Caused by a specific spirochaete, the Treponema pallidum. S. may be congenital or acquired. *Congenital* may be inherited from the mother. The chief symptoms in young babies: wasting, snuffles, rashes, enlargement of liver and spleen. If child survives, he may later show pallor, malnutrition, depressed bridge of nose, rhagades, square skull, thickening of tibiae, corneal opacities, Hutchinson's teeth (*see* RHAGADES, HUTCHINSON'S TEETH). *Acquired* is divided into three stages. (1) First stage or primary S. with local symptoms, two–three weeks after infection. Hard chancre on penis, vulva, or cervix. Inflamed glands in groin. Lesions infective (*see* CHANCRE). (2) Second stage or secondary S., one to two months after infection, with rashes, sore throat, mucous patches, condylomata, general enlargement of glands, anaemia, and fever. Infective (*see* CONDYLOMA). (2) Third stage or tertiary S., two to ten years or even longer after infection. Non-infective, giving, among other manifestations, gummata, tabes, GPI. *See* GENERAL PARALYSIS.

syringe (*si-rinj*). An instrument for injecting fluids, or for exploring and aspirating cavities.

syringomyelia (*se-rin'-go-mi-ēl'-i-a*). Progressive degenerative disease affecting the brain stem and spinal cord in which the tracts of the fibres subserving pain and temperature are mainly affected.

syringomyelocele (*si-rin-gō-mī-el'-ō-sēl*). A type of spina bifida. There is a communication between the projecting mass and the central canal of the spinal cord.

syringotomy (*sir-ing-got'-o-mi*). Cutting open a fistula.

system (*sis'-tem*). An organized scheme. A series of parts concerned in a basic function such as nutrition by the alimentary system.

systemic (*sis-te-mik*). Affecting the whole body.

systole (*sis'-tō-lē*). The period when the heart contracts. *See* DIASTOLE.

systolic blood pressure (*sis-to-lik blud pre-shor*). The force with which the left ventricle contracts and which is measured in the peripheral arteries.

systolic murmur (*sis-to-lik mer'-mer*). Murmur heard during systole. It may be due to aortic or tricuspid obstruction.

T

TAB. Triple vaccine to prevent typhoid, paratyphoid A and paratyphoid B.

T bandage. A special bandage used for keeping dressings on the perineum.

tabes (*tā-bēz*). Wasting. *T. dorsalis*, a disorder of the spinal cord, due to tertiary syphilis, also called locomotor ataxia, and characterized by loss of power over muscles. *See* SYPHILIS. *T. mesenterica*, tuberculosis of the mesenteric glands. Seen in children.

tachycardia (*tak-ē-kar'-di-a*). Abnormally rapid action of the heart, as in atrial fibrillation.

tactile (*tak'-tīl*). Relating to the touch. *T. corpuscles*. Cutaneous end organs of the tactile nerves.

taenia (*tē-ni-a*). A flat strip.

Taenia (*tē'-ni-a*). The tapeworm. The adult worm consists of a head and numerous segments. It has the appearance of jointed tape and may be several feet long. The *Taenia solium* is a common variety which gains entrance to the body through underdone infected pork. The head attaches itself to the mucous membrane of the intestines and the worm continues to grow. The treatment is (1) little food for several hours, (2) purge, (3) ext. filix mas, (4) purge.

talc. French chalk. Used as dusting powder.

talipes (*tal'-i-pēz*). Clubfoot. *Talipes valgus*, the foot turned outwards; *varus*, the foot turned inwards; *equinus*, the heel lifted from the ground; *calcaneus*, heel projected downwards.

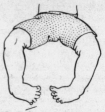

48 Talipes equino-varus

talus (*tāl'-us*). The ankle.

tampon (*tam'-pon*). A plug of wool or gauze introduced into the vagina.

tamponade (*tam-pō-nād*). Compression (usually *cardiac t.*) in which the action of the heart is impeded by the presence of fluid in the pericardium.

tantalum (*tan'-ta-lum*). A resistant metal sometimes used in bone surgery for plates or wire.

tapeworm (*tāp'-werm*). *See* TAENIA.

tapping. *See* ASPIRATION.

tar (*tah*). Dark liquid obtained from pine-wood. It has antipyretic and antiseptic properties. *Coal-t.* Black liquid distilled from coal. It contains benzene, phenol, cresols, naphthalene, etc.

tarsal (*tar-sal*). Bones of the

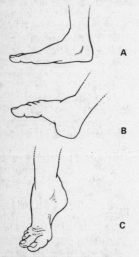

47 Types of talipes: A = talipes valgus B = talipes calcaneus with some cavus deformity C = talipes equinus

ankle, *cf.* carpal bones. There
are seven in man, forming a
group which articulate with
the tibia and fibula and the
metatarsal bones.

tarsalgia (*ta-sal'-ji-a*). Pain in
the foot.

tarsoplasty (*ta-sō-plas'-ti*). Plastic surgery of the eyelid.

tarsorrhaphy (*ta-so'-ra-fi*).
Stitching the eyelids
together.

tarsus (*tar'-sus*). (1) The seven
small bones of the foot. (2)
The cartilaginous framework
of the eyelid.

tartar (*tar'-ta*). Deposit on teeth
of calcium salts derived from
saliva.

tartaric acid (*tah-ta'-rik a'-sid*).
Used in making effervescent
preparations. It should be
taken well-diluted if not
neutralized.

tartrate (*tar'-trāt*). A salt of tartaric acid.

taste bud. Specialized sensory
end organ which is sensitive
to taste.

taurocholic acid (*taw-rō-kō-lik
a'-sid*). One of the bile acids.

taxis (*tak'-sis*). Hand-
manipulation for restoring a
part to its natural position,
such as reducing a hernia.

Tay-Sach's disease (*tā-saks*). A
rare genetically inherited
neurological condition which
also produces mental regression.

tears (*tārs*). Secretion of the lacrimal gland.

tease (*tēz*). To divide a tissue
into shreds.

teat (*tēt*). Nipple.

technetium (*tek-nē-tium*). Artificially produced radioactive material.

technique (*tek-nē'k*). The
method by which a process
may be carried out.

teeth, eruption of. The milk
teeth, or first dentition of the
infant, begin to erupt
between the sixth and twelfth

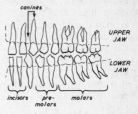

49 *First dentition or temporary
teeth*

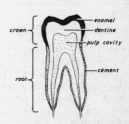

50 *Second dentition or
permanent teeth*

months. Occasionally they start to appear even earlier than the sixth month. The lower central incisors usually appear first, followed by the upper central incisors. As a rule there will be from eight to twelve teeth cut at a year old, and the twenty teeth which constitute the first dentition should be present at two years of age. The permanent teeth begin to erupt about the fifth or sixth year with the appearance of the first permanent molars; then about the seventh year there is shedding of the incisors. The numbers in the *top illustration* indicate the child's age in months when the teeth erupt.

Teflon (*tef'-lon*). Proprietary material used in heart surgery.

tegument (*teg'-ū-ment*). The skin.

tela (*tā-la*). Tissue formed like a web.

telangiectasis, telangioma (*te-lan-ji-ek'-ta-sis, te-lan-ji-ō'-ma*). Lesion consisting of a number of tortuous dilated capillaries which have a web-like appearance and a tendency to bleed. Often seen following a course of radiotherapy.

temper tantrums (*tem'-per tan'-trums*). Outburst of temper.

An infantile way of demanding that a need be satisfied.

temperament (*tem'-pe-ra-ment*). A person's mental outlook.

temperature (*tem'-per-a-tūr*). A measurement of the degree of heat. The average normal temperature of the human body is 98·4°F (37°C). The average temperature of a sick-room should be 60° to 65°F (16 to 18°C).

temples (*tem'-plz*). The part of the forehead between the outer corner of the eye and the hair.

temporal (*tem'-por-al*). Relating to the temple. Thus T. artery, T. bone, T. lobe of the brain.

temporal arteritis. *Giant cell arteritis*. A disease of unknown aetiology characterized by general malaise, aches and muscle pains and acute inflammation of the arteries, particularly those of the scalp.

tenaculum (*te-nak'-ū-lum*). An instrument like a vulsellum, but having only one pair of teeth for fixing the cervix uteri.

tendinitis (*ten-di-ni'-tis*). Inflammation of a tendon.

tendo Achilles (*ten-dō ak'-il-is*). The stout tendon of the calf muscles at the back of the heel.

tendon (*ten'-don*). A sinew, a cord of fibrous white tissue by which a muscle is attached to a bone or other structure.

tendovaginitis, stenosing (*tendō-va-gi-nī-tis stĕ'-nō-zing*). Stenosing tenosynovitis, de Quervain's disease. Fibrous thickening of tendon sheath most commonly affecting the tendons of the abductor muscles of the thumb.

tenesmus (*te-nes'-mus*). Continual desire to defaecate accompanied by painful straining.

tennis elbow (*ten'-nis el'-bō*). A condition characterized by pain at or near the insertion of the extensor muscles of the forearm at the lateral epicondyle of the humerus. Brought on by unusual and excessive use.

tenoplasty (*te-nō-plas'-ti*). Plastic surgery to a tendon.

tenorrhaphy (*te-no'-ra-fi*). Operation to suture a tendon.

tenosynovitis (*ten'-ō-sī-nō-vī'-tis*). Inflammation in the sheath of a tendon.

tenotomy (*te-not'-o-mi*). Cutting a tendon.

tension (*ten'-shon*). Stretching. A state of stress.

tentorium cerebelli (*ten-tor'-i-um se-ri-bel-li*). A septum of the dura mater which lies between the cerebrum and cerebellum. This may be torn in a breech delivery and may prove fatal to the child.

tepid (*te'-pid*). Just warm.

tepid sponging (*te-pid spun'-jing*). A method of bringing down high temperature by allowing tepid water to evaporate on the skin. During the treatment the patient must be watched carefully for signs of collapse and the temperature must not be allowed to drop by more than 1°C.

teratogen (*te-ra-tō-jen*). Any agent able to produce a fetal monster.

teratoma (*te-ra-tō-ma*). See EMBRYOMA.

teres (*te'-rās*). Round and smooth. *Ligamentum t.* Ligament of the head of the femur.

terminology (*ter-mi-no'-lo-ji*). Nomenclature. The science of the proper use of terms, as in medicine.

tertian (*ter'-shan*). A form of malaria with attacks every third day.

tertiary (*ter-she-ri*). Third.

tertiary syphilis. See SYPHILIS.

test. (1) Trial. (2) A reaction distinguishing one substance from another.

test meal. See FRACTIONAL TEST MEAL.

testicles (*tes'-ti-kls*). The two

glands of the scrotum, which secrete the semen.

testis (*tes'-tis*). A testicle.

testosterone (*tes-tos'-te-rōn*). Endocrine secretion of the testis. Promotes growth and secondary sexual development.

tetanus (*tet'-a-nus*). Lock-jaw. Disease caused by *clostridium tetani* characterized by rigidity and spasm of the muscles. The causative organism is anaerobic and thrives in wounds contaminated by soil or road dust containing the spores. A powerful toxin is produced by the clostridium which reaches the spinal cord by retrograde spread up the motor nerves, and is responsible for the clinical features.

tetany (*tet'-an-i*). A condition marked by spasms of the extremities, particularly of hands and feet (carpopedal spasm) due to faulty calcium metabolism. It may be due to dysfunction of the parathyroid glands, alkalosis, rickets.

tetralogy of Fallot (*te'-tra'-lo-ji*). A congenital heart disease. The aorta is displaced to the right so that it receives blood from the right ventricle, which is hypertrophied, as well as from the left ventricle. The interventricular septum

is patent and there is narrowing of the pulmonary artery.

tetraplegia (*te-tra-plē'-ji-a*). Paralysis of all four limbs. *Syn.* quadriplegia.

thalami (*thal-a-mī*). (Sing. **thalamus.**) Two areas of grey matter at the base of the brain; concerned with the appreciation of crude sensations.

thalassaemia (*tha-la-sē-mi-a*). Anaemia found in the Mediterranean area. The red cells contain some abnormal haemoglobin of the type usually found in the fetus. It is detected by the alkali resistance test.

theca (*thē'-ka*). A sheath. Examples are the meninges of the spinal cord, and the synovial sheaths of the flexor tendons of the fingers.

theine (*thē'-in*). The alkaloid of tea, same as caffeine.

thenar (*thē'-nar*). Relating to the palm of the hand at the base of the thumb.

Theobroma (*thē-o-brō'-ma*). A genus of trees. The seeds of *T. cacao* furnish cocoa and cocoa butter.

theory (*thē-o-ri*). (1) General principles of a subject. (2) A supposition.

therapeutics (*ther-a-pū'-tiks*). The branch of medicine which deals with treatment.

thermography. A means of

recording infra-red radiation from the body by the use of special cameras. A 'hot spot' suggests a malignant tumour.

thermolabile (*ther-mō-lā-bīl*). Substance which undergoes change with temperature.

thermometer (*ther-mom'-e-ter*). An instrument used to measure temperature. *Clinical thermometer*, a small thermometer used for taking the temperature of the body. It is generally graduated from 36° C to 42° C. It is made so that the mercury does not fall when the thermometer is taken from the patient. After the temperature has been recorded the mercury is shaken down. *See* ZERO, TEMPERATURE, and p. 14.

thermophilic (*ther-mō-fi-lik*). Applied to organism which flourishes at high temperatures.

thermostat (*ther'-mō-stat*). Apparatus which is made to regulate heat automatically.

thesis (*thē-sis*). Dissertation.

thiamine (*thī-a-min*). Synthetic vitamin B$_1$. also called aneurine. *See* VITAMINS.

Thiersch (*tersh*). Type of skin graft in which the epidermis and upper part of the dermis is employed. *See* GRAFT.

thigh (*thī*). The portion of the lower limb above the knee.

Thomas's splint. (1) Knee splint for immobilizing a fractured femur or tibia and fibula. It consists of two sidepieces of metal with a crosspiece at foot, and an oblique ring for fixation in groin. Leg is kept in position by pieces of material slung between sidepieces and adjusted to the fracture. (2) Arm splint.

thoracic (*thor-as'-sik*). Pertaining to the thorax.

thoracic duct. The largest lymphatic vessel. It receives the fat absorbed from the intestine and the lymph from the greater part of the body. It ascends from the abdomen through the thorax to the left side of the neck, where it empties itself into the angle of union between the left internal jugular vein and the subclavian vein.

thoracocentesis (*tho'-ra-kō-sen-tē'-sis*). Puncture of the thorax, *e.g.* aspiration of pleural effusion.

thoracolysis (*thor-a-kō-lī'-sis*). The severing of adhesions between the two layers of the pleura.

thoracoscopy (*tho-ra-kos'-ko-pi*). The pleural cavity is inspected by a thorascope.

thoracotomy (*tho-ra-ko'-to-mi*). Operation of opening the thorax.

thorax (*tho'-raks*). The chest; the cavity which holds the heart and lungs.

Thorium X (*thaw'-ri-um eks*). Radioactive isotope of radium (224 R) which is primarily an emitter of α particles which penetrate about 1mm in tissues.

threadworm (*thred'-werm*). Oxyuris vermicularis. Small parasitic worm in the rectum; common in children.

threonine (*thrē-ō-nin*). An amino-acid essential for protein metabolism.

threshold (*thresh'-hōld*). (1) The smallest stimulus which can yet produce a reaction. (2) The lowest level of concentration of a substance, such as sugar, in the blood. Above the level it is excreted in urine and this is called the renal threshold.

thrill (*thril*). A vibratory impulse perceived by palpation.

thrombectomy (*throm-bek'-to-mi*). Removal of a blood clot.

thrombin (*throm'-bin*). Enzyme necessary for the clotting of shed blood. It causes fibrinogen to become fibrin.

thromboangiitis (*throm-bō-an-ji-ī'-tis*). Inflamed blood vessel with formation of a blood clot. *T. obliterans.* Inflammatory, obliterative

disease of the blood vessels, especially in the limbs.

thrombo-arteritis (*throm-bō-ar-ter-ī'-tis*). Arteritis with thrombosis.

thrombocytes (*throm'-bō-sīts*). Blood platelets.

thrombocytopenia (*throm-bō-sī-tō-pē-ni-ah*). Deficiency of platelets in the blood.

thromboendarterectomy (*throm-bō-en-dar-te-rek'-to-mi*). Operation to remove a clot from a blood vessel.

thrombokinase (*throm-bō-kī'-nāz*). The active principle of a substance liberated when the blood platelets are disintegrated. It is necessary for the clotting of blood.

thrombolytic (*throm-bō-li-tik*). Causing a clot to disintegrate.

thrombophlebitis (*throm-bō-fle-bī'-tis*). Inflammation of a vein with thrombosis.

thromboplastin (*throm-bō-plas-tin*). *Syn.* thrombokinase.

thrombosis (*throm-bō'-sis*). Coagulation of blood in the vessels. The organized clot thus formed is termed a *thrombus.*

thrombus (*throm'-bus*). (Plu. **thrombi.**) A clot of blood found in the heart or in a blood vessel in the site in which it is formed, *cf.* infarct.

thrush (*thru'-sh*). Growth of

white patches of fungus (*oidium albicans*) in the mouth.

thymectomy (*thī-mek'-to-mi*). Operation to remove the thymus gland. Sometimes performed for myasthenia gravis.

thymol (*thī'-mol*). An antiseptic often used for mouthwashes and gargles.

thymoma (*thī-mō-ma*). Malignant neoplasm of the thymus.

thymus (*thī'-mus*). A gland at the root of the neck. It is largest in children and then gradually atrophies. The function of the thymus is not clear. It appears to be concerned with the immunological mechanisms of the body. It has been suggested that it acts as a 'priming station' for lymphocytes where they are selected for release into the general circulation. It is not yet possible to be certain of its function. The gland, which is situated in the anterior mediastinum, reaches its maximum size at puberty and thereafter atrophies slowly.

thyroglossal cyst (*thī'-rō-glos-al*). A type of dermoid cyst which appears in the midline of neck between hyoid bone and sternum.

thyroid cartilage (*thī'-royd*). The largest cartilage of the larynx. It forms an angle in front, more prominent in the male.

thyroid crisis. Acute severe thyrotoxicosis which may follow subtotal thyroidectomy in the absence of preoperative antithyroid treatment. Rarely occurs nowadays because of preoperative medication.

thyroidectomy (*thī-roy-dek'-to-mi*). Operative removal of the thyroid gland.

thyroid gland (*thī-'royd gland*). A bi-lobed ductless gland lying in front of the trachea. It secretes two thyroid hormones, thyroxine and triiodothyronine. These control metabolism, growth and development. Congenital lack causes cretinism. Under-secretion in later life

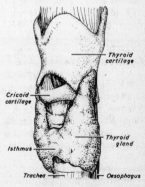

51 The thyroid gland

causes myxoedema. Excessive secretion causes thyrotoxicosis. A third hormone, calcitonin, plays a part in calcium metabolism.

thyroidism (*thī-royd-izm*). The symptoms caused by too rapid an absorption into the system of the secretion of the thyroid gland or by the administration by mouth of too large doses of thyroid extract. *Symptoms:* rapid pulse, sweating, diarrhoea, weight loss in spite of increased appetite, prominence of the eyeballs, fine tremor of the fingers and anxiety.

thyrotoxicosis (*thī-rō-tok-si-kō'-sis*). Condition produced by over-activity of thyroid gland. See THYROIDISM.

thyrotrophic (*thī-rō-trō-fik*). Stimulating the thyroid. *T. hormone* is produced by the anterior pituitary gland.

thyroxine (*thī-roks'-in*). One of the thyroid hormones. Known as T_4 because its molecule contains 4 iodine atoms.

tibia (*tib'-i-a*). The shin bone; the larger bone of the leg below the knee. See SKELETON.

tic. Spasmodic twitching of muscles; usually of face and neck.

tic douloureux (*tik doo-loo-rer*). Trigeminal neuralgia.

tick (*tik*). A blood-sucking parasite. *T. fever.* (1) Relapsing fever. (2) Rocky Mountain fever, a rickettsial fever.

tidal air (*tī-dal ā-r*). That which is inspired and expired during normal breathing.

tincture (*tink-tūr*). An alcoholic solution of a drug.

tinea (*tin'-e-a*). Disease of the skin due to a vegetable parasite. See RINGWORM.

tinnitus aurium (*tin-ni'-tus aw'-re-um*). A ringing in the ears.

tissue (*tish'-ū*). The arrangement of cells constituting the structure of an organ.

tissue culture. Method by which cells and tissues are grown under artificial conditions after their removal from the parent organism.

titration (*ti-trā'-shon*). Quantitative analysis by volume by means of standard solutions.

titre (*tē'-ter*). A standard of purity or strength.

tobacco amblyopia (*to-bak'-ō am-blē-ō'-pia*). Dimness of vision from excessive smoking.

tocography (*to-ko'-gra-fi*). Method of recording alterations in the intra-uterine pressure.

tocopheryl (*to-ko'-fe-ril*). Vitamin E. Its precise function is unknown but it is widely used as an antioxidant in medical preparations.

tolerance (*tol'-er-ans*). Capacity to take a certain drug in unusually large dosage. Sugar tolerance test for diabetic patients ascertains the degree of metabolism of sugar as shown by the blood-sugar curve and the amount of sugar in the urine.

tomography (*tom-og'-raf-i*). The technique in radiography which brings into focus only those objects lying in the plane of interest, while blurring structures on either side of the object's plane; also known as body section radiography.

tone (*tōn*). (1) State of tension as found in muscles. (2) Quality of sound.

tongue (*tung*). The muscular organ which lies in the floor of the mouth, and whose chief functions are to assist in the mastication and tasting of food and in vocalization.

tongue tie (*tung' tī*). When a fold of mucous membrane attaches the under surface of tongue to floor of mouth. It is very rare.

tonic (*to'-nik*). (1) A medicine which braces up the general health chiefly by increasing the appetite. (2) Term applied to continuous

spasms, in opposition to clonic.

tonometer (*to-no'-me-ter*). Instrument for measuring tensions such as that used to measure intra-ocular tension.

tonsillectomy (*ton-sil-ek'-to-mi*). The operation for removal of the tonsils.

tonsillitis (*ton-sil-ī'-tis*). Inflammation of tonsils.

tonsillotome (*ton-sil'-o-tōm*). An instrument for cutting off a tonsil.

tonsils (*ton'-sils*). Two oval bodies of lymphoid tissue on either side of the throat at the opening of the pharynx, and between the pillars of fauces.

toothed (*tootht*). Dentate. Possessing teeth.

tophus (*tō-fus*). (1) A gritty concretion due to gout, found most commonly on the edge of the auricle of the ear or in the joints. (2) A salivary calculus.

topical (*top'-ik-al*). Pertaining to a particular locality. Local.

topography (*to-po'-gra-fi*). A study of the various areas of the body.

torpor (*tor'-per*). Lethargy.

torsion (*tor'-shon*). Twisting.

torso (*tor'-sō*). The trunk.

torticollis (*tor-tē-kol'-lis*). Wry neck. The head is flexed and drawn to one side, due to damage to one of the sternomastoid muscles at birth.

tourniquet (*tor'-nē-kā*). An instrument used to exert pressure on an artery and so arrest bleeding.

toxaemia (*tok-sē'-mi-a*). Circulation of toxins in the blood. *Toxaemia of pregnancy.* The chief signs and symptoms are—oedema, rise in blood pressure, proteinuria, headache and vomiting. If not treated, eclampsia may result.

toxic (*tok'-sik*). Poisonous.

toxicology (*toks-i-kol-'o-ji*). Science of poisons.

toxicosis (*tok-si-kō'-sis*). Any disease due to poisoning.

toxin (*tok'-sin*). A poison, usually of bacterial origin,*i.e.* manufactured by the germs themselves.

toxoid (*tok'-soyd*). A non-poisonous modification of a toxin. Sometimes used to immunize against disease. *See* SCHICK TEST.

toxoid-antitoxin (*tok'-soyd-an-ti-tok'-sin*). A mixture of toxoid and its antitoxin.

toxoplasmosis (*tok-sō-plas-mō'-sis*). Infection caused by a parasite, the Toxoplasma, which can infect man as well as animals. If the fetus or young infant is infected encephalitis may occur. Other results of infection

include nephritis, pneumonia, rashes and lymphadenopathy.

trabecula (*tra-bek'-ū-la*). A septum extending into an organ from its capsule or wall.

trace elements (*trās e'-le-menz*). Mineral substances whose presence in minute amounts in the diet is necessary for the maintenance of health, *e.g.* cobalt, copper, manganese, etc.

tracer (*trā-ser*). Radioactive isotope or substance containing a radioactive isotope which enables the substance to be traced in metabolic systems.

trachea (*tra'-kē-a*). The windpipe; the air passage from the larynx to the bronchi. *See* BRONCHI.

tracheitis (*tra-kē-ī'-tis*). Inflammation of the trachea.

trachelorrhaphy (*trak-e-lor'-a-fi*). The operation of suturing a torn cervix uteri.

tracheobronchitis (*tra-ki-ō-bron-kī'-tis*). Inflammation of trachea and bronchi.

tracheostomy (*tra-kē-os'-to-mi*). The operation of making an opening into the trachea and inserting a tube. This may be performed in cases of respiratory obstruction and in cases where the patient is to be maintained on a ventilator.

trachoma (*trak-ō'-ma*). A contagious disease of the conjunctiva in which eyelids become red, rough and granular and the cornea becomes opaque.

traction (*trak'-shon*). The act of pulling or dragging. *Skeletal t.* Traction on a long bone to keep it in position after a fracture and to prevent muscle spasm.

tragus (*trā'-gus*). The small eminence just inside the ear.

trait (*trā*). A special characteristic of the individual.

trance (*trahn'-s*). State of unnatural sleep; catalepsy.

tranquillizer (*tran'-qwil-lī-zer*). Drug with sedative and tranquillizing action, such as chlorpromazine. Used to relieve anxiety, tension and agitation in psychotherapy. Whilst the patient is taking this drug, the action of a hypnotic or analgesic is made more powerful.

trans. Prefix meaning across, through.

transaminase (*tran-sa'-mi'-nāz*). Enzyme which transfers amino (—NH_2) groups from one substance to another. Enzymes of this type are liberated into the bloodstream from damaged cells, particularly muscle cells, and the estimation of the serum transaminases (glutamic-oxaloacetic transaminase, or GOT, and glutamic-pyruvic transaminase or GPT) is sometimes helpful in the diagnosis of conditions in which there is muscle damage, *e.g.* myocardial infarction, dermatomyositis, etc.

transference (*trans'-fe-renz*). A psychoanalytical term. The patient transfers his own emotions on to the analyst, *e.g.* he may develop an intense love or hatred of him. Also used if the patient transfers his own emotions on to someone else as when he blames someone else for what he has done himself.

transfusion (*trans-fū-zhon*). *See* BLOOD TRANSFUSION.

transillumination (*tranz-il-ū-min-ā'-shon*). The method whereby suppuration in the maxillary or frontal sinus is detected. The patient is placed in a completely darkened room, and a bright light placed in the mouth. The affected side is not so highly illuminated as the sound side.

transmigration (*tranz'-mī-grā'-shon*). The passage of cells through a membrane.

transperitoneal (*tranz-pe-rit-o-ne'-al*). Through the peritoneum.

transplantation (*tranz-plan-tā'-shon*). Operation to

remove a portion of tissue from one part of the body to another.

transposition of vessels. Defect of development in which the pulmonary artery arises from the left ventricle and the aorta from the right ventricle.

transudation (*tran-sū-dā'-shon*). Oozing of fluid through a membrane or from a tissue.

transurethral (*tranz-ū-rēth'-ral*). Via the urethra.

transverse (*trans'-vers*). Across. A transverse incision is from side to side. *T. process.* Lateral projection of the neural arch of a vertebra with which the head of a rib articulates.

transvestism (*trans'-ves-tizm*). Psychiatric condition in which there exists an anomaly of instinct. The patient wears clothes characteristic of the opposite sex. Transvestites may identify themselves completely with the opposite sex and develop delusional convictions of this kind.

trapezium (*tra-pē'-zi-um*). First bone in second row of carpal bones.

trapezius (*tra-pē'-zi-us*). A large muscle, running from the nape of the neck and the upper part of the spine, to the clavicle and scapula.

trapezoid (*tra-pē'-zoid*). Second bone in second row of carpal bones.

trauma (*traw'-ma*). A wound or injury. Thus *traumatic gangrene* is gangrene arising from an injury.

treatment (*trēt'-ment*). A way of curing a disease. *Conservative t.* Treatment by rest and drugs rather than by surgery. In dentistry, treatment of a tooth without extracting it. *Palliative t.* An attempt to alleviate pain, etc., but not a cure for the disease. *Prophylactic t.* A means of preventing the disease such as by immunization against it, or by avoiding the cause.

Trematoda (*trem-a-tō'-da*). Parasites which infect man, causing bilharzia.

tremor (*trem'-or*). Involuntary trembling.

Trendelenburg's operation (*tren-del'-en-bergs o-per-ā'-shon*). Used to treat varicose veins. The long saphenous vein is ligated in the groin.

Trendelenburg position (*tren-del'-en-berg poz-i'-shon*). A

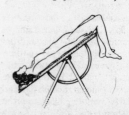

52 The Trendelenburg position

position often adopted for patients undergoing gynaecological operations, in which the head is at a lower level than the pelvis, and the latter is lower than the knees.

Trendelenburg's sign (*sīn*). Used to diagnose congenital dislocation of hip, etc. If the abductor muscles are not working properly, when the patient stands only on the affected leg the pelvis tilts downwards on the opposite side.

trephine (*tre-fīn*). An instrument for removing a disc of bone. *Elliot's t.* for removing a minute disc from the eyeball to relieve glaucoma.

trephining (*tre-fīn'-ing*). Removing a circular piece of tissue to gain access to an enclosed structure, *e.g.* trephining the bone of the skull.

Treponema pallidum (*trep-ō-nē'-ma pal'-i-dum*). The infecting agent of syphilis.

trial of labour. Attempt to achieve spontaneous delivery in case of disproportion.

triangular bandage (*trī-an'-gū-la*). Made by cutting a 36-inch square of linen diagonally across. It is very useful in emergencies and for minor casualties.

triceps (*trī'-seps*). Certain muscles with three heads,

especially the one at the back of the arm which extends the elbow.

trichiasis (*tri-kī-a-sis*). Inversion of the eyelashes towards the eye.

trichiniasis (*tri-ki-nī-a-sis*), **trichinosis** (*tri-ki-nō-sis*). Infection with a parasitic worm named *Trichina*. Trichina spiralis, which is parasitic in pigs and sometimes in man.

trichloroacetic acid (*trī-klo-rō-a-sē'-tik a'-sid*). An astringent and caustic used to remove warts.

Trichocephalus dispar (*trik-ō-kef'-a-lus*). The whipworm. A parasite of the human large intestine.

trichomonas vaginalis (*trik-ō-mōn-as' vag-ē-nā-lis*). A protozoon, motile by means of flagellae. It is a common cause of non-venereal vaginitis.

trichonosis, trichopathy (*trik-on-ō'-sis, trik-op'-a-thi*). Any disease of the hair

trichophytosis (*trī-kō-fī-tō'-sis*). Fungus infection of the hair caused by trichophyton.

trichuris (*tri-kū-ris*). Kind of whipworm.

tricuspid valve (*trī-kus'-pid*). Valve with three cusps, particularly the valve of the heart between the right atrium and right ventricle.

trigeminal (*trī-jem'-in-al*).
Triple.

trigeminal nerves (*trī-jem'-in-al*). Fifth pair of cranial
nerves. They are motor and
sensory and each has three
branches supplying the skin
and structures of the face,
tongue and teeth.

trigeminal neuralgia (*trī-jem'-in-al nū-ral'-jia*). Pain in the
face of unknown cause. The
distribution is confined to
branches of the trigeminal
nerve. The pain is parox-
ysmal and precipitated by
mild stimuli such as washing
the face or eating. Syn. tic
douloureux.

trigger finger (*trig'-ger fin'-ger*).
A thickening of the tendon
sheath at the metacarpo-
phalangeal joint often of
the first finger of the right
hand. The finger can be bent
but not straightened without
help.

trigone (*trī'-gōn*). A triangle, *T.
Vesicae*. Triangular space in
the bladder, immediately
behind the opening to the
urethra.

tri-iodothyronine. One of the
thyroid hormones. Known as
T_3 because its molecule contains 3 atoms of iodine.

trimester (*tri-mes'-ter*). A
three-month period.

trinitrin (*trī'-nī'-trin*). A name
for nitro-glycerin, given in

angina pectoris; it reduces
blood pressure.

trinitrotoluene (*trī-nī-tro-tol'-ū-ēn*). TNT. A high explo-
sive; harmful to workers with
it.

triplegia (*trī-plē-ji-a*). Paralysis
of three limbs.

triplets (*trip'-letz*). Three children resulting from a single
pregnancy. This occurs about
once in 7,800 labours.

trismus (*tris'-mus*). Lockjaw.
Occurs as a reflex in dental
caries. Is also a symptom of
tetanus.

trisomy (*tri-so-mi*). Division of
chromosome 21 into three as
in Down's syndrome.

trocar (*trō'-kar*). The perforating instrument used with a
cannula to draw off fluids
from the body.

trochanter (*tro-kan'-ter*). Two
processes (the greater and
the lesser), at the juncture of
the neck and shaft of femur.

trochlear (*trok'-lē-ar*). (1)
Relating to a pulley. (2)
Relating to the trochlear
nerve.

trochlear nerves (*trok'-lē-ar*).
The fourth pair of cranial
nerves. Motor nerves to the
eyes.

trophic (*trōf'-ik*). Relating to
nutrition. Trophic ulcers
occur where nutrition is poor,
particularly if there is paralysis.

trophoblast (*trō'-fō-blarst*). The outer ectodermal layer of the embedding ovum.

Trousseau's sign (*troo'-sōs sīn*). A spasm of the muscles, occurring in tetany, if pressure is applied over large arteries or nerves.

trunk. The torso.

truss (*trus*). An apparatus for retaining a hernia in place.

Trypanosoma (*trip'-an-o-sō-ma*). A genus of microscopic parasites which cause sleeping sickness and other diseases.

trypanosomiasis (*trip'-an-ō-so-mī'-a-sis*). Infection with trypanosomes.

trypsin. (*trip'-sin*). The digestive enzyme of the pancreatic juice; acts on proteins.

trypsinogen (*trip-sin'-ō-jen*). A precursor of trypsin.

tryptophane (*trip'-to-fān*). See AMINO-ACIDS.

tsetse (*tet-sē*). See SLEEPING SICKNESS.

tubal (*tū'-bal*). Relating to a tube, and especially to an oviduct. *T. gestation* or *T. pregnancy*, pregnancy in a Fallopian tube. *See* EXTRAUTERINE GESTATION.

Tubegauz (*tūb'-gawz*). Proprietary bandage of fine tubular cotton gauze made in many sizes from finger to body width. It is cool and light and does not ruck up.

tubercle (*tū'-ber-kl*). (1) A small eminence. (2) The small greyish nodule which is the specific lesion of the tubercle bacillus.

tuberculide (*tū-ber'-kū-līd*). Any skin rash due to tuberculous infection.

tuberculin (*tū-ber'-kū-lin*). A preparation from cultures of the tubercle bacillus used in the diagnosis of tuberculosis. Many different tuberculins have been prepared in many different ways, but few are in common use. Old tuberculin is used for the intradermal Mantoux test, and for tuberculin patch tests. Tuberculin PPD is also used for intradermal test. BCG vaccine is used for prophylaxis as an immunizing agent.

tuberculoma (*tū-ber-kū-lō'-ma*). Walled-off region of caseating tuberculosis.

tuberculosis (*tū-ber-kū-lō'-sis*). Infection with the Mycobacterium tuberculosis or tubercle bacillus. The human and bovine types attack man. Most infections enter by the respiratory tract and attack the lungs. Bovine bacilli, usually from infected milk, enter through the gastro-intestinal tract, causing lesions in the tonsils, glands of neck, lining of the intestinal tract and mesenteric glands. The tubercle bacillus acts slowly and a tiny nodule or tubercle forms in the affected area, which eventually calcifies. In most people, with good defences, no illness results from the primary infection and it probably serves to protect the patient against further attack. The person is termed *tuberculin positive* and this is ascertained by the Mantoux test (or other similar tests). BCG vaccination immunizes against tuberculosis by making a *tuberculin negative* person tuberculin positive. In a person who has contracted tuberculosis, the treatment is rest, good food and drug therapy, and the disease can be controlled, if diagnosed early, usually by x-ray.

tuberculous (*tū-ber′-kū-lus*). Connected with tuberculosis.

tuberosity (*tu-ber-os′-i-ti*). Bony eminence.

tuberous sclerosis (*tū′-be-rus skle-rō-sis*). *See* EPILOIA.

tubo-ovarian (*tū-bo-ō-vā′-ri-an*). Connected with both the Fallopian tube and the ovary (abscess, cyst).

tubule (*tū-būl*). Small tube.

tularaemia (*tu-lar-ē′-mē-a*). A disease transmitted to man from rabbits by a blood-sucking insect infected with *B. tularense*.

tumefaction (*tū-me-fak-shon*). Becoming swollen.

tumour (*tū′-mur*). A swelling; an abnormal enlargement. Tumours may be *simple* or *malignant*; in the first case, they are not dangerous in themselves; in the second case, they are cancerous and produce secondary deposits in distant organs. Also they may be *solid* or *cystic*.

tunica (*tū-nikā*). A term applied to several membranes, *e.g. T. vaginalis*, the serous coat of the testicle.

tuning fork (*tū′-ning fork*). An instrument used for testing hearing. Each tuning fork bears a figure giving number of vibrations per second when it is struck, and a letter indicating the musical pitch (*see* RINNE'S TEST). It is also applied to the skin of other parts of the body to test the sense of vibration.

turbinate bones (*ter′-bin-āt bōnz*). Three thin convoluted bones situated on the lateral wall of each nasal fossa.

turbinectomy (*ter-bi-nek-to-mi*). Operation to excise a turbinate bone.

turgid (*ter′-jid*). Swollen, distended.

Turner's syndrome (*ter-ners*

sin'-drōm). Ovarian agenesis. The patient is short in stature with webbed neck.

tussis (*tus'-sis*). A cough.

twin (*twi'n*). One of two individuals born at one birth.

tylosis (*tī-lō'-sis*). Thickening of the skin of the soles and palms.

tympanites (*tim-pan-ī'-tēz*). A distended state of the abdomen caused by gas in the intestines.

tympanitis (*tim-pa-nī-tis*). Otitis media.

tympanoplasty (*tim-pa-nō-plas-ti*). Operation to reconstruct the tympanum and the sound-conducting mechanism in middle ear.

tympanum (*tim'-pan-um*). Also called tympanic cavity. A part of the middle ear, and comprises a cavity in the temporal bone deep to the tympanic membrane. *T. membrane*. The membrane separating the middle from the external ear, commonly called the eardrum.

typhlitis (*tif-lī'tis*). Inflammation of the mucous surface of the caecum.

typhoid fever (*tī'-foyd fē-ver*). An acute infectious disease which flourishes where the standard of hygiene is poor. Caused by ingestion of the *Salmonella typhi* from contaminated food or water sup-

plies. The germs reach the intestines and through the lymph channels produce a bacteraemia. After the first week the germs settle in the spleen, liver and intestines, especially the ileum. Here the lymph follicles known as Peyer's patches are attacked. They become inflamed, raised, and eventually the tissue of the follicle sloughs off. It is at this stage that intestinal haemorrhage or perforation may occur. Incubation period for the disease is 12–14 days and the patient remains infectious until bacteriological tests are negative. The onset is gradual. For 4 or 5 days the temperature is of the step-ladder type. If untreated, the patient becomes very ill during the second week with high temperature and slow pulse and the stools are often pea-soup in character. Rose-coloured spots, in crops, appear on the abdomen, chest and between the shoulder blades. By the third week, if untreated, the patient is delirious. The treatment is chloramphenicol, usually with dramatic improvement. *See also* ENTERIC FEVER.

typhus fever (*tī'-fus fē-ver*). A highly infectious fever characterized by a petechial rash, high temperature and great prostration. It is caused by Rickettsia bodies from infected lice or rat fleas.

tyrosine (*tī'-rō-sin*). *See* AMINO-ACIDS.

U

ulcer (*ul'-ser*). Suppuration upon a surface. Ulcers can occur on skin or mucous membrane, and may be acute or chronic.

ulcerative (*ul'-se-ra-tiv*). Pertaining to ulceration. *U. colitis*. A disease with inflammation and ulceration of the colon. There is diarrhoea, and mucus and blood are passed in the stools. The patient is anaemic. The disease may be mild or severe and no pathogenic organisms can be found to cause it, though emotional stress seems to precipitate it.

ulna (*ul'-na*). The inner bone of the forearm. *See* SKELETON.

ulnar. The name of an artery, a vein and a nerve running beside the ulna.

ultramicroscopic (*ul-tra-mī-krō-sko'-pik*). Too small to be seen with a microscope.

ultrasonic (*ul-tru-so'-nik*). Of too high a frequency to be heard by the human ear.

ultraviolet rays. Beyond the visible (seven colour) spectrum into which white light is resolved by a prism, there are non-visible rays at each end, both below the red rays (infra-red) and above the violet rays (ultraviolet).

umbilical cord (*um-bil-ī-kal kord*). The funis; the cord connecting the fetus with the placenta.

umbilicated (*um-bil'-ik-ā'-ted*). Having a navel-like depression, e.g. the papules in smallpox.

umbilicus (*um-bi-lī'-kus*). Region of attachment of the placenta. A small depressed scar on the anterior abdominal wall.

unciform (*un'-si-form*). The hook-shaped bone of the wrist.

uncinariasis (*un'-sin-a-rī'-a-sis*). Infection with hookworm.

unconsciousness (*un-kon'-shus-nes*). A state of not responding to stimuli, *e.g.* as a result of anaesthesia.

undine (*un'-dēn*). A thin glass flask with two spouts. Used for irrigation of eye.

undulant (*un'-dū-lant*). Wavelike. *U. fever*, *Malta fever*. A specific febrile disease. It is transmitted through cow's or goat's milk and runs a prolonged course.

unguentum (*un-goo-en'-tum*). An ointment; abbreviation, *ung*.

unguis (*ung'-gwis*). A finger-nail.

unicellular (*ū-ni-sel'-lū-la*). An organism or structure composed of one cell only, *e.g.* ovum.

unilateral (*ū-ni-la'-te-ral*). Found only on one side.

uniocular (*ū-ni-ok'-ū-la*). Relating to one eye.

union (*ū'-nē-on*). Healing. The joining up of a bone after a fracture.

uniovular (*ū-ni-ov'-ū-la*). With one ovum. Identical twins come from the same ovum.

uniparous (*ū-nip'-a-rus*). Having borne only one child.

unit (*ū'-nit*). An individual thing or group forming a complete whole. A standard of measurement.

Unna's paste (*un'-az pāst*) Treatment for ulcers of leg seldom used nowadays. It consists of zinc oxide, gelatin, glycerin and water. It is liquefied in a pot of hot water, and painted over a layer of gauze wrapped round the limb; if necessary a second coat may be applied and then the limb is surrounded by a thin bandage soaked in the mixture. When dry, it gives a thin plaster-like covering which keeps the part at rest.

urachus (*ū'-rā-kus*). A fibrous cord in the fetus from the bladder to the umbilicus. It becomes the median umbilical ligament.

uraemia (*ū-rē'-m-ia*). Accumulation of unknown toxic substances in the blood together with an increase in the blood urea and electrolyte imbalance. It may be due to widespread renal disease or as a result of a greatly diminished fluid intake.

uraemic fit (*ū-rēm'-ik*). Epileptiform seizure resulting from a greatly raised blood urea.

uraniscorrhaphy (*ū-ra-nis-ko'-ra-fi*). Suture of a cleft palate.

uranium (*ū-rān'-ium*). A heavy white metallic element found in pitchblende. Radium is extracted from it.

urate (*ū-rāt*). Salt of uric acid.

urea (*ū-rē-a*). One of the end-products of protein metabolism; the chief solid constituent of urine. It is a diuretic.

urea concentration test (*ū'-rē-a kon-sen-trā'-shon test*). The normal amount of urea in urine is 2 per cent. If a definite quantity of urea, 15 grams in 100ml water, be given fasting—the amount of urea eliminated by the kidneys can be estimated by specimens taken 1, 2, and 3 hours after. The proper excretion of urea shows an adequately functioning kidney. The percentage should rise to 3 or 4. This test is used to estimate renal efficiency.

uresis (*ū-rē-sis*). Urination.

ureter (*ū-rē-ter*). The canal between the kidney and the bladder, down which the urine passes. *See illustration*, p. 192.

ureteral (*ū-rē'-ter-al*). Pertaining to the ureter.

ureterectomy (*ū-rē-te-rek'-to-mi*). Excision of a ureter.

ureteric (*ū-rē-te'-rik*). Pertaining to ureter.

ureteritis (*ū-rē-te-rī-tis*). Inflammation of a ureter.

ureterocele (*ū-rē-te-rō-sēl*). The result of congenital atresia of a ureteric orifice which causes a cystic enlargement of the portion of the ureter situated in the bladder wall.

ureterolith (*ū-rē'-te-r'o-lith'*). Stone in a ureter.

ureterolithotomy (*u-rē-te-rō-li-tho-to-mi*). Operation for the removal of a stone impacted in the ureter.

ureterosigmoidostomy (*ū-rē'-te-rō-sig-moy-dos'-to-mi*). Implantation of a ureter into the sigmoid colon. The operation may be performed in cases of bladder disease.

ureterovaginal (*ū-rē-te-rō-va-jī'-nal*). Pertaining to a ureter and the vagina.

ureterovesical (*ū-rē-te-rō-ve-si'-kal*). Pertaining to a ureter and the bladder.

urethra (*ū-rē'-thra*). The canal between the bladder and the exterior through which the urine is discharged.

urethral (*ū-rē'-thral*). Pertaining to the urethra.

urethritis (*ū-rē-thrī'-tis*). Inflammation of the urethra.

urethrocele (*ū-rē'-thrō-sēl*). Urethral diverticulum. A small pouch in the wall of the urethra more common in women than in men; the origin is probably the result of a developmental defect.

urethrography (*ū-rē-thro'-gra-fi*). X-ray examination of the urethra by means of retrograde injection of a radio-opaque dye.

urethroplasty (*ū-rē-thrō-plas'-ti*). Plastic repair to the urethra.

urethroscope (*ū-rē-thros-kōp*). An instrument for viewing the interior of the urethra.

urethrotomy (*ū-rē-throt'-o-mi*). Incision of the urethra to remedy stricture; the instrument used being a urethrotome.

uric acid (*ū'-rik as'-id*). Lithic acid; its presence in urine is discovered by its resemblance in colour to cayenne pepper. Frequently present in gout. Liquor potassae dissolves this red deposit.

urinalysis (*ū-ri-nal'-i-sis*). Analysis of urine.

urinary (*ū'-rin-a-ri*). Pertaining to the urine. *U. Organs.* These include the kidneys, ureters, bladder and urethra.

urination (*ū-ri-nā'-shon*). Micturition. The act of discharging urine.

urine (*ū'-rin*). The fluid secreted by the kidneys. The normal amount secreted in the twenty-four hours varies from 1 to 1½ litres in an adult, 300 to 400ml in a child, 250 to 300ml in an infant. The normal constituents are water, salts, urea, acid bodies.

uriniferous tubules (*ū-rin-if'-er-us*). Numerous minute tubules in the kidney which secrete urine.

urinometer (*ū-rin-om'-e-ter*). A small glass instrument with a graduated stem, used for measuring the specific gravity of urine.

urobilin (*ū-rō-bil'-in*). One of the pigments of the urine, derived from bile pigments.

urobilinogen (*ū-rō-bi'-li'-no-jen*). Derivative of bilirubin which is made in the intestine by the gut bacteria. Some of it is absorbed and, in circumstances in which there is impaired liver function, may be excreted in the urine.

urochrome (*ū-rō-krōm*). Pigment colouring urine.

urogenital (*ū-rō-je-ni-tal*). Relating to the urinary and genital organs.

urography (*ū-ro'-gra-fi*). X-ray of the urinary tract.

urokinase (*u-ro-kī-nāz*). Enzyme found in the urine. In disease states it can cause bleeding from the kidney.

urolith (*ū-rō-lith'*). A stone found in the urine.

urologist (*ū-ro'-lo-jist*). A specialist in urology.

urology (*ū-ro'-lo-ji*). The study of diseases of the urinary tract.

uroscopy (*ū-ros'-ko-pi*). Examination of the urine.

urticaria (*er-ti-kā'-ri-a*). Nettlerash; hives. Allergic reaction affecting the permeability of small blood vessels. Characterized by erythema and wheals.

uterine (*ū'-ter-īn*). Relating to the uterus.

uterogestation (*ū'-te-rō-jes-tā'-shon*). The period of pregnancy.

uterovesical (*ū-te-rō-ve-sī-kal*). Relating to the uterus and the bladder.

uterus (*ū'-ter-us*). Womb. Muscular hollow pelvic organ. In the resting state it measures about 7·5 × 5cm and is triangular in shape with a cervix about 2·5cm which projects into the vagina. It is connected bilaterally to the oviducts (Fallopian tubes). The uterus has a glandular epithelium lining it and the whole structure is under the control of sex hormones, in particular oestrogens and progesterone. *See* MENSTRUATION. The uterus is the normal site of implantation of the trophoblast. During pregnancy the uterus grows out of the pelvis to occupy much of the abdominal cavity.

utricle (*ū'-trikl*). (1) The larger sac of membrane in the vestibule of the internal ear. (2) The prostatic vesicle.

uvea (*ū-vē-a*), **uveal tract.** The middle coat of the eyeball. The choroid, ciliary body and iris as a whole.

uveitis (*ū-vi-ī'-tis*). Inflammation of the uvea.

uvula (*ū'-vū-la*). A small fleshy body hanging down at the back of the soft palate.

uvulectomy (*ū-vū-lek'-to-mi*). Excision of uvula.

uvulitis (*ū-vū-lī'-tis*). Inflammation of the uvula.

V

vaccination (*vak-sin-ā'-shon*). (1) Inoculation of cow-pox lymph into the arm as a protection from smallpox. (2) Protective inoculation with any vaccine.

vaccine (*vak'-sēn*). An extract or suspension of attenuated or killed organisms. The antigenic properties of the organism are retained and the vaccine is used to immunize the recipient.

vaccinia (*vak-sin'-ia*). Cowpox. In man, it gives immunity to smallpox and therefore used in vaccination against that disease.

vacuole (*vak'-ū-ōl*). Specialized region within a cell surrounded by plasma membrane.

vacuum extractor (**ventouse**). An alternative method to forceps in delivering a child. A cap is fixed to the fetal head by creating a vacuum and traction is applied to a chain attached to the cap.

vagal (*vā'-gal*). Pertaining to the vagus nerve.

vagina (*va-jī'-na*). The passage leading from the cervix uteri to the vulva. The lower limit of this canal is the hymen.

vaginal (*va-jī'-nal*). Pertaining to the vagina.

vaginismus (*vaj-in-iz'-mus*). Spasmodic contraction of vagina whenever the vulva or vagina is touched.

vaginitis (*va-jin-ī'-tis*). Inflammation of the vagina.

vagotomy (*vā-go'-to-mi*). Surgical division of the vagus nerve sometimes performed on patients with peptic or duodenal ulcers.

vagus (*vā'-gus*). The pneumogastric nerve.

valgus (*val'-gus*). Turned outward. (Bow legged.) *Talipes v. See* p. 318.

valine (*vā'-lēn*). One of the essential amino-acids.

valve (*va'-lv*). A fold across a channel allowing flow in one direction only.

valvotomy (*val-vo'-to-mi*). Incision into a valve, especially heart valve. The purpose of the operation is to widen the orifice of a stenosed valve.

valvulae conniventes (*val-vū-lē kon-i-ven-tāz*). Transverse folds of mucous membrane in the upper part of the small intestine.

valvulitis (*val-vū-lī'-tis*). Inflammation of a valve.

valvulotomy (*val-vū-lo'-to-mi*). *See* VALVOTOMY.

van den Bergh's test (*van' den bergs*). Performed to discover the presence of bile pigment in the blood. It also differentiates between the pigment retained in the blood from obstruction of the bile passages, and that due to haemolysis.

Vaquez's disease (*vak-kāz' dis-sēz*). *See* POLYCYTHAEMIA.

varicella (*var-i-sel'-la*). Chicken-pox.

varices (*va'-ri-sēz*). Dilated, twisted veins. Sing. varix.

varicocele (*var'-ē-kō-sēl*). A varicose condition of the veins of the spermatic cord.

varicose ulcer. Ulceration of the lower legs due to reduction in the blood supply resulting from increased venous pressure.

varicose veins (*var'-i-kōs vānz*). Dilated veins in which the valves have become incompetent. As a result the blood flow may become reversed or static. Most common in the legs where the blood pools by gravitation. Other examples are piles and oesophageal varices.

varicotomy (*va-ri-ko-to-mi*). Excision of varicose vein.

variola (*va-ri'-ō-la*). *See* SMALL-POX. *V. minor.* Much less severe disease than that of smallpox which it resembles.

varioloid (*va-ri-ō'-loyd*). A mild form of smallpox, sometimes seen in person who have been previously vaccinated.

varix (*vā'-riks*). An enlarged and tortuous vein.

varus (*vā'-rus*). Turned inward. (Knock-kneed). *Talipes v. See* p. 318.

vas. A vessel, or duct of the body; as *vas deferens*, the duct of the testis.

vascular (*vas'-kū-lar*). Possessing many blood vessels.

vascular system. System of blood vessels.

vasectomy (*va-sek'-to-mi*). Removal of a part of the vas deferens.

vasoconstriction (*vā'-zō-kon-strik'-shon*). Contraction of blood vessels.

vasodilatation (*vā'-zō-di-la-tā'-shon*). Dilatation of blood vessels.

vasomotor (*vā-zō-mō'-tor*). Concerned with constriction of blood vessels. *V. nerves.* Sympathetic nerves which control the tone of smooth muscle in the walls of blood vessels.

vasospasm (*vā'-zo-spasm*). Spasm of the blood vessels.

vasovagal syndrome (*vā-zō-vā'-gal sin'-drōm*). Slowing of the heart rate with a feeling of nausea and grave distress. The attack may last a few minutes or an hour. The cause is unknown.

Vater's ampulla (*va'-ters am-poo'-la*). Small dilation in the terminal portion of the common bile duct where it empties into the duodenum.

vector (*vek'-tor*). A carrier. One who conveys the infection to another person.

vegetations (*ve-je-tā'-shons*). Concretion of organic debris on the diseased valves of the heart which occurs in endocarditis.

vegetative (*ve'-je-tā-tiv*). Having the power of growth.

vein (*vān*). A vessel carrying the blood to the heart.

vena cava (*vē-na kā'-va*). The superior vena cava and the inferior vena cava are two large veins which return blood from the head and body and empty it into the right atrium of the heart.

venepuncture (*ve-nē-punk'-tūr*). Inserting a needle into a vein.

venereal (*ve-nē'-re-al*). Relating to sexual intercourse. *V. disease.* Infectious diseases transmitted during sexual intercourse, *e.g.* gonorrhoea, syphilis.

venereology (*ve-nār-ē-ol'-o-ji*). The study of venereal disease.

venesection (*vē-nē-sek'-shon*). Blood-letting. A vein is opened and blood drained off from it. Frequently performed in the past for almost any ailment. There are very few present-day indications for venesection.

venography (*ve-no'-gra-fi*). X-ray examination of veins following injection of contrast medium.

venous (*vē'-nus*). Relating to the veins.

ventilation (*ven-ti-lā'-shon*). (1)

Supply of fresh air. (2) Process of breathing.

ventral (*ven'-tral*). Relating to the belly. *V. root.* Anterior root, motor root. The nerve root containing the motor fibres.

ventricles (*ven'-tri-kls*). The two lower chambers of the heart are known as the right and left ventricles. The cavities in the brain also are known as ventricles.

ventriculography (*ven-tri-kū-log'-raf-i*). X-ray examination of the ventricles of the brain. Air or a radio-opaque dye is introduced into the ventricles, enabling their size and position to be observed.

ventrofixation (*ven'-tro-fik-sā-shon*). The operation to suture an abdominal viscus to the anterior abdominal wall.

ventrosuspension (*ven-trō-sus-pen'-shon*). Another operation having the same object as ventrofixation, but fixing the round ligaments instead of the uterus to the abdominal wall.

venule (*ve'-nūl*). Small vein.

vermicide (*ver'-mi-sīd*). Substance able to kill worms in the intestine.

vermiform appendix (*ver'-mi-form*). See APPENDIX VERMIFORMIS.

vermifuge (*ver-mi-fūj*). Substance used to dispel worms.

verminous (*ver'-min-us*). Infested with animal parasites.

vernix caseosa (*ver'-niks kā-sē-ō'-sah*). The sebaceous material which covers the skin of the fetus.

verruca (*ver'-ū'-ka*). A wart.

version (*ver'-shon*). The operation of altering the presentation of the fetus in the uterus so as to facilitate its delivery. *Cephalic version* is turning the fetus, so that the head presents, while *podalic version* brings about a breech presentation. *Bipolar version*, version by acting upon both poles of the fetus.

vertebrae (*ver'-te-brē*). The thirty-three small bones which form the backbone, or spinal column. See SKELETON, p. 299.

vertex (*ver'-teks*). The crown of the head.

vertigo (*ver-tī'-gō*). Giddiness.

vesica (*ves'-i-ka*). The bladder.

vesical (*ve-sī'-kal*). Relating to the bladder.

vesicant (*vēs'-i-kant*). A blistering agent.

vesicle (*vēs'-i-kl*). A blister. Blisters of greater diameter than 5mm are termed bullae. Blisters contain serum.

vesicovaginal (*ve-sī-kō-va-jī-nal*). Relating to the bladder and the vagina.

vesicular mole (*ve-sik'-ū-lar*). See MOLE.

vesicular breathing (*ve-sik'-ū-lar brē-thing*). The normal sound of inspiration heard on auscultation.

vesiculitis (*ve-si-kū-lī-tis*). Inflammation of seminal vesicles.

vestibular neuronitis (*ves-ti-bū-la nū-rō-nī-tis*). Disorder affecting the vestibular nerve which is characterized by extreme vertigo while hearing is unaffected. May result from streptomycin toxicity.

vestibule (*ves'-ti-būl*). (1) A small cavity of the ear into which the cochlea opens. (2) The space between the labia minora.

vestigial (*ves-ti'-ji-al*). Rudimentary. Bearing a trace of something now vanished or degenerate.

viable (*vī'-ab-l*). Capable of living. An obstetrical term implying that an unborn child is sufficiently developed to survive its birth.

Vibrio (*vi-brē-ō*). A genus of micro-organisms shaped like a bacillus but curved. One causes cholera.

vicarious (*vi-kā'-ri-us*). When one organ performs the work of another. *V. menstruation.* Menstruation from a passage other than the uterus.

villi (*vil-lī*) (sing. **villus**). Fine soft processes of living cells. *Intestinal v.* in the small intes-

tines each contain a central vessel or lacteal, surrounded by a plexus of capillaries. Their function is to increase the surface area of the small intestine thereby aiding absorption. *Chorionic v.* Processes arising from the chorion, the outer membrane of the developing ovum. Specialization of a mass of villi ultimately forms the placenta.

villous (*vil'-us*). Having the nature of villi, thus a villous tumour of the bladder is a growth consisting of long slender processes of cells.

Vincent's angina (*vin'-sents an-jī'-na*). Infection of the mucous epithelium of the mouth by a symbiotic (*see* SYMBIOSIS) association of a spirochaete Borrelia vincenti and a fusiform Gram-negative bacterium Fusobacterium planti-vincenti.

vinegar (*vin'-e-gah*). A weak solution of acetic acid formed by fermentation of wine and other alcoholic liquids.

vinum (*vē'-num*). Wine.

viraemia (*vī-rē-mi-a*). Viruses present in the blood stream.

virilism (*vi'ri-lism*). The appearance of masculine characteristics in the female.

virology (*vī-ro'-lo-ji*). The study of viruses and the diseases caused by them.

virulent (*vir'-ū-lent*). Violent. *V. infection.* One with severe symptoms.

virus (*vī'-rus*). Infecting agent that will pass through the finest filter known, *e.g.* the cause of mumps, anterior poliomyelitis and other infectious diseases.

viscera (*vis'-se-ra*). The internal organs of the great cavities of the body, the term being generally applied to the abdomen. *Sing.* viscus.

visceroptosis (*vis-e-rop-tō-sis*). Prolapse of the abdominal viscera.

viscid (*vis'-kid*), **viscous** (*vis'-kus*). Sticky, thick, adhesive.

Viscopaste (*vis'-kō-pāst*). A proprietary zinc paste bandage.

viscus (*vis'-kus*). See VISCERA.

vision (*vi-zhon*). The act or faculty of seeing. *Binocular vision*, use of both eyes without seeing double. *Central vision, direct vision*, that performed through the centre of the retina. *Double vision, diplopia*, a failure to fuse the images thrown upon the two retinae at the same time: two images are therefore seen and objects appear double. May be due to defect in muscles of the eye or an error of refraction. It is also a symptom of some nervous diseases, *e.g.* encephalitis

lethargica. *Peripheral vision, indirect vision*, that performed by the peripheral or circumferential portion of the retina. *Stereoscopic vision*, that which gives perception of distance and solidity.

visual (*vi'-zū-al*). Pertaining to vision. *V. field.* The total area which can be seen at the same time without turning the head.

vital (*vī-tal*). Pertaining to life. *V. capacity.* The amount of air that can be breathed out after a complete inspiration. *V. statistics.* Statistics of births, marriages, deaths and diseases in a population.

vitallium (*vi-ta'-li-um*). An alloy used in bone surgery for nails, screws, plates, etc.

vitamins (*vi'-ta-mins*). Chemical substances present in food, necessary for health and development. Those at present known are:

A. Anti-infective, fat soluble; found in animal fat such as butter, cream, milk, fish oil and derived from carotin, the colouring matter of carrots and tomatoes. Lack of A causes a lowered resistance to infection, night blindness and opacity of the cornea.

B complex (has different parts). Water soluble, found in whole-meal cereals, yeast,

Marmite, liver, lean meat. B_1, or thiamine, anti-neuritic; prevents polyneuritis and beriberi. B_2, or riboflavin; deficiency causes a syndrome which includes visual disturbances. B_6, or pyridoxine: no deficiency symptoms are known, but the drug has been used in irradiation and pregnancy sickness. B_{12}, or cyanocobalamin, the specific anti-anaemia principle of liver. Nicotinic acid is also a constituent of the B complex.

C. Anti-scorbutic; found in rose hips, black currants, oranges, tomatoes, raw vegetables. Lack of C causes scurvy.

D. Anti-rachitic; found in animal fats and fish oils. The action of ultraviolet rays on certain fats, known as sterols, produces vitamin D. It is necessary for the metabolism of calcium. Lack of vitamin D causes rickets.

E. Anti-sterility; found in wheat germ oil, an ingredient of whole wheat. Lack of E causes sterility and insecurity of pregnancy.

K. The 'Koagulation Vitamin'. Fat soluble. Occurs in the green part of plants, particularly alfalfa grass, spinach, kale, carrot tops, and vegetable oils. It may be formed by bacterial action from food in the lower part of the intestine and absorbed. Bile salts in the intestine are necessary for absorption. Lack of vitamin K causes a deficiency of prothrombin in the blood, which is necessary for the clotting of blood. Prescribed in cases of obstructive jaundice.

vitelline (*vi'-te-lēn*). Pertaining to the vitellus, or yolk.

vitiate (*vi-shē-āt*). To make a substance less efficient.

vitiligo (*vit-il-i'-go*). Disorder of pigment cells in which patches of depigmented skin arise, often in a symmetrical distribution.

vitreous chamber of the eye (*vi'-trē-us chăm'-ber*). The posterior five-sixths of the eyeball, that part behind the lens. It is filled with a clear jelly-like substance called the *vitreous humour*.

vitriol (*vit'-rē-ol*). Any crystalline sulphate. *Blue vitriol*, copper sulphate or blue stone. Sometimes applied to granulation tissue on the eyelids. *Oil of v.* Sulphuric acid.

vivisection (*viv-i-sek'-shon*). Scientific examination of a living animal.

vocal cords (*vō'-kal kor'dz*). Two folds of mucous membrane in the larynx attached behind to the arytenoid cartilages, and in front to the back of the thyroid cartilage. Voice is produced by variation in position of these cords when acted on by small muscles of the larynx, and at the same time forcing through them an expiratory blast of air.

volatile (*vol'-a-tīl*). That which evaporates quickly.

volition (*vo-lish'-on*). The act or power of willing.

Volkmann's paralysis (*volk-munz*), **V. contracture.** A muscular paralysis caused by applying splints too tightly so that the blood supply is impaired. Most commonly seen in the forearm after fractures about the elbow joint.

Volkmann's spoon (*volk-munz*). A sharp spoon used for scraping a septic cavity.

volsellum (*vol'-sel-um*). *See* VULSELLUM.

volt (*vōlt*). A unit of electrical potential.

voluntary (*vol'-un-ta-ri*). Free. Regulated by choice and desire. *V. worker.* One who gives his services free.

volvulus (*vol'-vū'-lus*). A twisting of a piece of intestine on its mesenteric attachment. Acute intestinal obstruction is the result.

vomer (*vō'-mer*). A bone of the septum of the nose.

vomit (*vo'-mit*). To eject the contents of the stomach through the mouth. *Projectile v.* Forcible ejection of gastric contents without warning.

vomiting of pregnancy. The vomiting to which about two-thirds of pregnant women are subject at some time or other during the period of gestation. Occurs usually about the second, third and fourth months, and is commonest in the morning. In most cases no ill results follow, but occasionally the vomiting becomes so frequent and severe that a grave condition is produced, called the *intractable*, or *pernicious vomiting of pregnancy*, or *hyperemesis gravidarum*. Vomiting is also a symptom of toxaemia of pregnancy. *See* TOXAEMIA.

von Gierke's disease (*von gerkes di-sēz*). Glycogen storage disease. Recessively inherited defect in the metabolism of glycogen so that it cannot be used. The tissues become stuffed with glycogen while hypoglycaemia occurs.

von Recklinghausen's disease (*von rek'-ling-how-zenz*). Characterized by multiple tumours along cutaneous nerves of trunk and scalp, with areas of pigmentation. *See also* OSTEITIS FIBROSA.

vulnerable (*vul'-ne-rubl*). Susceptible.

vulsellum (*vul-sel'-um*), (plu. **vulsella**). Catch forceps with toothed blades.

vulva (*vul'-va*). The external organs of generation of the female.

vulvectomy (*vul-vek'-to-mi*). Excision of vulva.

vulvitis (*vul-vī'-tis*). Inflammation of the vulva.

vulvovaginal (*vul-vō-va-ji-nal*). Pertaining to the vulva and the vagina.

vulvovaginitis (*vul-vō-va-ji-nī-tis*). Inflammation of both the vulva and the vagina.

W

Waldeyer's ring (*vul-dā'-yers ring*). Circle of adenoid tissue in the pharynx formed by the faucial, lingual and pharyngeal tonsils.

Wallerian degeneration (*va-lār-i-an dē-je-ne-rā'-shon*). Degeneration of a nerve after it has been cut or severed.

wart (*wawt*). Small horny tumour from the skin. The *common wart* is due to a virus infection. A *plantar wart* is found on the sole of the foot. *Venereal warts* are common warts on the genitalia and not to be confused with flat con-dylomata of secondary syphilis.

washing soda (*wo'-shing sō'-dah*). Sodium carbonate.

Wassermann reaction (*vas'-er-man*). A blood test which shows whether the individual from whom the blood is taken is or is not the subject of active syphilis. Sometimes the cerebrospinal fluid is taken instead of blood. *See* KAHN TEST.

water beds. Rubber mattress filled with warm water and used to prevent pressure sores.

water-borne (*waw'-ter-bawn*). Spread by water, such as certain diseases, *e.g.* typhoid fever.

water-brash. Regurgitation of stomach acid into the oesophagus and thence to the mouth.

water-hammer pulse. *See* CORRIGAN'S PULSE.

Waterhouse Friderichsen syndrome (*waw-te-hows fri-de-rik'-sen sin'-drōm*). Syndrome resulting from bilateral adrenal haemorrhage accompanying the purpura of acute septicaemia, usually meningococcal.

watt (*wot*). The amount of power developed by an electrical current of one ampere having an electromotive force of one volt.

wave length. The distance between two adjacent crests of any wave motion.

weal (*wēl*). A white or pinkish elevation on the skin, as in urticaria.

wean (*wēn*). To cease feeding a baby at the breast.

Weber syndrome. Hemianopia caused by posterior cerebral aneurysm.

Weil's disese (*vīls*). Epidemic spirochaetal jaundice. Disease caused by a Leptospira characterized by fever, headache, and pains in the limbs. Many patients develop jaundice and a purpuric rash.

Weil-Felix reaction (*vīl-fē'-liks rē-ak'-shon*). An agglutination reaction for typhus.

Welch's bacillus (*wel'-shes ba-si'-lus*). Clostridium perfringens, a spore-forming organism found in gas gangrene.

wen. See SEBACEOUS CYST.

Wernicke's encephalopathy (*ver-ni-kers en-ke-fa-lo-pa-thi*). Syndrome occurring in association with alcoholic polyneuritis, characterized by vertigo, nystagmus, ataxia and stupor. Considered to be due to thiamine deficiency.

Wertheim's operation (*vār'-tīms*). A radical operation for uterine cancer, whereby the uterus, tubes, ovaries, broad ligaments, pelvic lymph nodes and cellular tissue around ureters are removed *en masse*.

Wharton's duct (*wor'-tonz*). The duct of the submaxillary gland.

Wharton's jelly. A special tissue of the umbilical cord.

Wheelhouse's operation. External (perineal) urethrotomy for stricture of the urethra.

whey (*whā*). The liquid left after milk has been clotted with rennin.

Whipple's disease (*wi-pels di-sēz*). Intestinal lipodystrophy. Disease of unknown cause. There is progressive deposition of mucoprotein material in the wall of the small intestine.

whipworm (*wip'-werm*). See TRICHOCEPHALUS.

white cell (*wīt sel*). See BLOOD.

white leg (*wīt leg*). See PHLEGMASIA ALBA DOLENS.

whites (*wītz*). A popular term for leucorrhoea.

Whitfield's ointment (*wit'-fēldz oynt'-ment*). Contains salicylic and benzoic acids. Used for athlete's foot and ringworm.

whitlow (*wit'-lō*). Inflammation near a finger-nail, with suppuration. See ONYCHIA.

whooping cough (*hoop'-ing kof*). Pertussis.

Widal reaction (*vē'-dal*). A

blood test for typhoid fever. Not available until patient has been ill for about ten days.

Willebrand's disease (*wi-lē-brans di-sēz*). Inherited defect of blood vessels and clotting mechanism.

willpower (*wil'-pow-er*). A voluntary effort which directs our actions and can overcome some primary impulse such as fear.

Wilms' tumour (*wilms tū'-mer*). A congenital tumour of the kidney which is malignant.

Wilson's disease (*wil'-sons di'-sēz*). A rare metabolic disorder (hepatolenticular degeneration) in which copper accumulates in the liver and certain nuclei of the brain.

windpipe (*wind'-pīp*). The trachea.

Winslow's foramen (*winz'-lōz for-ā-men*). An aperture between the stomach and liver formed by folds of peritoneum. It forms a communication between the greater and lesser peritoneal cavities.

wisdom teeth (*wiz'-dom tēth*). The posterior molars. They erupt last, usually when a person is about 21 years old.

withdrawal (*with-draw'-al*). In psychology meaning to 'shrink into oneself'. A normal method of adjustment in a frightening situation. *W. symptoms*. Symptoms which appear when a drug, to which a person has become addicted, is withheld from him.

womb (*woom*). The uterus.

Wood's glass. Glass which contains nickel oxide. It causes fluorescence of certain objects and is used to detect ringworm.

woolsorter's disease (*wool'-sor-terz*). See ANTHRAX.

word salad (*werd sal'-ad*). A jumble of disconnected words heard when certain schizophrenic patients speak.

worms (*werms*). Invertebrate animal. See ASCARIS, TAENIA, TRICHURIS AND TRICHO-CEPHALUS DISPAR.

Woulfe's bottle (*woolfs bot'-tel*). Bottle in which a gas (*e.g.* oxygen) passes through water to moisten it.

wound (*woond*). Injury.

wrist (*rist*). The joint between the hand and the forearm. The carpus.

writer's cramp (*ri'-terz kramp*). Spasm of the hand and forearm brought on by efforts to write. Largely due to defective posture when writing.

wry-neck (*rī'-nek*). See TORTICOLLIS.

X

X chromosome (*eks krō-mō-sōm*). The sex chromosome which is paired in the homogametic sex. Unlike the Y chromosome it carries many major genes.

xanthelasma (*zan-the-las'-ma*). A condition in which yellow patches or nodules occur on the skin, especially in the eyelids.

xanthine (*zan'-thin*). A nitrogenous substance produced in the body. Sometimes found in the urine.

xanthochromia (*zan-thō-krō-mi-a*). The distinctive yellow colour of cerebrospinal fluid following a subarachnoid haemorrhage. It is due to haemolysis of the blood in the subarachnoid space, and indicates that subarachnoid haemorrhage has occurred.

xanthoderma (*zan-thō-der'-ma*). Yellowness of the skin.

xanthoma (*zan-thō'-mah*). The same as xanthelasma.

xenopsylla cheopis (*zen-op-si'-la chē-ō'-pis*). A rat flea which can transmit plague and typhus.

xenopus test (*zen-'ō-pus test*). Test for pregnancy. The mother's urine is injected into the lymph sac of a female toad. If the woman is pregnant, the toad will pass ova, in from 24–48 hours. Now obsolete.

xeroderma (*ze-rō-der'-ma*). A dry state of the skin.

xerophthalmia (*ze-rof-thal-mi-a*). Ulceration of the cornea occurring in vitamin A deficiency.

xeroradiography. The technique for soft tissue radiography using special equipment giving a positive print.

xerosis (*zer-ō'-sis*). Abnormal dryness, *e.g.* of the conjunctiva or the skin.

xerostomia (*ze-ro-stō'-mi-a*). Dryness of the mouth.

xiphoid process (*zif'-oyd prō-ses*). A sword-shaped cartilage attached to the breast-bone. Also called the ensiform cartilage.

x-rays (*eks'-rāz*). One of the radiations capable of penetrating many substances impervious to ordinary light. These rays are used (1) diagnostically, as in showing injury to bone, or the condition of hollow organs after they have been rendered opaque, and (2) therapeutically: (*a*) less penetrating rays are used for superficial skin lesions, such as warts or rodent ulcers; (*b*) deep x-ray therapy is used generally under a high voltage for the cure of cancer. *See* RÖNTGEN RAYS.

Xylene (*zī-lēn*). Xylol. Used as a solvent and also in microscopy.

Y

Y chromosome (*wī krō-mō-sōm*). Sex chromosome found only in the heterogametic sex (male). It is shorter than the X chromosome and usually carries few major genes.

yaws (*yaws*). Framboesia. Tropical disease, resembling syphilis, caused by Treponema pertenue.

yeast (*yē-st*). Unicellular fungi, Ascomycetes, which possess enzymes capable of converting sugars into ethanol with the release of carbon dioxide. Yeasts are also used as sources of protein and vitamins.

yellow fever (*ye'-lō fē-ver*). Virus-mediated disease transmitted by mosquitoes. Characterized by fever, prostration, jaundice and gastro-intestinal haemorrhage.

Z

zero (*zē'-rō*). The point on a temperature scale at which positive and negative temperatures begin. The zero of the Centigrade (Celsius) and Réaumur thermometer is the melting-point of ice. That of the Fahrenheit is 32 degrees below the melting-point of ice.

Ziehl-Neelsen's stain (*zēl-nēl-sens stān*). Staining technique used to identify tubercle bacilli by their ability to retain the stain when treated with acid; hence acid-fast bacilli.

zinc (*zi'nk*). A metallic element. The chloride is used as a caustic and disinfectant. Zinc oxide ointment is used for dressing minor ulcerations of the skin.

Zollinger-Ellison syndrome (*zo-ling-er e-li-son sin'-drōm*). Increased production of acid gastric juice in response to gastrin secreted by pancreatic neoplasm, resulting in peptic ulceration and inactivation of enzymes of small intestine which operate only in the alkaline range.

zona (*zō'-na*). Literally a girdle and applied to mean shingles. *See* HERPES. *Z. pellucida.* Membrane surrounding the ovum.

Zondek-Aschheim test (*zon-dek-ash'-hīm*). To diagnose pregnancy. The urine of a pregnant woman contains a counterpart of the luteinizing hormone of the pituitary gland. Where the diagnosis is uncertain, the urine is injected into immature mice. A few days later the mice are killed and if the generative organs of the mice have undergone the changes characteristic of puberty the woman is known to be pregnant.

zonula ciliaris (*zo-nŭ-la si-li-a-ris*). Suspensory ligament of lens of the eye.

zoogloea layer (*zō-ō-glē-a lā-er*). Colonies of bacteria in a jelly-like layer. Found on the top of a sand filter bed. This layer contains algae and pro-

tozoa and helps in water purification.

zoology (*zō-ol'-o-ji*). That part of biology which deals with the study of animal life.

zoosperm (*zō'-o-sperm*). Same as spermatozoon.

zoster (*zos'-ter*). Shingles. *See* HERPES.

zygoma (*zīg-ō'-ma*). The cheekbone.

zygote (*zī-gōt*). The cell formed by combination of ovum with spermatozoon.

zymotic (*zī-mot'-ik*). A term which includes all epidemic, endemic and contagious diseases arising from germs.

Appendix 1

BLOOD

The figures given below represent the approximate range of values for the constituents of the peripheral blood. ('Same' in the S.I. units column implies that the traditional measurement is used.)

Red Cells

	S.I. Units	Traditional Units
Haemoglobin	12·0 to 18·0 g/dl	12 to 16g per 100ml
Red cells	3·9 to 6·5 × 10^{12}/l	4·5 to 6·0 million per cu mm or mm^3
Reticulocytes (newly formed red cells)	same	less than 1 per cent of total red cells
Mean cell volume (MCV)	same	75 to 95 cuμ is the average volume of a single red cell
Packed cell volume (PCV or haematocrit)	same	35 to 55 per cent
Mean cell diameter (MCD)	same	7·2μ
Mean cell haemoglobin (MCH)	same	20 to 32μg

White Cells

	S.I. Units	Traditional Units
Total white cells	5·0 to 10·0 × 10⁹/l	5,000 to 10,000 per cu mm or mm³
Neutrophils	same	60 to 70 per cent
Lymphocytes	same	25 to 35 per cent
Basophils	same	1 per cent
Eosinophils	same	1 to 4 per cent
Monocytes	same	4 to 8 per cent
Platelets (thrombocytes)	2·5 to 3·5 × 10¹¹/l	250,000 to 350,000 per cu mm or mm³

Blood Chemistry

	S.I. Units	Traditional Units
pH	same	7·35 to 7·45
Urea	2 to 3 mmol/2	20 to 40mg per 100ml
Uric acid	0·10 to 0·40 mmol/l	1·5 to 6·5mg per cent
Cholesterol	3·9 to 7·8 mmol/l	1·5 to 6·5mg per cent
Bilirubin	3 to 20 μmol/l	0·2 to 1·2mg per cent
Calcium	2·3 to 2·6 mmol/l	9·0 to 10·2mg per cent
Phosphate	0·8 to 1·46 mmol/	2·5 to 4·5mg per cent

Bicarbonate	20 to 28 mmol/l	20 to 28 mEq/litre
Fasting blood glucose	2·3 to 5·0 mmol/l	45 to 90mg per cent
Potassium	3·5 to 5·5 mmol/l	3·3 to 5·5 mEq/litre
Sodium	135 to 145 mmol/l	135 to 145 mEq/litre
Total Plasma Proteins	60 to 80g/l	6·0 to 8·0g per cent
Albumin	35 to 55g/l	3·5 to 5·5g per cent
Globulin	15 to 30g/l	1·5 to 3·0g per cent
Fibrinogen	2 to 4g/l	0·2 to 0·4g per cent

Appendix 2

URINE TESTING

1. COLOUR: Normal, straw to light amber.

(a) Pale. Low specific gravity urines are usually very pale.
1. After drinking much fluid.
2. In cold weather.
3. Diabetes insipidus.
4. Chronic nephritis.
5. Diabetes mellitus (high specific gravity).

(b) High colour. Concentrated urine.
Concentration occurs:
1. Reduced fluid intake.
2. Febrile disease, e.g. pneumonia, rheumatic fever.
3. Profuse vomiting.
4. Profuse diarrhoea.
5. Profuse sweating.
6. Heart disease.

(c) When coloured by blood it may be:
1. Bright red } if blood is present in large
2. The colour of a dark beer } amounts.
3. Brownish if there is only a small amount of blood.

(d) When coloured by bile it may be:
Mahogany or greenish-brown, frothy.

2. QUANTITY: During 24 hours the normal output of urine is about 1500ml.

3. SPECIFIC GRAVITY of water is taken as $1 \cdot 0$ (formerly 1000).
The specific gravity of urine depends on the amount of soluble solid matter, e.g. salts, urates, etc.
Normal specific gravity varies from $1 \cdot 010$ to $1 \cdot 025$.

Light-coloured urines, except in diabetes mellitus, as given in list under *colour*, are of low specific gravity and there is usually an increased amount of urine passed.

Concentrated urines are of high specific gravity, and in diabetes mellitus may be 1·025 to 1·060.

With concentrated urine the quantity is usually decreased.

4. REACTION: Normal reaction slightly acid, due to acid phosphates:

1. May be neutral.
2. May become alkaline:
   a. In cystitis.
   b. After taking alkalis.
   c. Specimen stale when tested.

5. SMELL: Normal, sweet.
In diabetes mellitus—very sweet, like new-mown hay.
In cystitis—ammoniacal, and often 'fishy'.

6. NAKED-EYE DEPOSITS:

1. *Urates*. Fawn, pink, or brick-red deposits occur in concentrated urines when the urine becomes cold.
2. *Uric acid*. Small red grains, like cayenne pepper.
3. *Mucus*. Light flocculent deposit.
4. *Pus*. Thick yellow or greenish-yellow.
5. *Blood*. Clots or brownish deposit.
6. *Phosphates*. Thick white deposit.

To test a specimen of urine

1. Note the colour.
2. Note the specific gravity.
3. Note the reaction. This is tested with blue or red litmus paper.
   a. Blue litmus turns red = acid reaction.
   b. Red litmus turns blue = alkaline reaction.
   c. Red and blue litmus do not change = neutral.
4. Note the smell.
5. Note the naked-eye deposits.

In many cases a bacteriological examination of the urine is required.

Tests for albumin
(a) Albustix Reagent Strips

Proceed according to instructions on bottle.

Tests (b) or (c) may be carried out if Albustix is not available.

(b) Heat
1. Fill $\frac{2}{3}$ test tube with urine.
2. If not acid, add 2 or 3 drops of acetic acid.
3. Heat the upper $\frac{1}{3}$ of the urine until it boils.
4. The part heated becomes white and opaque.
5. Add 2 or 3 drops of acetic acid.
   a. The deposit remains = albumin.
   b. The deposit clears up = phosphates.

A cloudy urine which becomes clear on heating = urates.

(c) Salicyl-sulphonic acid
Take 10 drops of urine in a test tube. If alkaline, add 3 drops of acetic acid. Add 1 drop of salicyl-sulphonic acid 25%. If a cloud forms albumin is present.

(d) Estimation of quantity of albumin by an Esbach's albumino-meter
Render the urine acid if not already so.

If the specific gravity is higher than 1·010 dilute with an equal quantity of water.

Take a graduated Esbach's tube and put in urine up to the mark U. Add Esbach's solution up to mark R. Cork tube and mix by carefully inverting. Carefully label tube with patient's name and date and time. Let it stand for twenty-four hours. Read off the height of deposit in tube and record as grams per litre.

If the urine was diluted, the result must be multiplied by 2.

Tests for blood

(a) Occultest Reagent Tablets
Proceed according to instructions on bottle.

Test (b) may be carried out if Occultest tablets are not available.

(b) Tincture of guaiacum and ozonic ether
1. Stir the specimen.
2. Pour about 5ml of urine into a test tube.
3. Add 2 drops of tincture of guaiacum.
4. Shake and mix.
5. Add slowly 3 to 4ml of ozonic ether.

A blue ring appears at the junction of the fluids when blood is present. (A similar result is obtained if a patient is taking potassium iodide.)

Tests for sugar

(a) Clinitest Reagent Tablets
This is a test for all sugars. Proceed according to instructions on bottle.

(b) Clinistix Reagent Strips
This is a test for glucose only. Proceed according to instructions on bottle.

(c) Benedict's test
This test is only carried out if Clinitest tablets are not available.
1. Take 5ml of Benedict's solution and to this add 8 drops of urine with a pipette.
2. Boil for three minutes.
If sugar is present the colour will change. Greenish-yellow denotes a trace of sugar; yellow: some sugar; and orange-brown: much sugar.

Tests for acetone

(a) Acetest Reagent Tablets
Proceed according to instructions on bottle.

(b) Rothera's test
This test is only carried out if Acetest tablets are not available.
1. To half a test tube full of urine add ammonium sulphate crystals until the liquid is saturated.
2. Dissolve two or three nitro-prusside crystals in 8ml of water and add four drops of this to the urine.
3. Shake well.
4. Add ten drops of strong ammonia.
There will be a purple colour in 15 minutes if acetone or diacetic acid is present.

Tests for bilirubin

(a) Ictotest Reagent Tablets
Proceed according to instructions on bottle.

(b) Iodine test
This test is only used if Ictotest tablets are not available. To 5ml of

urine add a few drops of tincture of iodine which has been diluted with equal parts of water.

A green ring will form where the two liquids join if bilirubin is present.

Special reagent strips may be available which give a combined test for a number of abnormalities in the urine. The given procedure should be followed meticulously, particularly the timing of the reading of results.

Any nurse who knows that she is colourblind should have her tests checked.

Appendix 3

DIET

The human does not eat nutrients but food and the type of food eaten varies a great deal from culture to culture. However, certain basic nutrients are necessary for the production of energy, for adequate growth, the replacement of tissues and the maintenance of health.

The basic nutrients include:

1. Carbohydrates
2. Proteins
3. Fats
4. Vitamins
5. Minerals

The first three groups of these nutrients are energy-giving foods and the energy value of a diet is measured in kilojoules (SI unit). 4.186 kilojoules = 1 Calorie (kilocalorie). Energy requirements vary greatly according to sex, age and degree of activity.

Composition of some common foodstuffs per ounce (approx. 30 grams)

	kilojoules	Protein grams	Fat grams	Carbohydrate grams
Bread	306	2·2	0·2	15·5
Potato	87	0·6	–	4·6
Sugar	452	–	–	26·9
Butter	883	0·1	23·4	–
Cheese	490	7·1	9·8	–
Egg	188	3·5	3·3	0·3
Milk	71	0·9	1·0	1·2
Bacon	536	3·1	12·8	–
Beef	373	4·2	8·0	–
Apple	50	0·1	–	3·0
Orange	42	0·2	–	2·2

1. Carbohydrates

These contain carbon, hydrogen, and oxygen. Carbohydrates may be eaten as starch or as sugars. Sugars may be disaccharides or monosaccharides. The disaccharides are sucrose, containing one molecule of glucose and one of fructose; maltose, which contains two molecules of glucose; and lactose, which contains glucose and galactose. During digestion carbohydrates are broken down to the monosaccharides glucose, fructose and galactose. These are used in the body for the production of energy or stored as glycogen.

Carbohydrate is the only nutrient in sugar but is also present in such foods as bread, potatoes, rice and pasta. In these foods there are other nutrients including protein and vitamins.

The carbohydrates in the food supply from 50% to 80% of the total daily intake of energy. In wealthier countries fat and protein account for a relatively greater proportion but in poorer countries a larger proportion of energy is obtained from carbohydrates.

1 gram carbohydrate gives 17kJ

2. Proteins

These contain oxygen, hydrogen, nitrogen and sometimes sulphur. They are necessary to the body for growth and repair. Opinions about the amount of protein necessary daily for a human differ widely and the amount suggested has varied from 40 grams to 100 grams. At present in the United Kingdom it is recommended that a fully grown adult should eat between 60 and 70 grams of protein a day which will supply about 10% of his total daily intake of calories. It is possible that humans would be healthier with a smaller amount of protein in the diet. Pregnant and lactating mothers need more protein than other adults.

Protein is made up of 23 amino-acids and of these 8 are called 'essential' amino-acids and a further two are 'essential' in children. The term 'essential' is used because the body is unable to synthesise these amino-acids and must have them in the food. Proteins were formerly known as first class or animal proteins which contained all the essential amino-acids and second class or vegetable proteins which contained some of the essential amino-acids. This categorisation has now stopped because it is realised that a varied intake of vegetable proteins including cereals and pulses can contain all the essential amino-acids. The quantity of vegetable protein that needs to be eaten is very much greater than animal protein and this can be a disadvantage.

Protein is used in the body for growth and repair and any excess is used up for energy or stored as fat.

1 gram protein gives 17kJ

3. Fats

All fats are made up of a mixture of glycerol and fatty acids but the characteristics of the fatty acids differ. A fatty acid is formed from a chain of carbon atoms with hydrogen and oxygen. A saturated fatty acid is one in which all the bonds between the carbon atoms are single. A mono-saturated fatty acid is one in which one bond is double; a poly-unsaturated fatty acid is one in which there are two or more double bonds.

Fat is found in dairy products such as milk, cream, cheese and butter; but it is also present in and around meat, in nuts, pulses and in some fish including herring and salmon.

There are three poly-unsaturated fatty acids essential for health and these are linoleic acid, linolenic acid and arachidonic acid.

The amount of fat that is necessary in the diet for health is not known. Cultural factors and the family income cause a wide variation in intake.

Fats are emulsified by the bile salts in the digestive tract and then broken down by lipase into glycerides, glycerol and fatty acids.

Fats form the main supply of stored energy in the body. When it is metabolised one gram of fat produces twice as many calories as a gram of protein or a gram of carbohydrate. Fat is also a source of vitamins A, D, E and K.

1 gram fat gives 38kJ

4. Vitamins

These are a small but necessary part of the diet. The results of vitamin deficiencies were recognised in most cases before the chemical structure of the vitamin had been established. They were called A, B, C, etc. but this, in the light of later knowledge, has led to some confusion in the nomenclature.

FAT SOLUBLE VITAMINS

Vitamin A is supplied to the body in food as retinol and carotene. It is present in animal fats such as halibut and cod liver oil, milk, butter and cheese. It is also present in carrots and green vegetables with dark green leaves such as spinach.

2,500 International Units (IU) are necessary each day. Deficiency causes night blindness, hardening of the skin and the covering of the eye which can cause blindness. A deficiency is rare in the developed countries.

An excess of vitamin A, which can occur if children are given too large an amount, can cause irritability, loss of appetite, an itching skin and swellings over the bones.

Vitamin D is supplied to the body in animal fats including milk, butter and cheese. It can also be made by the body when the skin is exposed to ultraviolet light.

The recommended daily intake of vitamin D for infants is 400 International Units and for adults 100 International Units.

A deficiency of vitamin D in children causes rickets; and in malnourished women who have a number of pregnancies it can cause osteomalacia.

An excess of vitamin D occurs through overdosage of small children and can cause irritability, loss of appetite, loss of weight and occasionally death.

Vitamin E is associated with fertility in rats but in humans its use is still uncertain.

Vitamin K. A deficiency of vitamin K in the human is associated with impaired clotting of the blood. The deficiency is unlikely to be caused by a low intake and is probably due to a defect in its use by the body.

THE WATER SOLUBLE VITAMINS

Vitamin B is now known to be a collection of different vitamins.

1. *Vitamin B_1* or thiamine is necessary for the metabolism of glucose in the body and is probably of particular importance in the nourishment of nerve cells. A regular supply of this vitamin is needed because very little is stored in the body. It is present in a wide variety of foods including unrefined cereals, potatoes, green vegetables and milk. A deficiency of this vitamin is very rare in the United Kingdom unless a patient is not taking food. A deficiency is common in poorer countries particularly if rice or other cereals are refined. Beriberi is the result of deficiency.

2. There used to be a vitamin known as *vitamin B_2* but it is now known to be a group of vitamins of which the most important is riboflavine. Its source and use are similar to those of thiamine. Deficiency, which is rare in the United Kingdom, causes cracks at the corners of the mouth, a sore, red tongue and a dry, scaly skin.

3. *Nicotinic acid* is present in unrefined cereals and dairy products. Deficiency is most common in rice eating countries and causes pellagra. Exposed areas of the skin become pigmented and scaly, there is diarrhoea and there may be severe mental symptoms including depression.

4. *Vitamin B_6* is rather like vitamin E. Its use is established in animals but in humans it is not yet understood. It is widely available in vegetables.

5. *Vitamin B_{12}* is present in meat and is necessary for the formation of blood cells. A deficiency occurs because it is not absorbed through the stomach wall and its lack causes pernicious anaemia. Replacement must be by repeated injections.

6. *Folic acid* is also necessary for the formation of blood cells and it is widely available in vegetables. A deficiency may occur in pregnant women and iron and folic acid may be given routinely during pregnancy to prevent anaemia.

Vitamin C or ascorbic acid is necessary for the healthy development of collagen in the body; this includes bones, teeth and the lining of blood vessels. It is present in all fruits and vegetables but a good source is citrus fruits. The human adult needs about 30mg a day and in the United Kingdom a quarter of this amount is normally supplied by potatoes. A deficiency of vitamin C causes scurvy and the disease is most commonly seen in elderly people who have an insufficient dietary intake.

5. Minerals

These, like vitamins, are essential in the human diet for normal development and health; less, however, is known about many of them than about some vitamins.

1. *Sodium* or salt. All body fluids contain this mineral and the greater amount of it is in the extracellular fluid. The amount remains constant in the healthy adult. Sodium acts with potassium to stabilise the acid base balance. The daily intake necessary is about 1g but some people who like salty food may eat up to 10g.

2. *Potassium* acts with sodium to keep a constant acid base balance in the body. Potassium is found mostly in intracellular fluid. Potassium is present in most foods that humans eat including fruit, vegetables and cereals. A deficiency is unlikely to be due to a low intake but to an excessive loss from the body as may occur in severe diarrhoea or while taking diuretics.

3. *Calcium* is present in the greatest quantity of all minerals in the body. Most of it is in the teeth and bones. The daily intake necessary is probably about 500mg but it has been suggested that 1,000mg could be necessary. It is present in large amounts in dairy foods particularly cheese and in 'hard' water and in many vegetables. A deficiency of calcium is seldom due to a lack in the dietary intake but to a failure of absorption as may occur in steatorrhoea; or to defective use in the body as may occur in diseases of the parathyroid.

4. *Phosphorus* forms compounds with calcium in the bones and teeth. It also takes part in cell metabolism and reproduction. It is widely available in the diet and the body can deal with an excess by excretion in the stools or urine.

5. *Iron* is necessary in the body for the formation of haemoglobin. The daily intake needs to be about 10mg and probably up to 20mg in pregnant women. It is present in meat, liver, bread and vegetables. A deficient intake causes one type of anaemia but in the United Kingdom this type of anaemia is more often due to an acute or chronic loss of blood than to a low intake of iron.

6. *Iodine* is vital to the body for the production of thyroxin by the thyroid gland. In most parts of the world it is present in the earth and water and vegetables in the diet have absorbed it. In areas where there is a shortage of iodine in the soil, humans may develop enlargement of the thyroid gland.

7. *Fluorine* occurs naturally in some soils and therefore in some water supplies. If it is present in a quantity of about one part per million of water it lessens the incidence of dental caries. If present in amounts of 4 or 5 p.p.m. it can cause mottling of the teeth.

DIET FOR OBESITY

The problem of being overweight is largely one of more affluent countries. It is usually caused by eating more than is necessary coupled with a sedentary way of life. Crash diets are of little use and a change in eating habits is necessary for the maintenance of permanent weight reduction.

During weight reduction the total intake of calories should be limited to 4,200kJ (1,000 calories) a day and a steady weight loss of 0·5–1·0kg a week is sufficient.

A normal pattern of eating should be observed and the total calories divided between three or four meals.

The following foods should be omitted entirely:

Sugar, cakes, biscuits, sweet puddings
Alcohol
Fried foods
Chocolate, sweets, etc.
Jam, honey, marmalade, syrup, etc.
Dried fruits
Potato crisps
Sweet canned or bottled drinks

When the target weight has been reached the daily diet may be increased but the above foods are better omitted. A weekly check should be kept and a stricter diet started if the weight is increasing.

DIABETIC DIETS

A detailed description of a diabetic diet will not be given because physicians managing diabetes usually have their own methods of controlling diet.

The principles of any diabetic diet are the restriction of starches and sugars. The quantity allowed in the diet each day must be eaten and at regular intervals; this is particularly important if insulin is being used. In children it is more difficult to keep an exact control of these foods but it is best to encourage the diabetic child to take an early, responsible share in the management of his diet.

In all diabetic diets it is usual to aim at a daily fixed total calorie intake which may be about 7,500kJ. This amount will vary with the sex, size and occupation of the patient. The diet is usually made up of about 210g of carbohydrate, 80g of protein and 70g of fat.

Carbohydrate is the nutrient which must be most carefully controlled and it is common to work out a system of dietary 'exchanges' based on the quantity of a food which contains 10g of carbohydrate.

The daily intake of milk will be controlled at about ¾ pint and of butter at ½oz.

It is usual to give the patient guidance about the following groups of foods which may also be controlled by the 'exchange' system:

1. Foods which may be eaten in an unlimited quantity including tea and coffee without sugar and with milk from the daily allowance, clear soups, cheese, fish, meat, eggs and most vegetables.
2. Foods which may be eaten in moderation including all carbohydrate foods, fresh and dried fruit, pasta, thick soups, 'diabetic' foods and dry wines and sherry.
3. Foods to be avoided include sugar, sweets, jam, syrup, sweet puddings, ice-cream, sweet wines and sherry, spirits and liqueurs.

EQUIVALENTS FOR USE IN DIABETIC DIETS

Bread: The equivalent to 1oz of bread (i.e. 15 grams of carbohydrate) is found in the following:

2 Ryvita or Vita-Weat
3 Cream Crackers or Water Biscuits
3 semi-sweet biscuits
¾ cupful cornflakes or other breakfast cereal
3 tablespoons porridge
1 medium-sized potato (3oz)
2 tablespoons boiled rice, spaghetti or macaroni
½ pint of milk

Drinks: The following are equivalent to 20 grams of carbohydrate:

1 glassful milk (7oz) and
2 teaspoons Horlicks, Ovaltine or Bournvita.

⅔ cupful fresh orange juice (4oz) and
2 lumps or 2 teaspoonfuls of sugar.

Diabetic fruit squash and
4 lumps or 4 teaspoons of sugar.

½ cup milk (3oz) in tea or coffee and
1oz bread (or equivalent).

Fruit: The following portions of fruit are equivalent to 10 grams of carbohydrate:

Apple, dessert	1 small
Apple, stewed	1½ cups
Apricots, dried	6 halves
Apricots, fresh	2 medium
Banana	1 small
Cherries	10 large
Dates	2
Figs, dried	1 small
Figs, fresh	2 large
Gooseberries	6 large
Grapefruit	1 medium
Grapes	12
Greengages	4 medium
Melon	1 slice, 2in thick
Orange	1 small
Orange juice	⅔ cup
Peach	1 medium
Pear	1 medium
Pineapple, fresh	1 slice, 1in thick
Plums, dessert	2 large
Plums, stewed	3 medium
Prunes	6 small
Raspberries	1 cup
Strawberries	1 cup
Tangerine	1 large

FOODS TO BE AVOIDED IN A DIABETIC DIET

The following foods contain a high percentage of carbohydrate, and are therefore to be avoided by the diabetic: sugar, sweets and chocolate; jam, marmalade, honey or syrup; puddings, cakes and pastries; biscuits (except as equivalents to bread); sweetened fruit drinks and minerals.

FOODS ALLOWED AT WILL IN A DIABETIC DIET

The following foods may be taken as desired by the diabetic: coffee, tea or soda water; clear broth, Bovril, Oxo or Marmite, and the following vegetables:

artichokes	chicory	lettuce	radishes
asparagus	cucumber	marrow	rhubarb
broccoli	endive	mustard and cress	runner beans
Brussels sprouts	French beans	mushrooms	sauerkraut
cabbage	kale	onions	spinach
cauliflower	leeks	parsley	swedes
celery	lemons	pepper, green	tomatoes
			watercress

HIGH FIBRE DIET

This diet is increasingly used in constipation and in diverticulitis. It should include a large proportion of foods which are rich in fibres and relatively low in calories. These foods include:

Porridge and muesli
Bran which can be used in baking
Wholemeal flour and bread
Fresh and dried fruit
Vegetables and pulses
Unrefined rice

GLUTEN FREE DIET

This diet is used in the management of coeliac disease and in other conditions in which the bowel is unable to deal with gluten. Gluten, a plant protein, is found in wheat, rye and barley. It is made of two parts which are glutenin and gliadin and it is the latter which is harmful. Flour can be produced which is free of gluten and this flour must be used in all baking for a patient who is unable to tolerate gluten. Very small amounts of gluten can be harmful and the diet must be strictly adhered to. All cereals which are not gluten free, e.g. cakes, biscuits, tinned foods, sauces, etc. which contain normal flour, must be excluded from the diet.

LOW SATURATED FAT DIET

This diet may be used in the management of diseases of the blood
vessels and in multiple sclerosis. Fats to be avoided are those of
animal origin and those which are solid at room temperature.
Structurally the fats to be avoided are those that are saturated and
the fats to be included in the diet are the mono-unsaturated or
preferably the poly-unsaturated fats. The fats to be avoided are fat
on meat, butter, lard, cream, cheese and bacon. Milk should be
skimmed and not more than two eggs should be eaten a week.

Sunflower seed oil is the best oil to use in the preparation of food
and one of the varieties of poly-unsaturated margarine must be
used instead of butter on bread and in baking.

Fatty fishes to be avoided include mackerel, herring and salmon;
also all fish canned in oil such as sardines and tuna fish.

LOW RESIDUE AND HIGH PROTEIN DIET

This diet may be used in the management of ulcerative colitis. All
foods that are high in fibre content should be avoided. These
include unrefined cereals, wholemeal bread, vegetables except
potato, fruit and dried fruit and nuts. Fried food should also be
avoided.

There should be an increased intake of lean meat, milk, fish,
cheese (apart from cream cheese), eggs and refined cereals. Fruit
juices and fruit jellies should be included in the diet to ensure an
adequate intake of vitamin C.

LOW SODIUM DIET
(Used chiefly for cardiac failure)

Avoid adding salt to food at meal times, and only *very* small
quantities may be used in cooking.

The following food should be avoided: soups made from ham or
salt meat; Oxo, Bovril; tinned and preserved meats; smoked and
dried products such as ham and bacon; salt fish and offal (although
heart and liver may be taken).

The patient should also avoid cheese; beetroot, celery and

spinach; puddings made with baking powder or soda; and anything made with self-raising flour.

He should not take meat sauces, pickles, salad cream or mayonnaise.

LOW FAT DIET
(For liver and gallbladder disease)

Butter should be replaced by honey or golden syrup. No cheese. No nuts, chocolate or cocoa. Eggs are best avoided. No pastry or cakes, except small amounts of fatless sponge.

Lean meat is allowed: all fat should be carefully separated by the patient. Fat meat, ham, bacon and pork to be avoided. No suet. No sausages, liver, kidneys or offal. No fish or meat pastes.

Haddock, cod, whiting, turbot, brill and plaice are allowed, but no other fish.

The patient should have skimmed milk.

Appendix 4

FIRST AID

The AIMS of first aid are;

1. To save life.
2. To prevent the injury and the effects of the injury getting worse.
3. To get a live patient to hospital or into other medical care.
4. To reduce the anxiety of the patient.

First aid may be carried out by a doctor but it can also be carried out effectively by anybody trained in the art of giving first aid and practised in applying it.

ALCOHOL should never be given.

NO DRINKS should be given to any patient apart from the conscious severely burned adult.

Priorities

The first aider must identify and treat urgently all life-threatening conditions. To this end the following questions should be asked about each casualty and answered as rapidly and accurately as possible in order that the appropriate steps may be instigated.

1. Should the patient be removed from a position of danger such as a live source of electricity?
2. Is the patient breathing or not breathing? The brain can live for only about four minutes without a supply of oxygen reaching it in the blood. Do not waste time splinting or bandaging a patient who is not breathing. A hospital can treat a live casualty but not a dead one.
3. Is the patient bleeding severely? Both internal and external bleeding need to be recognized and immediate attention paid to stopping any visible bleeding; a casualty with internal bleeding needs urgent transfer to hospital.

4. Is the patient conscious or unconscious? Diagnosing the cause of unconsciousness is not of immediate concern to the first aider but the correct positioning of the patient will save life and must be practised by all those who study first aid.

REMOVING THE PATIENT FROM A POSITION OF DANGER

This may involve turning off an electric supply with a well-insulated device or dragging the patient out of water. A casualty trapped in a car should be left until a doctor and, if possible, the fire brigade arrive. The first aider should only attempt to carry out this manoeuvre if the car is on fire. If you are dragging a casualty out of water, artificial respiration can and should be started before you have the patient in an ideal place and position.

IS THE PATIENT BREATHING?

If the casualty is not breathing artificial respiration should be started with the minimum delay. The following measures should be carried out as rapidly as possible because there is no time to waste.

a. Put the casualty flat on his back, arch his neck and lift his lower jaw upwards and forwards. This will lift his tongue away from the back of his throat and provide an airway (Figs. 53 & 54).
b. Clear the mouth of any debris including pieces of food and false teeth.

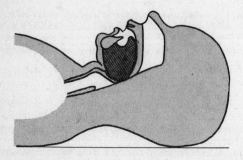

53 The tongue blocking the throat of an unconscious patient

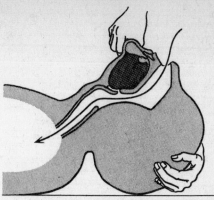

54 *The lower jaw lifted upwards and forwards thus lifting the tongue from the back of the throat*

c. Keeping the jaw in the correct position with one hand under the patient's chin, take a deep breath in. Place your open mouth firmly over the patient's nose while keeping his mouth shut with upward pressure under his chin. Breathe out steadily and firmly until you see the patient's chest rise. Lift your head, turn it to one side, take a deep breath in and repeat the manoeuvre (Figs. 55 & 56). If mouth-to-nose respiration is impossible mouth-to-mouth respiration should be carried on.

d. Artificial respiration should be continued until either the patient breathes spontaneously, a doctor says that he is dead, or if a doctor is not available it should be continued for at least an hour.

The most common cause of difficulty in getting air into the lungs is an obstruction in the air passages; the most common obstruction is the tongue which due to the malpositioning of the head falls backwards and effectively blocks the passage at the back of the nose and mouth. Have a quick look in the mouth to make sure that no further debris has appeared and then lift the lower jaw and pull it

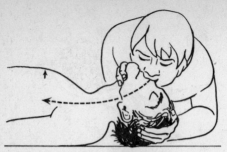

55 *Mouth-to-nose respiration. The chest of the casualty rises as it fills with air*

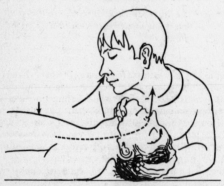

56 *Operator takes away his mouth and breathes in himself. The chest of the casualty falls on expiration*

forward. Correct the extension of the neck by putting one hand under the nape of the neck and pulling the head backwards with the other hand. Continue mouth-to-nose or mouth-to-mouth respiration.

If you are using this method of artificial respiration on a child, care must be taken in the amount of air blown into the lungs. The chest must be watched constantly because damage can be done to the lungs by over-vigorous inflation. If the patient is a small child it is usually easier for the first aider to put his mouth over the child's nose and mouth.

Vomiting may occur while artificial respiration is being carried out. The patient's head should be turned immediately to one side and the mouth rapidly cleaned out before artificial respiration is continued.

Mouth-to-nose or mouth-to-mouth respiration is the most effective method of artificial respiration available to the first aider. It is impossible to practise on a live person but should be practised on one of the models available for this purpose.

IS THE PATIENT BLEEDING SEVERELY?

Bleeding may be external or internal.

External bleeding can be seen on the outside of the body.

Internal bleeding may be hidden within the body or show its presence when passed in the urine, coughed up, etc. Internal bleeding may be severe around a fracture particularly that of the femur or thigh bone.

The diagnosis of severe bleeding must be made quickly because the loss of a litre of blood is serious.

External bleeding will be seen if looked for. Press on the area from which the blood is coming. A sterile pad is best but a bare hand is better than nothing. Put a pad over the area and bandage firmly. Raise the limb which is injured in order to decrease the blood supply to it. If blood appears through the bandage, do not remove the dressing but put another pad on top and bandage again more firmly.

If there are pieces of glass or other foreign bodies in a wound remove the loose ones but do not touch those that are firmly embedded. If you think that there may be a fracture under the wound build up a pad around the wound before bandaging firmly.

Internal bleeding. The patient will be pale, cold and sweating. There may be swelling from an injury such as a fractured femur. No time should be lost trying to make an accurate diagnosis. The casualty should be sent to hospital because he will need replacement of the blood lost as well as treatment of his injuries.

IS THE PATIENT CONSCIOUS OR UNCONSCIOUS?

A conscious patient makes some effort to answer a question or obey a command.

If a casualty is breathing but unconscious he should be put in the unconscious position (Fig. 57). Clear any debris from the patient's mouth. Turn the patient on to his front and his face towards you. Bend his leg, nearest to you, at the knee and bring it towards you

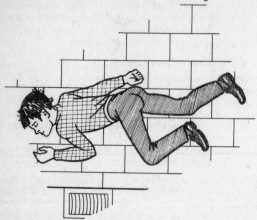

57 The unconscious position

over the other leg. Bend the arm nearest to you, at the elbow and bring the forearm towards you and let it rest on the ground parallel to the casualty's face. Finally lift his chin upwards. If possible arrange the casualty so that he has a slight head down tip.

An unconscious patient must not be left alone. A constant watch must be kept to make sure that he continues to breathe, does not choke and is gently controlled if he becomes restless.

If a patient is unconscious and not breathing artificial respiration must be initiated immediately. If he starts breathing but remains unconscious he must then be put in the unconscious position.

ALL CASUALTIES who have needed treatment for FAILURE TO BREATHE or for UNCONSCIOUSNESS must be seen by a doctor at a hospital.

Organization

At some point while dealing with a number of casualties who have life-threatening conditions you must also get an estimate of the total number of casualties and send somebody to arrange for ambulances and a doctor if possible. You will need to decide which patients need hospital treatment most urgently. Use all the available help in carrying out this organization. Calm organization is an important function of a trained first aider.

Burns

After life-saving measures have been applied, burns must be given first aid treatment. The seriousness of a burn depends to a large extent on the amount of the surface area of the body affected.

TREATMENT

1. *Extinguish the fire.* If necessary lay the casualty down and roll him in a blanket or rug to put out flames.
2. *Cool* the burnt area with cold water, if available, for at least ten minutes. This procedure lessens the damage done to the body tissues by the burn and also relieves the pain.
3. *Cover the burnt area.* Use a sterile dressing if possible; if such dressings are not available use any clean pieces of cloth.

DO NOT USE ANY OINTMENT OR LOTION.
DO NOT BURST ANY BLISTERS.

Keep the casualty lying down until he reaches hospital. A large amount of fluid is lost from burnt areas and to remedy this loss conscious adult casualties should be given frequent small drinks of liquid.

DO NOT GIVE ALCOHOL

Burns of the eye should be washed under running water for at least ten minutes and then covered with a clean dry dressing until medical help can be obtained.

A SEVERELY BURNT PATIENT NEEDS QUIET, CALM HANDLING AND
A GREAT DEAL OF REASSURANCE.

Fractures and dislocations

A fracture is any break or crack in a bone. A fracture may be either
closed or open.

1. *A closed fracture.* The skin is intact over the area of the fracture.
2. *An open fracture.* The skin is broken over the area of the
   fracture. This is important because germs can enter and cause
   infection.

   A dislocation is the disruption of a joint and occurs most commonly at the shoulder joint and the jaw. Again this may be closed or
open.
   Diagnosis of a fracture or dislocation can only be made conclu-
sively by an x-ray. This is beyond the scope of the first aider but the
following signs are suggestive.

1. History of a fall or other violent injury.
2. Pain.
3. Tenderness on examination.
4. Swelling.
5. Loss of power.
6. Deformity.

TREATMENT

Always remember that the fracture of a large bone such as the
femur can be a major cause of blood loss and a blood transfusion
may be the most urgent treatment. Never waste time on elaborate
splinting; concentrate on getting a live patient to hospital but
remember the following principles:

1. A closed fracture must never become an open fracture through
   careless handling.
2. An open fracture must be covered to prevent infection.
3. The fracture must be prevented from getting worse during the
   journey to hospital.
4. *Never* cause the casualty greater pain during the diagnosis or
   treatment. The fractured area will be very tender and must be
   handled with great care.

5. No attempt must be made to restore a dislocated joint to its normal position.

The two basic principles to be observed in the treatment of all fractures and dislocations are:

1. Immobilization to increase the comfort of the patient and prevent the injury getting worse.
2. Speedy removal to hospital for expert diagnosis and treatment.

If you are in doubt about the diagnosis of a fracture treat the injury as a fracture.

If one arm or one leg is fractured the uninjured limb can be used as a standard of normality and the injured limb compared with it for size and shape. Elaborate splinting is unnecessary and may do more harm than good by causing undue movement of the casualty and delaying his removal to hospital.

BASIC PRINCIPLES OF SPLINTING

1. The site of the fracture must be immobilized together with the joints above and below it.
2. The natural contours of the body should be levelled out by soft padding or a rolled up woollen scarf, rags, etc.
3. No bandages should be put on so tightly that the blood circulation is hindered.

Fractures of the shoulder blade and upper arm: Loose padding should be put between the arm and the body. The chest can be used as a splint and the arm placed in the most comfortable position against it—usually with the elbow bent and the forearm in a sling. This position immobilizes both the shoulder and elbow joints.

Fractures of the elbow and lower arm: Padding should be placed between the arm and the body but the elbow should not be bent. The casualty will usually be more comfortable lying on a stretcher with the injured arm tied gently to the side of his body.

Fractures of the wrist and hand: The elbow can be bent and a sling used to keep the forearm and hand immobilized against the front of the chest.

Fractures of the thigh bone or femur: These are serious injuries because of the large amount of blood that can be lost around the site of the fracture. It is important that the casualty should be sent to hospital as soon as possible. Lay the casualty flat on a stretcher. Put padding between the knees, ankles and contours of the legs. Gentleness is important. Tie the feet together with a figure of eight bandage (Fig. 58). Tie the knees together and place bandages around both legs above and below the fracture. Always remember that the casualty will be severely ill with this fracture and be gentle, calm and reassuring.

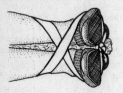

58 Figure of eight
     bandage for lower
     limb fracture

Fractures below the knee: Remember that in all fractures of the shin bone or tibia the injury is likely to be or to become an open fracture. If one leg is fractured the sound leg may be used as a splint for the injured one. Lay the casualty flat. Place padding between the thighs, knees and ankles. Tie the feet together with a figure of eight bandage. Tie the knees together and both legs together with bandages above and below the fracture.

If both legs are fractured the injury is a very severe one. If possible two long splints should be used, one on each side of the body, long enough to reach from the armpits to beyond the feet. If such splints are not available one splint should be used from the level of the groin to beyond the feet and put between the two legs. Padding should be placed between the long splints or the shorter splint and the contours of the body and around the knees and ankles. The feet should be tied together with a figure of eight bandage. Tie the knees together and put bandages around both legs and the splints above and below the levels of the fractures. If two long splints are being used additional bandages should be put around the hips and chest.

Fractures of the jaw: Bandaging is unnecessary. If both sides of the jaw are fractured passage of air into the lungs may be affected. An unconscious casualty should be put in the unconscious position. A conscious casualty should be in a sitting position with the head tilted slightly forward. The casualty must be taken to hospital.

Fracture of the hip bone or pelvis: This can be a serious injury depending on the amount of damage that is done inside the body. The casualty must be put on his back on a stretcher. Put padding between his knees and ankles. Tie his feet together with a figure of eight bandage. Warn the casualty not to pass water on his way to hospital.

Fracture of the spine: This can be a very serious injury and be both life-threatening and the cause of paralysis below the site of the fracture. Send for help, a stretcher and an ambulance.

No attempt should be made to move the casualty until at least four and preferably five people are present. The movement of the casualty on to a stretcher is a job for an expert because the position of the spine must not be changed at any time during the manoeuvre. Minor flexion or bending forward of the spine is the most dangerous change of position because it can compress the spinal cord and cause irreversible damage to the nerves below the level of the fracture.

Dislocations: Any dislocation is a very painful and frightening injury and the casualty needs reassurance and calm treatment.

No attempt must be made to restore the joint to its normal position. The injured area must be supported in the position which is most comfortable for the casualty. The casualty must be taken to hospital.

Poisoning

Poisoning is a hazard that should be prevented rather than treated. There are so many poisonous substances now in general use that it is impracticable to give the treatment of each one. A general outline will be given. In the United Kingdom there are poison reference centres to which an urgent telephone call can be made for information. The numbers are as follows:

TELEPHONE NUMBERS OF POISON REFERENCE CENTRES

Belfast	0232 40503	*London*	01 407 7600
Cardiff	0222 33101	*Manchester*	061 740 2254
Edinburgh	031 229 2477	*Newcastle*	0632 25131
Leeds	0532 32799		

ALWAYS KEEP A CONTAINER FROM WHICH THE POISON IS BELIEVED

TO HAVE BEEN TAKEN AND SEND IT TO HOSPITAL WITH THE PATIENT.

If the patient is not breathing artificial respiration must be given. When the patient starts breathing put him in the unconscious position. Send him to hospital.

If the casualty is conscious but shows signs of burning in or around the mouth send him urgently to hospital and do not make him vomit.

If the casualty is conscious and shows no signs of burning in or around his mouth make him vomit. This can usually be achieved by giving him two tablespoons of salt in a cup of warm water or putting your finger down the back of his throat. If you are trying to make a child vomit put a spoon handle down the back of his throat and not your finger. After he has vomited give him at least a litre of water, milk, weak tea or coffee while waiting for him to be taken to hospital or on the way.

Miscellaneous mishaps

FOREIGN BODIES IN THE EYE

A loose foreign body in the eye may be moved by rapid blinking of the eye or by pulling the upper lid outwards and downwards over the lower lid. No attempt should be made to remove a foreign body forcibly even if it can be clearly seen. A pad should be put over the eye and medical help obtained.

FOREIGN BODIES IN THE NOSE AND EAR

These are usually self-inflicted accidents by small children. The presence of the foreign body may only be suspected by the observation of a one sided blood or pus stained discharge. No attempt should be made to remove the object and medical advice should be obtained.

NOSE BLEEDS

A nose bleed may follow an injury to the nose and is sometimes associated with a fracture. More often a nose bleed occurs spontaneously. The casualty should then be made to sit leaning slightly forwards and hold a pad of handkerchief or soft paper firmly around the end of his nose. Sniffing must be discouraged and the pad should be held in place for ten minutes after the bleeding has stopped.

SNAKE BITES

In the United Kingdom the only poisonous snake is the adder. Its bite is seldom dangerous or fatal but the anxiety it produces is very great. The casualty should be lain down and the bitten limb raised. No attempt should be made to cut or suck the bite. The casualty should be taken to hospital.

In parts of the world where snake bites can be fatal the same initial treatment should be given and transport to hospital arranged as speedily as possible. It may be helpful if the species of the snake can be identified so that appropriate treatment can be given.

Appendix 5

ABBREVIATIONS OF SOME DEGREES, DIPLOMAS, OTHER TITLES AND ORGANIZATIONS

AHA	Area Health Authority
AIMSW	Associate of the Institute of Medical Social Workers
ANO	Area Nursing Officer
ARRC	Associate of the Royal Red Cross
ARSH	Associate of the Royal Society of Health
BA	Bachelor of Arts
BCh, BS, BChir	Bachelor of Surgery
BChD, BDS	Bachelor of Dental Surgery
BM	Bachelor of Medicine
BSc	Bachelor of Science
CHC	Community Health Council
CM, ChM	Master in Surgery
CMB	Central Midwives Board
CNAA	Council for National Academic Awards
CQSW	Certificate of Qualification in Social Work
DA	Diploma in Anaesthetics
DCH	Diploma in Child Health
DCP	District Community Physician
DDS	Doctor of Dental Surgery
DHSS	Department of Health and Social Security
DM	Doctor of Medicine
DMRD	Diploma in Medical Radiology: Diagnostic
DMRT	Diploma in Medical Radiology: Therapy

DMT	District Management Team
DN, DipN	Diploma in Nursing
DNE	Director of Nurse Education
DNO	District Nursing Officer
DO	Diploma in Ophthalmology
BObstRCOG	Diploma in Obstetrics of the Royal College of Obstetricians and Gynaecologists
DON	Diploma in Orthopaedic Nursing
DPH	Diploma in Public Health
DPM	Diploma in Psychological Medicine
DipPhysMed	Diploma of Physical Medicine
DSc	Doctor of Science
DTM&H	Diploma in Tropical Medicine and Hygiene
DivNO	Divisional Nursing Officer
FCSP	Fellow of the Chartered Society of Physiotherapy
FChS	Fellow of the Society of Chiropodists
FFARCS	Fellow of the Faculty of Anaesthetists of the Royal College of Surgeons
FPS	Fellow of the Pharmaceutical Society
FRCGP	Fellow of the Royal College of General Practitioners
FRCN	Fellow of the Royal College of Nursing
FRCOG	Fellow of the Royal College of Obstetricians and Gynaecologists
FRCP	Fellow of the Royal College of Physicians
FRCPath	Fellow of the Royal College of Pathologists
FRCPE, FRCP(Ed)	Fellow of the Royal College of Physicians, Edinburgh
FRCPI	Fellow of the Royal College of Physicians of Ireland
FRCPsych	Fellow of the Royal College of Psychiatrists
FRCR	Fellow of the Royal College of Radiologists

FRCS	Fellow of the Royal College of Surgeons
FRCSE, FRCS(Ed)	Fellow of the Royal College of Surgeons, Edinburgh
FRCSI	Fellow of the Royal College of Surgeons of Ireland
FRFPSG	Fellow of the Royal Faculty of Physicians and Surgeons, Glasgow
FRS	Fellow of the Royal Society
FRSE	Fellow of the Royal Society, Edinburgh
GNC	General Nursing Council
HV	Health Visitor
JBCNS	Joint Board of Clinical Nursing Studies
LDS	Licentiate in Dental Surgery
LMSSA	Licentiate in Medicine and Surgery, Society of Apothecaries, London
LRCP	Licentiate of the Royal College of Physicians
LSA	Licentiate of the Society of Apothecaries, London
MA	Master of Arts
MAO	Master of the Art of Obstetrics
MB	Bachelor of Medicine
MBAOT	Member of the British Association of Occupational Therapy
MC, MS, MCh, MChir	Master of Surgery
MChD, MDS	Master of Dental Surgery
MChS	Member of the Society of Chiropodists
MCSP	Member of the Chartered Society of Physiotherapy
MD	Doctor of Medicine
MPS	Member of the Pharmaceutical Society
MRCGP	Member of the Royal College of General Practitioners
MRCOG	Member of the Royal College of Obstetricians and Gynaecologists